LATER EDITION AVAILABLE JUNE 2017

Th

Ex

an

OF01032

ERRATUM

There is a dosage error in Chapter 5 which contains the questions for the module on postpartum problems; in the option list for Questions 5.36 to 5.40 inclusive.

The dose of Ergometrine (which is option C) should read Ergometrine 500 micrograms IM instead of Ergometrine 500 milligrams IM.

The principal author would like to apologise for this error, which is entirely her fault.

The DRCOG Revision Guide
Examination Preparation and Practice Questions

SUSAN WARD
Consultant Obstetrician and Gynaecologist,
Kings Mill Hospital, Sherwood Forest Hospitals Trust,
Sutton-in-Ashfield, Nottinghamshire, UK

With contributions from:
LISA JOELS
Consultant Obstetrician and Gynaecologist,
Royal Devon and Exeter NHS Foundation Trust,
Exeter, Devon, UK

ELAINE MELROSE
Retired Consultant Obstetrician and Gynaecologist
Ayrshire Maternity Unit and Crosshouse Hospitals,
Kilmarnock, Ayrshire, UK

SRINIVAS VINDLA
Consultant Obstetrician and Gynaecologist,
Kings Mill Hospital, Sherwood Forest Hospitals Trust,
Sutton-in-Ashfield, Nottinghamshire, UK

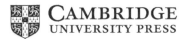

CAMBRIDGE
UNIVERSITY PRESS

CAMBRIDGE
UNIVERSITY PRESS

University Printing House, Cambridge CB2 8BS, United Kingdom

Cambridge University Press is part of the University of Cambridge.

It furthers the University's mission by disseminating knowledge in the pursuit of education, learning and research at the highest international levels of excellence.

www.cambridge.org
Information on this title: www.cambridge.org/9781107422957

© Susan Ward, Lisa Joels, Elaine Melrose and Srinivas Vindla 2014

First published 2014

Printed in the United Kingdom by Clays, St Ives plc

A catalogue record for this publication is available from the British Library

Library of Congress Cataloguing in Publication data
Ward, Susan, 1957– author.
The DRCOG revision guide : examination preparation and practice questions / Susan Ward ; with contributions from Lisa Joels, Elaine Melrose, Srinivas Vindla.
     p.   ;   cm.
Includes index.
ISBN 978-1-107-42295-7 (pbk.)
I. Joels, Lisa, author.   II. Melrose, Elaine B., author.   III. Vindla, Srinivas, author.   IV. Title.
[DNLM: 1. Gynecologic Surgical Procedures – methods – Examination Questions. 2. Obstetric Surgical Procedures – Examination Questions.   3. Perinatal Care – methods – Examination Questions.   4. Pregnancy Complications – Examination Questions. WQ 18.2]
RG111
618.10076–dc23

                                                              2014005353

ISBN 978-1-107-42295-7 Paperback

....

Contents

Foreword

This up-to-date revision text for the DRCOG examination fills a well-recognized gap in the market for potential candidates. The authors have taken a structured approach to the layout with an initial short section providing guidance on how to answer the different types of question found in the examination. For each of the seven modules in the women's health syllabus a bank of questions has been written as multiple choice questions (MCQs), single best answers (SBAs) and extended matching questions (EMQs) to ensure the candidate is tested on relevant knowledge, while becoming familiar with the question styles. The rationale for the correct answer is then concisely explained in the answer section.

In addition, there are two complete mock examination papers in the same format as the actual examination to enable candidates to test their time management. All four authors have been members of the DRCOG subcommittee, so that the questions have been produced in the same way as questions in the actual examination – by a committee – which is a unique selling point when compared to other books on the market. The questions have been tested with real candidates sitting the DRCOG examination within the last year to check that the level of difficulty is appropriate.

I am delighted that this book has been produced at this time and I am sure that it will become the required reading for all DRCOG candidates.

Corinne Hargreaves, MRCOG
Consultant in Obstetrics and Gynaecology
Chair of the DRCOG Subcommittee 2011–2014

Introduction

This volume is intended as a guide for candidates studying for the DRCOG examination. It is set out in a format aligned to the DRCOG syllabus with each chapter relating to one of the seven modules, containing examples of the type of questions that could be asked about that particular subject. Examination candidates can use the specimen questions to check their knowledge about that section of the syllabus and discover where to concentrate their revision efforts.

The Diploma of the Royal College of Obstetricians and Gynaecologists is a clinically orientated rather than just a theoretical examination. Any doctor who has spent a few months in a busy obstetric and gynaecology post will have a good chance of passing the examination after spending some time studying. When choosing which books to use for revision it is important to realize that the examination is intended to be relevant to doctors working in General Practice in the UK, where women's health issues represent a large proportion of the workload of the average GP. There are many books on the market aimed at candidates revising for DRCOG and also many books written for GPs with an interest in women's health.

The questions in this book have been written by four consultants who have all been on the DRCOG Examination Subcommittee and have written questions for the actual examination. As well as making suggestions regarding strategy and technique for answering the questions, we have included lots of examples of each type of question for each section of the syllabus to give you some idea of the form, content and level of difficulty of the questions you might encounter in the examination.

The chapters represent each of the seven sections of the syllabus. In each chapter there are ten multiple choice question (MCQ) stems with five parts each, ten single best answer (SBA) questions and six extended matching questions (EMQs) with five parts to each question – a total of 350 MCQs, 70 SBAs and 210 EMQs within the main part of the book. This should give you plenty of practice!

In addition there is a separate mock exam in the two-paper format currently used for the DRCOG examination that you could use to practise time management if you would find that helpful.

As each of the authors has participated in the setting of the actual examination over the last few years, we have tried to give you some idea of the thought processes behind the answers provided. These comments are representative of the discussions around the table at the DRCOG Examination Subcommittee meetings where the examination is constructed. The committee consists of a group of obstetricians and gynaecologists with different special interests and a general practitioner. Every time a new question is added to the question bank, the GP member is asked to assess whether the content is 'reasonable knowledge that could be expected of a GP with an interest in women's health in the UK' as the committee is keen to avoid setting questions that test MRCOG-level knowledge.

We have also tried to give you some suggestions as to where to find the knowledge being tested in the examination. During the meetings where the questions are set, the committee has at its disposal a wide range of textbooks and resources such as the British National Formulary, along with the NICE guidelines and the 'green-top' guidelines produced by the College. These guidelines can be accessed from the RCOG website and are now collected into a rather thick compendium available in book form, on a data stick or on an 'app' for your mobile telephone or computer tablet. The guidelines would be a good starting point for your revision since some of the questions are set directly from there. It is also worth being familiar with the triennial report on Confidential Enquiries into Maternal Deaths in the UK; the most recent edition before this book went to press was the eighth report covering the 2006 to 2008 deaths (accessible from the RCOG website) but a new report is expected soon. We have also provided a list of other websites where you can find useful information to guide your revision.

We hope you enjoy studying for this examination: your patients will certainly benefit from the knowledge you acquire. Good luck!

The DRCOG examination

In this chapter we explain the format of the exam and discuss the three different styles of questions as a foundation for giving you hints and tips about how to approach the questions and apply your knowledge logically in order to answer correctly. This will be consolidated in subsequent chapters as we explain each of the examples.

The exam format

The format of the examination was altered a few years ago with the first new-style paper appearing in April 2007. The OSCE has been replaced by two written papers lasting 90 minutes each with a short break in between. The first exam paper consists of ten extended matching questions (EMQs) with three parts to each question and 18 single best answer (SBA) questions. The EMQs and SBAs test the ability to interpret information and apply knowledge. After a short break this is followed by a multiple choice question (MCQ) paper consisting of 40 questions, each with five parts (200 questions in total). The MCQs are good for testing recall of core knowledge.

The questions are weighted differently. The EMQs score 3.5 for each correct answer and give you 30% of your total marks. The SBAs score 2.5 each and comprise 12.9% of your marks, whereas the MCQs are worth 1 point each and 57.1% of your total. The reason for this is that there is a lot more reasoning and application of knowledge needed when answering an EMQ so it is worth more. The RCOG recommends that you spend the majority of the time allowed – 60 minutes – on the EMQ and the rest on the SBA part of the paper. You will get a time warning 30 minutes before the end of the examination. In this book there is a complete mock examination – paper 1 and paper 2 – which you could use to practise time management under examination conditions, not forgetting that your answers must be transferred to the computer-marked answer paper before leaving the exam hall on the actual examination day.

The rationale for changing the exam was to improve reliability and validity by removing the subjective aspects of assessment in both the written and face-to-face elements of the OSCE. The whole paper is now marked by computer, significantly improving validity by standardisation. The exam is further improved by a standard-setting process whereby 'more difficult' exams will have a lower pass mark than 'easier' exams, ensuring that the pass mark constantly reflects a competent candidate with the necessary knowledge, skills and attitudes.

In reality the pass mark is somewhere between 60 and 70%, usually towards the upper part of the range. It differs between exams because of the standard setting but if you are scoring over 70% in your revision practice, you are probably doing well enough to pass. The top mark is usually between 85 and 95% and the highest scoring candidate is awarded the DRCOG Prize Medal. Could this be you?

Extended matching questions

It is likely that you will have come across extended matching questions (EMQs) before during your training. The exam has ten EMQs, each with three parts. In order to help you prepare for the examination we have provided you with two additional questions for each EMQ in the chapters of this book. This increases the breadth and depth of material covered to help your revision and your understanding of exam technique.

The format of the EMQs in the DRCOG examination is shown in this example:

OPTION LIST

A.	Continue shopping
B.	Walk out of the shop
C.	Call the police
D.	Lie on the floor and scream
E.	Smack the child
F.	Pick up the child and walk out
G.	Ignore the child till she stops screaming
H.	Pour water over the child
I.	Ask a shop assistant for help
J.	Give the child a bag of crisps

INSTRUCTIONS

Each of the following situations relate to parenting skills. For each situation select the single most appropriate course of action. Each answer may be used once, more than once or not at all.

1. A 29-year-old woman is carrying out her weekly shopping with her two-year-old child. Halfway round the supermarket the child becomes fractious and asks for a bag of crisps. When the woman says no, the child throws a temper tantrum lying on the floor, screaming and crying. Other shoppers are beginning to point and stare.

Don't worry, parenting skills aren't part of the DRCOG curriculum but this example can be used to show how knowledge, skills and attitudes can be applied to ensure the correct answer is selected.

How to tackle this question:

The best way of tackling the EMQs is to read very briefly down the list of options but then cover up the options and use your knowledge, skills and attitudes to work out the answer as if you were answering the questions verbally.

If the first answer that comes in to your head is on the list of options, it is very likely that this is the correct option. Now read the whole option list very carefully and double check that your chosen option is the 'single correct answer'.

Double check the question again to make sure you haven't missed a subtle fact and that you've interpreted the situation correctly. You should be aware that there is usually at least one 'distractor' on each list, i.e. an option that is nearly correct but good candidates will know why the distractor is not the correct option.

So how should you answer this question? Firstly use your experience; if you have looked after a toddler (i.e. for a clinical question you will be using your experience of working in obstetrics and gynaecology) this will be a familiar situation. You will need some knowledge of the psychology of parenting (clinical knowledge gained from reading textbooks) and you will need to be aware of child protection issues and safety concerns (ethics and law). Applying your skills/experience, knowledge and attitudes you can correctly select the answer G – ignore the child till she stops screaming – which will ensure you finish your shopping and avoid child protection services.

The EMQs are specifically designed to test interpretation of a scenario and demonstrate application of knowledge, skills and attitudes and therefore are unlikely to be found as a paragraph in a textbook. We have deliberately constructed the questions to reflect potential clinical scenarios that could be encountered by a GP or GP trainee.

Three questions follow each option list. Each option may be used more than once or not at all, i.e. it is possible that one of the options could be the correct answer for two of the questions. If the list of options looks a bit unusual, the reason for this is that the committee writes many more questions to go with each option list so that there is a large bank of questions available looking at various aspects of a clinical scenario. Each year only three of them are selected from the bank for the examination paper, so an unusual option may belong to another question on the bank. Don't fall into the trap of assuming that because it's an unusual option that you hadn't thought of, then it must be the correct answer.

Single best answer questions

Single best answer (SBA) questions – used to be called 'best of fives' – are similar to EMQs in requiring application of knowledge as opposed to direct recall of facts. The majority of SBAs are also based on a clinical scenario which requires interpretation of facts in order to select the single best answer but this can be either the most appropriate or the least appropriate answer depending on how the question is phrased. For example, an SBA based on a similar scenario to that above might be:

A 29-year-old woman is trying to cope with her two-year-old child who is having a temper tantrum in the middle of a supermarket. Which of the following is the most appropriate course of action?

1. To pacify the child with sweets
2. To remove the child to a safe place
3. To ignore the child until she calms down
4. To leave the store and go home
5. To distract the child with something interesting to look at

These options initially all look plausible and very similar, however if you reflect on your reading of parenting manuals (textbooks) you will recall that bribing with sweets will set up a vicious cycle resulting in worsening behaviour and your experience tells you that a toddler in a full-blown tantrum is not distractible. Leaving the store rewards bad behaviour and if you review carefully the scenario it's hard to imagine a supermarket as being a particularly dangerous place (experience) unless you 'over think' the question and imagine the child to be next to an unstable display of baked bean cans or something similar. Again the answer is 3 – ignore the child till she calms down.

The message here is: carefully assess the information given but don't read complexity into the scenario where there is none.

Multiple choice questions

Multiple choice questions (MCQs) are best for testing factual recall, hence our advice that you will need to do some revision before the exam. It is extremely unlikely that you can get all the background knowledge you need to be sure of passing this examination just by working in an obstetrics and gynaecology department.

Continuing our theme of parenting skills, the same scenario written as an MCQ might look like:

Regarding the management of toddler tantrums in public:

1.	Police intervention may be necessary	[F]
2.	Smacking will reduce crying by 90%	[F]
3.	Withdrawing attention is a useful strategy	[T]
4.	Child safety must be considered	[T]
5.	Bribes help to establish good behaviour patterns	[F]

The MCQ format is the one most of us are familiar with and the good news for candidates sitting the DRCOG exam is that the MCQs are not marked negatively. The answer is either unequivocally true or false; no marks are deducted for incorrect responses. You don't need to miss out questions where you really don't know the answer as you lose nothing by guessing.

In the actual examination, you can use the question booklet to write on and make notes (as it is not read when it is returned to the RCOG) but you must transfer your answers to the computer-marked sheet before the examination finishes. The risk of leaving gaps on the answer sheet as you progress through the examination is that you might incorrectly transcribe your answers and lose marks when your answers were originally correct. You are supplied with an eraser to make corrections and you must be very careful when you've finally chosen your answers to make sure that you complete the answer sheet correctly.

Another common mistake is to assume that not all five answers can be correct (or incorrect). The examiners try hard to avoid predictable patterns when selecting the questions. Great care is also taken to avoid questions that have 'always' or 'never' as these are obviously incorrect given the nature of clinical medicine. If a question looks like an 'always or never' scenario, re-read it as you may have missed a crucial part of the question.

Revising for the exam

The DRCOG exam strives to be relevant to General Practice and therefore focuses on core knowledge rather than rarities and minutiae; however facts such as maternal mortality rates, prevalence and incidence rates are considered core knowledge and may feature in the exam. These facts are unlikely to be the topic of your ward rounds, handovers or reflective practice sessions so it really does pay to revise.

The DRCOG is blueprinted to ensure that all areas of the syllabus are covered, so the best advice is to ensure that you have covered the whole syllabus in your reading and revision, rather than trying to 'spot' questions.

In addition to the textbooks you used as an undergraduate, there are several books on the market covering issues relevant to women's health in General Practice and we suggest that you also access specific texts on contraception and genitourinary medicine. We have provided a list of websites where you will find helpful information about some topics which could come up in the examination and although this list is not exhaustive, we think you will find that they contain interesting revision material.

Doing exam questions is a very good way to revise and it is highly recommended that you re-read a topic where your score is disappointing – you will be even more disappointed if it comes up in the examination and you have neglected to revisit that topic and top up your knowledge.

While you are revising don't forget to eat, sleep and relax too – all these things will improve your performance!

Conclusions

The DRCOG uses three different question formats to test objectively the knowledge, skills and attitudes of all areas of the syllabus to the standard of a GP practising in the UK. To pass the exam, reading and revision is required but understanding the style of questions and practising questions will improve your chance of success.

Curriculum module 1

Basic clinical skills

Syllabus

- You will be expected to understand the patterns of symptoms in patients presenting with obstetric problems, gynaecological problems, sexually transmitted infections and patients in a family planning setting.
- You will be expected to demonstrate an understanding of the pathophysiological basis of physical signs and understand the indications, risks, benefits and effectiveness of investigations in a clinical setting.
- You will be required to demonstrate an understanding of the components of effective verbal and non-verbal communication.
- You will need to be aware of relevant ethical and legal issues including the implications of the legal status of the unborn child, the legal issues relating to medical certification and issues related to medical confidentiality. You will be expected to understand the issues surrounding consent in all clinical situations including postmortem examination and termination of pregnancy.

Learning outcomes

This module covers history taking, clinical examination and investigation, note keeping, legal issues relating to medical certification, time management and decision making, communication, ethics and legal issues. It is easy to set clinical questions on history, examination or investigation but quite a challenge to set written questions to test the other areas. Previously viva voce examinations such as the OSCE were used to test communication skills. The OSCE component of the DRCOG has now been abandoned because in reality nobody ever failed due to poor communication skills.

Although you might imagine that attributes such as 'good time management' could not be tested in a written format, we can test this to some extent – for example whether a candidate can prioritize clinical cases safely – using both EMQ and SBA formats.

We have also tried to look at attitudes and behaviour using written questions concentrating on issues such as consent, domestic violence and confidentiality. We recommend that you have a look at the GMC website (especially *Duties of a Doctor*) to find information about these attitudinal and ethical issues, and of course you should discuss cases with your supervisors in both O&G and General Practice.

MULTIPLE CHOICE QUESTIONS

1.1   Concerning symptoms caused by endometriosis:

A.   Patients often complain of deep dyspareunia   [T]   [F]
B.   There is a correlation between the severity of pain symptoms and [T]   [F]
the extent of the endometriotic lesions found at laparoscopy
C.   Dyschezia is caused by endometriosis in the rectovaginal septum [T]   [F]
D.   Patients with endometriosis may suffer from chronic fatigue   [T]   [F]
E.   Primary dysmenorrhoea is a common symptom of endometriosis [T]   [F]

1.2   Regarding early pregnancy complications:

A.   Diarrhoea may be due to intra-abdominal bleeding   [T]   [F]
B.   Hyperemesis is a recognized presentation of hydatidiform mole   [T]   [F]
C.   Missed abortion usually presents with light bleeding   [T]   [F]
D.   Pain in the shoulder indicates that the patient may have an ectopic [T]   [F]
pregnancy
E.   A patient with an ectopic pregnancy may not have missed a period [T]   [F]

1.3   Considering domestic abuse in an O&G setting:

A.   Pregnancy is known to provoke episodes of domestic violence   [T]   [F]
B.   Community midwives are required to ask about domestic violence [T]   [F]
during routine antenatal care even if it seems unlikely (e.g. the
patient works as a doctor)
C.   Female relatives can be used to translate when asking about   [T]   [F]
domestic violence to ensure a non-English speaker has understood
the question
D.   There is a recognized association between domestic violence and [T]   [F]
repeated requests for termination of unwanted pregnancy
E.   Domestic abuse may involve control of a woman's finances   [T]   [F]

1.4   These conditions may cause amenorrhoea:

A.   Polycystic ovarian syndrome   [T]   [F]
B.   Endometrial hyperplasia   [T]   [F]
C.   Mullerian agenesis   [T]   [F]
D.   Asherman syndrome   [T]   [F]
E.   Anorexia nervosa   [T]   [F]

1.5   A 37-year-old woman attends your surgery to inform you that she is six weeks pregnant. She has a BMI of 38 and has had four previous caesarean sections, delivering babies of over 4 kg each time.

She is at increased risk of the following pregnancy complications:

A.   Placenta accreta   [T]   [F]
B.   Postpartum haemorrhage   [T]   [F]
C.   Intrauterine growth retardation   [T]   [F]
D.   Gestational diabetes   [T]   [F]
E.   Pre-eclampsia   [T]   [F]

1.6 The following factors contribute to the 'Risk of malignancy index' when evaluating the likelihood of an ovarian cyst being malignant in nature:

A. Solid areas in the cyst on ultrasound scan [T] [F]
B. The age of the woman [T] [F]
C. The CA125 tumour marker level [T] [F]
D. The menopausal status of the woman [T] [F]
E. A family history of ovarian cancer [T] [F]

1.7 A 42-year-old nulliparous woman consults you in the surgery about her urinary problems. She has been suffering with urinary frequency and urge incontinence for over a year. The following should be considered as a possible cause of her symptoms:

A. Uterine fibroid [T] [F]
B. Multiple sclerosis [T] [F]
C. Urinary tract infection [T] [F]
D. Detrusor instability [T] [F]
E. Interstitial cystitis [T] [F]

1.8 When assessing a gynaecological patient with pelvic pain, these examination findings are recognized signs of endometriosis:

A. Fixed retroversion of the uterus [T] [F]
B. Palpable nodules in the rectovaginal septum [T] [F]
C. A tender swelling situated within the umbilicus [T] [F]
D. Adnexal tenderness [T] [F]
E. Contact bleeding of the cervix [T] [F]

1.9 Non-sensitized, Rhesus-negative women should receive anti-D immunoglobulin in the following situations:

A. Miscarriage below 12 weeks when the uterus is evacuated surgically [T] [F]
B. Ectopic pregnancy [T] [F]
C. Incomplete miscarriage over 12 weeks [T] [F]
D. Complete miscarriage under 12 weeks when bleeding is heavy [T] [F]
E. Threatened miscarriage below 12 weeks when the fetus is viable [T] [F]

1.10 Concerning maternal death:

A. The maternal mortality rate is lower in the UK than in the USA [T] [F]
B. Reducing the number of maternal deaths worldwide by the year 2050 is a 'millennium development goal' [T] [F]
C. The maternal mortality ratio is defined as the number of maternal deaths per 100 000 pregnancies [T] [F]
D. The details of every maternal death in the UK are scrutinized to look for elements of substandard care [T] [F]
E. There has been an increase in maternal deaths from sepsis related to sore throats [T] [F]

SINGLE BEST ANSWER QUESTIONS

1.11 Taking over the gynaecology on-call duties one evening, you are given this list of tasks to be done. Which one would you do first?

A. Site an intravenous infusion for a severely dehydrated patient with hyperemesis

B. Sign a death certificate as a patient's husband is waiting on the ward for it

C. Review the scan report of a woman with a suspected ectopic pregnancy

D. Review a woman who has just miscarried an 18-week fetus but not delivered the placenta

E. Clerk a new patient that the GP has sent in to hospital with a suspected torted ovarian cyst

Answer [   ]

1.12 You are trying to persuade a postoperative woman with a haemoglobin of 55 g/l that she would not be so breathless if she had a blood transfusion, but she is concerned about the risk of acquiring HIV. The chance of acquiring HIV infection as a result of blood transfusion in the UK is approximately:

A. 1 in 6000

B. 1 in 60 000

C. 1 in 600 000

D. 1 in 6 million

E. 1 in 60 million

Answer [   ]

1.13 The community midwife doing an antenatal clinic in your GP surgery asks you to see a 37-year-old obese woman who has come for a routine check-up at 32 weeks gestation in her first pregnancy. Her booking blood pressure in the first trimester was 130/88 but it is now 160/95 and the midwife has checked the blood pressure twice. The woman is asymptomatic. Which is the most appropriate course of action?

A. Urinalysis and prescribe antihypertensives if no proteinuria

B. Send urgent full blood count, urate and liver function test

C. Refer her urgently to hospital for further investigation and treatment

D. Urinalysis and request urgent antenatal appointment if no proteinuria

E. Twenty-four hour urine collection for protein analysis

Answer [   ]

1.14 A 52-year-old woman presents to your surgery with a very sore vulva. On examination you find thickening of the labia minora with a couple of shallow ulcers on both sides and a split area at the fourchette. What is the most likely diagnosis in her case?

A. Eczema

B. Genital herpes

C. Lichen planus

D. Lichen sclerosus

E. Vulval intraepithelial neoplasia

Answer [   ]

1.15 The clinical scenarios detailed below describe gynaecological patients admitted as an emergency. Which patient is most likely to have a diagnosis of ectopic pregnancy?

A. Acute onset of central abdominal pain and nausea at 12 weeks gestation. On examination severe lower abdominal tenderness with generalized guarding and rebound, also fetor oris. White cell count is $18 \times 10^9/l$ and urinalysis is negative

B. History of 11 weeks amenorrhoea and brown vaginal discharge but no pain. Pelvic examination reveals no tenderness but uterus is small for dates and the cervical os is closed. Serum βhCG is 2010 IU/ml and scan is awaited

C. Seven weeks amenorrhoea and vaginal bleeding. Pelvic examination reveals no tenderness. Uterus is soft and slightly enlarged with an open cervical os

D. Admitted with bleeding and lower abdominal pain at eight weeks gestation. Transvaginal ultrasound scan shows intrauterine sac with a fetal pole but no heart pulsation detected. Serum βhCG is 150 000 IU/ml

E. Patient with lower abdominal and shoulder tip pain who has a copper coil fitted. Last menstrual period was two weeks ago and on examination has a tender abdomen with guarding. Urinary hCG test positive in A&E

Answer [   ]

1.16 A 46-year-old woman presents to her GP seeking help with her period problems which date back almost a year. Her cycles are still regular with a cycle of 26 days but the bleeding is now very heavy with clots. She complains of severe secondary dysmenorrhoea but no other pelvic pain. On examination there are no masses palpable in the pelvis. The uterus is enlarged to the size of an orange, smooth and very tender but mobile with no adnexal tenderness.

Select the most likely gynaecological cause of this clinical picture:

A. Adenomyosis
B. Chronic pelvic inflammatory disease
C. Endometriosis
D. Endometrial hyperplasia
E. Fibroids

Answer [   ]

1.17 A 39-year-old woman asks for a hospital referral so that she can be investigated for recurrent miscarriage, having suffered three first-trimester pregnancy losses. She believes that her miscarriages are due to stress. She works long hours as a computer programmer and smokes 15 cigarettes a day. Which of the following factors is the most likely cause of her recurrent miscarriages?

A. Working with visual display units
B. Smoking
C. Advanced maternal age
D. Natural killer cells
E. Bacterial vaginosis

Answer [   ]

1.18 In your GP surgery the practice nurse asks you to see a 25-year-old woman who is unable to tolerate speculum examination for her first smear test. The patient tells you that she has experienced severe dyspareunia since her marriage two years ago and discloses that she was sexually abused as a child. Which of the following statements about child abuse is untrue?

A. Abuse in childhood predisposes to depressive illness in later life which does not respond to treatment

B. Child abuse encompasses neglect as well as physical and sexual abuse

C. Somatization as an adult can be a result of child abuse

D. Women who have been abused as children rarely disclose such a history

E. Abuse in childhood is known to be associated with illicit drug use as an adult

Answer [ ]

1.19 The mother of a 13-year-old girl attends the surgery for advice. Her daughter has been offered human papilloma virus (HPV) vaccine at school but did not bring an information leaflet home, so she wants to know more about it. Which of these statements about the bivalent vaccine (Cervarix®) is correct?

A. She will require two doses of the vaccine over six months

B. The vaccine will reduce the chance of her developing genital warts as well as cervical intraepithelial neoplasia

C. If she completes the course of vaccinations she will not need cervical smears in the future

D. The duration of protection offered by the vaccine is unknown

E. The vaccine is made from live attenuated human papilloma virus

Answer [ ]

1.20 Which of the following statements is true in relation to women with Turner syndrome?

A. They have no problems with learning difficulties

B. Estrogen therapy may result in spontaneous fertility

C. There is a high prevalence of left-sided congenital heart malformation

D. Administration of growth hormone will not produce any extra height

E. They all have karyotype 46XO

Answer [ ]

EXTENDED MATCHING QUESTIONS

A.	CT scan of the pelvis
B.	Cystoscopy
C.	Diagnostic laparoscopy
D.	Dye laparoscopy
E.	High vaginal swab for chlamydia
F.	Hysterosalpingogram
G.	MRI scan of the pelvis
H.	Serum CA125 level
I.	Transvaginal ultrasound scan
J.	Urodynamic study

Each of these clinical scenarios describes a woman presenting with symptoms of pelvic pain; for each case pick the most appropriate initial investigation, given the information that you are presented with.

Each option may be used once, more than once or not at all.

1.21 Secondary dysmenorrhoea in a 40-year-old obese woman with a BMI of 48. Over the last year her periods have become heavier and she is not currently sexually active

Answer [   ]

1.22 A 38-year-old woman complains of premenstrual pain, severe secondary dysmenorrhoea and dyschezia

Answer [   ]

1.23 A 24-year-old secretary with non-cyclical pain and deep dyspareunia who has been trying to get pregnant for two years

Answer [   ]

1.24 A perimenopausal woman with left iliac fossa pain radiating down her leg, whose abdominal ultrasound shows a 9 cm septated cyst adjacent to the uterus on the left side with free fluid around it

Answer [   ]

1.25 A 62-year-old woman with severe urinary frequency for eight weeks associated with dyspareunia

Answer [   ]

A.	Bleeding corpus luteum cyst
B.	Ectopic pregnancy
C.	Gastroenteritis
D.	Heterotopic pregnancy
E.	Ovarian hyperstimulation syndrome
F.	Ovarian torsion
G.	Pelvic sepsis
H.	Pulmonary embolism
I.	Threatened miscarriage

These women have all undergone assisted conception treatment with IVF and have developed complications. For each clinical scenario select the most likely diagnosis.

Each option may be used once, more than once or not at all.

1.26 Following a cycle of IVF six weeks ago, a young woman is pregnant for the first time. She presents to A&E with increasing lower abdominal pain and diarrhoea. She has had brown vaginal loss for a couple of days. On examination she is pale with a tachycardia of 100 beats per minute but her blood pressure is normal. An urgent ultrasound scan shows an endometrial thickness of 12 mm but no gestation sac is seen.

Answer [   ]

1.27 A slightly obese woman with polycystic ovarian syndrome is admitted a week after an IVF cycle during which 12 oocytes were collected. She had an embryo transfer five days previously and now has shortness of breath, nausea and abdominal pain. Her abdomen is distended on examination.

Answer [   ]

1.28 A 27-year-old woman is admitted to the gynaecology ward as an emergency with severe abdominal pain and vomiting. She is unable to lie still and scores her pain 9 out of 10. On examination she is apyrexial, tachycardic and normotensive. She has a tender mass on the left side of the pelvis. She had a cycle of IVF recently with oocyte recovery ten days previously, followed by embryo transfer two days later.

Answer [   ]

1.29 Three weeks after a cycle of IVF a 34-year-old woman presents to her GP with increasing pain in the lower abdomen and rigors. She only had one embryo replaced in the uterus because only one of the oocytes that were retrieved actually fertilized.

Answer [   ]

1.30 A pregnant woman is rushed to A&E in the UK having collapsed at the airport. She had a cycle of IVF in another country seven weeks ago, during which three embryos were replaced in the uterus. She has a scan picture with her showing an intrauterine pregnancy with a viable six-week fetus. Her blood pressure is 85/45 mmHg, her pulse is 120 bpm, her temperature is 36.5 °C and on abdominal examination she has rigidity, rebound tenderness and guarding. Pelvic examination reveals tenderness in the left adnexa and she has cervical excitation. Her haemoglobin is 95 g/l and her white cell count is 8×10^9/l.

Answer [ ]

A.	Bacterial vaginosis
B.	Beta-haemolytic streptococcus
C.	Candida
D.	Chlamydia
E.	Gonorrhoea
F.	Herpes genitalis
G.	Primary syphilis
H.	Streptococcus A (*Streptococcus pyogenes*)
I.	Trichomonas vaginalis

These clinical scenarios relate to women presenting to a hospital clinic or general practice surgery. Select the most likely infecting organism given the clinical information for each woman.

Each option may be used once, more than once or not at all.

1.31 A 23-year-old woman admitted two days postpartum with severe sepsis. Her temperature is 38 °C, pulse 110 bpm, her respiratory rate is raised and her uterus is enlarged and tender. She has a sore throat with a red pharynx and white spots on her tonsils on examination.

Answer [ ]

1.32 A 55-year-old diabetic woman presents to her GP with a six-week history of a sore vulva. On examination her vulva is red and excoriated.

Answer [ ]

1.33 A 19-year-old presents to the practice nurse with postcoital bleeding and on speculum examination her cervix bleeds on contact.

Answer [ ]

1.34 A primigravid woman is admitted in labour at term. Her uterus is tender and a diagnosis of chorioamnionitis is made. Postnatally the baby develops meningitis.

Answer [ ]

1.35 A 22-year-old woman is admitted to the gynaecology ward with acute retention of urine. On examination she has a sore vulva.

Answer [   ]

A.	Colposcopy
B.	Colposcopy and cervical biopsy
C.	Dilatation and curettage
D.	Endometrial biopsy using sampling device
E.	Hysteroscopy and endometrial biopsy
F.	Human papilloma virus typing
G.	Liquid-based cervical cytology
H.	MRI scan of abdomen and pelvis
I.	Transvaginal ultrasound scan

The scenarios described below relate to women whose GP suspects that they might have cancer so they have been referred to the gynaecology clinic with an urgent 'two-week wait' appointment. For each patient select the most appropriate investigation given the clinical information described in each case.

Each option may be used once, more than once or not at all.

1.36 A 48-year-old diabetic woman with a BMI of 48 presents with a history of irregular periods and intermenstrual bleeding. She is nulliparous.

Answer [   ]

1.37 A 26-year-old woman attends for her first smear at the GP's surgery and mentions that she has experienced postcoital bleeding for the last six months. While taking the smear, a friable 3 mm diameter red lesion is noted on her cervix, which bleeds profusely.

Answer [   ]

1.38 A 57-year-old woman goes to see her GP complaining of indigestion and abdominal distension. She has had a CA125 blood test done privately and the result is 60 IU/l.

Answer [   ]

1.39 A worried 31-year-old refugee woman presents to the surgery a few weeks after arrival in the country saying that her younger sister has just died of cervical cancer back home. She wishes to be reassured that she does not have it too.

Answer [   ]

1.40 A 32-year-old nulliparous woman presents with lower abdominal pain and severe dysmenorrhoea three years after radiotherapy treatment for cancer of the cervix. On examination her cervix looks normal but atrophic with radiotherapy changes and an ultrasound scan shows that the cavity of the uterus is distended with blood.

Answer [   ]

A.	Discuss with on-call consultant
B.	Discuss with on-call registrar (Specialty Trainee year 4)
C.	Leave for consultant to deal with on his return
D.	No action required
E.	Phone GP
F.	Phone patient
G.	Post a prescription to patient
H.	Recall urgently to gynaecology clinic next week
I.	Refer to gynae-oncology multidisciplinary team (MDT) meeting
J.	Routine gynaecology clinic follow-up
K.	Write to GP
L.	Write to patient

The rest of your clinical team are away and your consultant's secretary has asked you to go through some messages and results in her in-tray. For each of the scenarios below select the most appropriate course of action to ensure the best use of NHS time and resources, as well as considering the most safe and convenient solution for the patient.

Each option may be used once, more than once or not at all.

1.41 A 28-year-old woman attended the antenatal clinic a few days ago for a growth scan at 28 weeks gestation and gave a history of an offensive vaginal discharge for the last week. The result of the high vaginal swab is reported as showing clue cells on microscopy and profuse anaerobes on culture.

Answer [   ]

1.42 An 18-year-old woman attended the emergency gynaecology clinic two days ago with pelvic pain, discharge and postcoital bleeding for the preceding fortnight. The endocervical swab result shows *Chlamydia trachomatis* detected by PCR.

Answer [   ]

1.43 A GP has written a letter about a 30-year-old woman with a two-year history of pelvic pain. She has been previously seen in the gynaecology clinic by your consultant and was advised to start the combined oral contraceptive pill. She is getting headaches so has discontinued the pill but is still getting pelvic pain.

Answer [   ]

1.44 A 23-year-old woman was seen in the gynaecology clinic two weeks ago with a three-month history of pelvic pain throughout the cycle. Examination showed no abnormality, in particular no tenderness on vaginal examination and the high vaginal and endocervical swabs were negative. In clinic, you gave her an advice leaflet about irritable bowel syndrome and organized an ultrasound scan. The scan result shows a normal-sized anteverted uterus, both ovaries are clearly seen and are normal. There is no free fluid and there are no adnexal masses.

Answer [   ]

1.45 A 22-year-old woman was admitted as an emergency one week ago. She was found to have a torted ovarian cyst and had a laparoscopic oophorectomy. The rest of her pelvis was normal and she was given that information before discharge. The histology report on the cyst shows a mature cystic teratoma (dermoid cyst).

Answer [   ]

A.	Appendicitis
B.	Complete mole
C.	Ectopic pregnancy
D.	Hyperemesis gravidarum
E.	Incomplete miscarriage
F.	Missed miscarriage
G.	Partial hydatidiform mole
H.	Threatened miscarriage
I.	Urinary tract infection

The clinical scenarios below describe pregnant women presenting with acute problems. In each case select the most likely diagnosis.

Each option may be used once, more than once or not at all.

1.46 Having had a positive pregnancy test two weeks after her missed period, a 29-year-old primigravid woman is referred to have a scan because of vaginal bleeding. On arrival in the Early Pregnancy Unit the bleeding is noted to be heavy and when you insert a speculum you find that the cervical os is open.

Answer [   ]

1.47 A 28-year-old woman has a transvaginal ultrasound scan on the Early Pregnancy Unit at eight weeks gestation because of vaginal bleeding. The uterus is larger than expected with a closed os. The scan shows an abnormal looking intrauterine sac with a fetal pole but no heart pulsation detected. Her serum βhCG is 150 000 IU/ml.

Answer [   ]

1.48 A 28-year-old woman attends her GP's surgery asking for a pregnancy test after 14 weeks of amenorrhoea. She feels unwell and has been vomiting throughout the day. On examination she is tachycardic, sweaty and has a tremor. Her uterus is easily palpable and the fundus is just below the umbilicus.

Answer [   ]

1.49 Having reached 11 weeks gestation, a 22-year-old woman is relieved when her morning sickness disappears. A week later she is devastated when her booking scan shows an irregular sac which is ten weeks size. A fetal pole is present but cardiac activity is absent.

Answer [   ]

1.50 A GP asks you to admit a pregnant 19-year-old at 14 weeks gestation because she has been vomiting for the last week. She has no diarrhoea but is clinically very dehydrated. Urine dip is positive for ketones, nitrites and protein.

Answer [   ]

Curriculum module 2

Basic surgical skills and surgical procedures

Syllabus

- You will be expected to demonstrate an understanding of commonly performed obstetric and gynaecological surgical procedures including their complications and the legal issues around consent to surgical procedures.
- You will need to be aware of commonly encountered infections, including an understanding of the principles of infection control.
- You will be expected to interpret preoperative investigations and be aware of the principles involved in appropriate preoperative and postoperative care.

Learning outcomes

Although you might think that this topic is not relevant to GPs with little or no involvement in surgical events happening in secondary care, we feel that some core knowledge is necessary. For example, patients often wish to be able to discuss their proposed treatment with their GP or they may develop a surgical complication after they have left hospital. Increasingly, GPs are taking on postoperative follow-up for patients in an attempt to move care out of hospital into the community. It is usually the GP who is asked to supply certification for time off work or who is asked for information about driving, resuming intercourse etc.

Therefore, although you would not be expected to actually perform the operations yourself, a basic knowledge of the technicalities of gynaecological and obstetric operations is useful in this context and you may have picked up some of this if you have worked as a junior doctor in O&G. Some of the knowledge is transferable from other surgical specialties and everyone will have had some exposure to some sort of surgery during their previous training.

You may need to refer back to your undergraduate textbooks, or there may be some guidelines on the RCOG website that you might find useful, e.g. 'birth after previous caesarean', 'blood transfusion in obstetrics'. There are also a set of Clinical Governance guidelines on the RCOG website (accessible to non-members) which cover obtaining consent for many obstetric and gynaecological operations and procedures. These are full of useful information such as the possible complications and these are highly recommended source material.

MULTIPLE CHOICE QUESTIONS

2.1 Potential complications of delivery by elective caesarean section include:

A. Placenta accreta in the next pregnancy   [T] [F]
B. Urinary tract infection   [T] [F]
C. Arterial thromboembolism   [T] [F]
D. Subsequent subfertility   [T] [F]
E. Prolonged ileus   [T] [F]

2.2 An 'alert' notice should be added to the operating list to warn theatre staff in advance of patients with the following issues as they may need to change the order of the list or arrange special equipment:

A. Latex allergy   [T] [F]
B. HIV infection   [T] [F]
C. Previous abdominal surgery in a patient undergoing laparoscopy [T] [F]
D. BMI over 50   [T] [F]
E. A Jehovah's Witness 'advance directive' refusing transfusion   [T] [F]

2.3 The following operations are likely to result in primary haemorrhage needing transfusion, so cross-matched blood should be available rather than just 'group and save' being requested:

A. Hysterectomy for dysfunctional uterine bleeding   [T] [F]
B. Posterior vaginal repair   [T] [F]
C. Salpingectomy for ruptured ectopic pregnancy   [T] [F]
D. Adhesiolysis   [T] [F]
E. Laparotomy for ovarian cancer   [T] [F]

2.4 Perioperative antibiotic prophylaxis is advisable for patients undergoing:

A. Caesarean section   [T] [F]
B. Vaginal hysterectomy   [T] [F]
C. Laparoscopic removal of ectopic pregnancy   [T] [F]
D. Anterior vaginal repair   [T] [F]
E. Oophorectomy for ovarian cyst   [T] [F]

2.5 The following are possible causes of pyrexia on the third day following an open (laparotomy) operation to remove an adherent endometrioma of the ovary:

A. Chest infection   [T] [F]
B. Deep vein thrombosis   [T] [F]
C. Ureteric injury   [T] [F]
D. Urinary tract infection   [T] [F]
E. Small bowel obstruction   [T] [F]

2.6 The risk of ureteric injury at hysterectomy is higher if:

A. There is heavy bleeding during the operation   [T] [F]
B. The patient has a duplex kidney   [T] [F]
C. The ovaries are being conserved   [T] [F]
D. The patient's obstetric history involves caesarean deliveries   [T] [F]
E. The operation is being done for endometriosis   [T] [F]

2.7 The following situations might render laparoscopic sterilization more difficult:

A. A woman with a BMI less than 20   [T]   [F]
B. A woman with a BMI over 40   [T]   [F]
C. Previous diagnostic laparoscopy   [T]   [F]
D. Previous caesarean section   [T]   [F]
E. A woman with a history of endometriosis   [T]   [F]

2.8 When looking after elderly women on a postoperative gynaecology ward, wound dehiscence is an important complication to look out for. Following a hysterectomy, postoperative dehiscence of an abdominal wound is more likely to occur if:

A. The patient is being treated for cancer   [T]   [F]
B. The wound becomes infected   [T]   [F]
C. The patient develops a postoperative ileus   [T]   [F]
D. The wound is transverse rather than vertical   [T]   [F]
E. The patient develops a vault haematoma   [T]   [F]

2.9 A clinically appropriate reason for advising a woman to have her ovaries removed at the time of hysterectomy is:

A. So she can have postoperative estrogen replacement therapy   [T]   [F]
B. The hysterectomy is treatment for carcinoma of the endometrium [T]   [F]
C. Oophorectomy eliminates premenstrual syndrome   [T]   [F]
D. She has a strong family history of ovarian cancer   [T]   [F]
E. To prevent metabolic effects of polycystic ovarian syndrome, e.g. diabetes   [T]   [F]

2.10 Surgery can be carried out without written consent if:

A. Permission is obtained via a court order   [T]   [F]
B. The patient is unconscious and it is in her best interests   [T]   [F]
C. The patient is a child who is Fraser-competent   [T]   [F]
D. The woman's husband agrees to it   [T]   [F]
E. The operation is a dire emergency, e.g. caesarean for fetal bradycardia   [T]   [F]

SINGLE BEST ANSWER QUESTIONS

2.11 You are about to sign a consent form with a patient who is having a caesarean section. After you have listed the complications for her, she asks you which is the most common:

A. Wound dehiscence
B. Subsequent subfertility
C. Pseudo-obstruction of the bowel
D. Excess blood loss during surgery
E. Fetal laceration

Answer [   ]

2.12 In the antenatal clinic you see a primigravid woman who has been referred by her community midwife at 37 weeks because the fetus is lying transversely. You organize an ultrasound scan which shows that the reason for the abnormal lie is an 8 cm diameter ovarian cyst filling her pelvis. Your consultant tells you to arrange a caesarean section and the woman asks you about the management of the cyst. Select the most appropriate advice in this clinical situation:

A. It will be dealt with later as ovaries are not accessible during a caesarean

B. Spontaneous resolution of the cyst is likely after delivery

C. Removing the cyst at the time of caesarean will require a general anaesthetic

D. Caesarean and removal of the cyst should take place now in case the cyst torts

E. Ovarian cystectomy during a caesarean at 39 weeks is appropriate

Answer [　]

2.13 You have seen a woman in preoperative assessment clinic who is due to undergo hysterectomy for prolapse in a few weeks time. Which one of these is the most important factor to warn the anaesthetist about from her case notes?

A. She lives alone and has no postoperative social arrangements for care

B. Her mother had a DVT during chemotherapy many years ago

C. She has hypertension which is adequately treated with bendrofluazide

D. She is allergic to penicillin

E. There is a family history of suxamethonium apnoea

Answer [　]

2.14 You are filling out a thromboprophylaxis risk form in the preoperative assessment clinic for a woman about to undergo pelvic floor repair. Which of the following does **not** contribute to her risk score for venous thromboembolism?

A. The woman has a BMI of 44

B. The woman has inflammatory bowel disease

C. The woman has essential hypertension

D. The woman has protein S deficiency

E. The woman has a history of recent breast cancer

Answer [　]

2.15 A 45-year-old woman has been put on the waiting list for endometrial ablation to treat her menorrhagia. She visits the surgery to ask for further information as she wasn't given adequate time to discuss the procedure in gynaecology clinic. Which one of the following statements about endometrial ablation is correct?

A. Endometrial ablation is always done under general anaesthetic

B. Endometrial sampling is not required prior to the procedure

C. It cannot be undertaken in the presence of a caesarean scar

D. She should continue using contraception afterwards

E. The operation has a 90% chance of producing amenorrhoea

Answer [　]

2.16 A woman attends A&E due to heavy vaginal bleeding a week after having a large loop excision of the transformation zone (LLETZ procedure) for CIN 3. Her pulse and blood pressure are normal and her haemoglobin is 120 g/l. On speculum examination there is active bleeding from the cervix. What is the most appropriate initial management in this case?

A. Arrange the operating theatre immediately for suturing of the cervix
B. Pack the vagina and give broad-spectrum antibiotics
C. Prescribe oral norethisterone and allow home
D. Prescribe tranexamic acid and allow home
E. Take a swab and commence broad-spectrum oral antibiotics

Answer [　]

2.17 You would have concerns about the legitimacy of one of these patients signing their consent form for surgery. Which patient?

A. A girl aged 15 years requesting termination of pregnancy
B. An elderly woman who has had a stroke
C. A woman requesting sterilization whose husband did not agree
D. A Jehovah's Witness who needs a caesarean for placenta praevia
E. A non-English speaking woman whose husband is translating for her

Answer [　]

2.18 An 86-year-old woman presents to the gynaecology outpatient clinic with postmenopausal bleeding. Having examined her, the consultant decides that hysteroscopy and cervical biopsy are necessary but she is currently taking warfarin on account of an artificial heart valve. Select the most appropriate option regarding her anticoagulation:

A. Continue with current dose of warfarin
B. Change to heparin and omit dose on morning of surgery
C. Omit warfarin for three days before surgery and check INR
D. Omit anticoagulation on morning of surgery
E. Postpone surgery until anticoagulant therapy completed

Answer [　]

2.19 You are asked to review a woman on the Day Case Unit who had a laparoscopic sterilization yesterday. She has had four children between the ages of six months and four years, all delivered by caesarean section via a Pfannenstiel incision. The nurses are concerned because she has abdominal pain and she is still not well enough to go home, although your consultant saw her last night after the operating list had finished and discharged her. When you examine her you notice some watery discharge from her suprapubic incision which is soaking through the dressing.

Which one of the following statements applies to this case?

A. Bowel damage is unlikely because her previous incision was suprapubic
B. She is probably evading being discharged because the children exhaust her
C. She should be sent home because your consultant discharged her
D. There could be a hole in her bladder
E. Unrecognized laparoscopic bowel injury produces peritonitis very quickly

Answer [　]

2.20 An asthmatic woman is breathless on return to the Day Case Unit from the operating theatre recovery room and you are asked for advice. She has had an uncomplicated evacuation of uterus performed, but the hospital notes mention that she did have a coughing fit as she was being anaesthetized. Select the most appropriate immediate course of action in this situation:

A. Send her for an urgent chest x-ray
B. Organize a peak flow estimation
C. Prescribe nebulized salbutamol
D. Ask the anaesthetist to review her at the end of the list
E. Check her airway and give her oxygen by face mask

Answer [ ]

EXTENDED MATCHING QUESTIONS

A.	CA125 level
B.	Chest x-ray
C.	Clotting screen
D.	CT scan of abdomen and pelvis
E.	Electrocardiogram
F.	Endocervical chlamydia swab
G.	Ferritin
H.	Haemoglobin
I.	High vaginal swab
J.	Plain abdominal x-ray
K.	Pregnancy test
L.	Thrombophilia screen
M.	Ultrasound guided biopsy
N.	Ultrasound scan of the pelvis

The clinical scenarios below describe women who are on the waiting list for various gynaecological operations. Select the single most appropriate preoperative investigation for each case.

Each option may be used once, more than once or not at all.

2.21 A 31-year-old woman requesting fertility investigations is to be admitted to the Day Case Unit on day 8 of her next menstrual cycle for a laparoscopy and dye test to check tubal patency because she has a past history of pelvic inflammatory disease.

Answer [ ]

2.22 To investigate her severe long-standing menorrhagia a 49-year-old woman is going to undergo hysteroscopy and endometrial biopsy and she has chosen to have it done under general anaesthetic.

Answer [　]

2.23 A woman aged 42 years has an ultrasound scan revealing a left ovarian cyst measuring 9 cm with solid elements in it. The right ovary seems normal on the scan and there is no ascites. Your consultant is trying to decide whether to remove the uterus and other ovary as well as the diseased ovary.

Answer [　]

2.24 A 32-year-old multiparous woman is admitted as a day case for laparoscopic sterilization. She has been using a copper coil for contraception but you cannot see the strings and she thinks it was extruded from the uterus during an unusually heavy period four weeks ago.

Answer [　]

2.25 A 40-year-old woman is going to have a hysterectomy for endometriosis. The preoperative ultrasound scan reveals bilateral chocolate cysts on the ovaries. She has not had any surgery before but her mother had a DVT following hysterectomy at the same age.

Answer [　]

A.	Chest x-ray
B.	CT scan of abdomen and pelvis
C.	Electrocardiogram
D.	Haemoglobin
E.	High vaginal swab
F.	Intravenous pyelogram (IVP) x-ray
G.	Plain abdominal x-ray
H.	Serum calcium
I.	Ultrasound scan of kidneys
J.	Urea and electrolytes
K.	Urine culture

These clinical scenarios describe women developing complications after gynaecological operations. Select the most appropriate investigation for each case.

Each option may be used once, more than once or not at all.

2.26 Three days after a hysterectomy for endometrial cancer, a 60-year-old woman still has a distended abdomen with no bowel sounds. Which investigation will help you most with planning her management?

Answer [　]

2.27 An obese 58-year-old woman who normally smokes 20 cigarettes a day develops severe left-sided chest pain two days after a prolapse operation. She is tachycardic and tachypnoeic. On examination you find an inspiratory wheeze but normal air entry all over the chest. Which investigation would you carry out initially?

Answer [   ]

2.28 Having undergone hysteroscopy and insertion of a levonorgestrel intrauterine system (Mirena®) for menorrhagia under general anaesthetic, a 42-year-old woman was not well enough to be discharged home and has stayed in hospital overnight because of severe lower abdominal pain. The next morning she is still in pain and has a temperature of 38 °C. You cannot locate the coil strings on speculum examination.

Answer [   ]

2.29 On the fourth day following a difficult hysterectomy and bilateral salpingo-oophorectomy operation for endometriosis a 38-year-old woman has a swinging pyrexia and unilateral loin pain. She is still nauseous and seems to have a persistent ileus.

Answer [   ]

2.30 Six days after leaving hospital following a vaginal hysterectomy operation, an anaemic woman is readmitted with further vaginal discharge and pain. She was sent home on iron tablets and analgesics. On readmission she is pyrexial and bimanual pelvic examination reveals a palpable tender mass at the vault with offensive brown blood in the vagina.

Answer [   ]

A.	A guardian with Power of Attorney should sign the consent form
B.	Consent from the patient is valid
C.	Defer the operation until a court order can be obtained
D.	Defer the operation until an independent interpreter is available
E.	Defer the operation until the woman is fully recovered
F.	The consent already given is not valid
G.	The clinician could go ahead with surgery in the patient's best interests
H.	The woman has a right to refuse consent
I.	The woman should not be asked to participate in the research
J.	Verbal consent from the patient is adequate
K.	Written consent could be obtained from the patient's husband

These clinical scenarios describe women in different situations where consent may be an issue. Select the most appropriate advice for each case.

Each option may be used once, more than once or not at all.

2.31 A 51-year-old woman with severe learning difficulties is brought into A&E as an emergency with prolonged heavy bleeding. On admission her haemoglobin is 93 g/l. She needs a hysteroscopy to investigate the problem but cannot understand what is being proposed.

Answer [   ]

2.32 On the labour ward a primigravid woman has reluctantly had a fetal blood sample done at 4 cm dilatation and the result shows that the baby is hypoxic. She has a needle phobia and adamantly refuses caesarean section to deliver the baby quickly. Both the obstetric consultant and the paediatrician have explained the possible consequences to her.

Answer [   ]

2.33 A Jehovah's Witness has a hysterectomy operation for endometrial cancer. She specifically states that she will not accept blood transfusion and signs a disclaimer form preoperatively. In the recovery room it becomes apparent that she has internal bleeding and the consultant decides to take her back to theatre. She has had a lot of opiates to control her pain and is very drowsy.

Answer [   ]

2.34 On the labour ward a new research project is underway comparing two different drugs to treat postpartum haemorrhage. You are called in to put a drip up for a woman who has lost 400 ml of blood already and the blood loss seems to be ongoing. Although it has not been discussed previously with the patient, the midwife mentions the possibility of the patient being asked to participate in the research project.

Answer [   ]

2.35 A 15-year-old schoolgirl presents to clinic requesting surgical termination of pregnancy accompanied by her 15-year-old boyfriend. She will not tell her parents about the pregnancy and after much discussion she is thought to be able to understand the risks of the procedure.

Answer [   ]

A.	Cancel the operation as it is not the correct procedure for this patient
B.	Go ahead with the operation as planned
C.	Postpone the operation and arrange counselling
D.	Postpone the operation and arrange review in the genitourinary medicine clinic
E.	Postpone the operation and arrange routine gynaecology clinic review
F.	Postpone the operation and arrange urgent gynaecology clinic review
G.	Postpone the operation and organize an ultrasound scan
H.	Postpone the operation until you can arrange further tests
I.	Refer her urgently to her GP for a prescription
J.	Suggest that the patient has a spinal anaesthetic

The patients that you are seeing in the preoperative clinic are about to undergo gynaecological operations and unfortunately your consultant is not immediately available for advice.

Select the most appropriate management plan for each clinical scenario.

Each option may be used once, more than once or not at all.

2.36 The waiting list clerk has arranged for a 49-year-old woman to fill a cancelled slot on the operating list at short notice. She is due to have an abdominal hysterectomy in three days' time and you are doing her preoperative check. She had a hysteroscopy done under local anaesthetic for irregular heavy bleeding recently but the histology on the endometrium from that operation is not yet available.

Answer [   ]

2.37 A 37-year-old woman presented to clinic with left iliac fossa pain radiating down her left leg several weeks ago and ultrasound scan revealed a 7 cm simple left ovarian cyst. She was put on the waiting list for an ovarian cystectomy but her symptoms have now disappeared.

Answer [   ]

2.38 A healthy 62-year-old woman is due to be admitted for a prolapse repair. She mentions a family history of 'difficulty waking up' after anaesthetics but is not sure of the clinical details.

Answer [   ]

2.39 A 33-year-old woman is to be admitted for endometrial ablation to treat her menorrhagia. She has turned down the option of a Mirena® intrauterine system because she wishes to have another baby within the next couple of years.

Answer [   ]

2.40 When she was seen in the fertility clinic a couple of weeks ago, a 29-year-old woman had a speculum examination during which some routine swabs were taken. You look up the results before signing her consent form for a laparoscopy and dye test only to discover that the chlamydia swab is positive.

Answer [   ]

A.	Acute primary haemorrhage
B.	Chest infection
C.	Deep vein thrombosis
D.	Haemolysis
E.	Intestinal obstruction
F.	Pelvic haematoma
G.	Pulmonary embolus
H.	Secondary haemorrhage due to vault infection
I.	Ureteric injury
J.	Urinary tract infection
K.	Urinary retention
L.	Vault granulations
M.	Vault dehiscence

Each of these clinical scenarios describes a woman presenting with complications after a hysterectomy operation; for each patient pick the most likely diagnosis given the information that you are presented with.

Each option may be used once, more than once or not at all.

2.41 You are called to see a morbidly obese 40-year-old woman who had a hysterectomy for endometrial cancer three days ago. She has gradually become more breathless over the previous 24 hours and now seems a little confused. She is hypoxic and expresses discomfort when you ask for deep breaths to auscultate her chest but there is normal air entry. Her temperature is normal and you do not see any abnormality on her chest x-ray.

Answer [   ]

2.42 Three days after a hysterectomy for endometriosis, a 35-year-old woman is found to have a mild pyrexia and a tachycardia of 100 beats per minute. There is a moderate amount of old blood coming from the vagina and her haemoglobin has dropped from 127 g/l preoperatively to 82 g/l now. The estimated blood loss at operation was described as 250 ml.

Answer [   ]

2.43 A 30-year-old woman has had a hysterectomy and left salpingo-oophorectomy for chronic pelvic inflammatory disease with hydrosalpinx. The operation notes document dense adhesions on the left side of the pelvis and there was a perioperative blood loss of 900 ml. Two days later she is very unwell with swinging pyrexia, a prolonged ileus and severe left loin pain.

Answer [   ]

2.44 A woman who had a hysterectomy ten weeks ago comes to your surgery because she has just started to bleed vaginally again. She has not seen any blood since a week after her hysterectomy but has not been examined following the operation as she did not go to the hospital for her postoperative check-up.

Answer [   ]

2.45 On her fluid balance chart on the first postoperative day, you notice that a woman has not passed urine since she returned from theatre in spite of having received over 2 litres of fluid intravenously. She has a pelvic drain *in situ* which contains 400 ml. The nurses report that she asked for a bedpan twice during the night.

Answer [   ]

A.	Advise alternative method of contraception four weeks before surgery
B.	Continue using current contraceptive method
C.	Prescribe full therapeutic anticoagulation therapy
D.	Prescribe local vaginal estrogen instead of systemic HRT
E.	Switch HRT to transdermal method before surgery
F.	Stop HRT four weeks before surgery
G.	Stop HRT 12 weeks before surgery
H.	Stopping HRT is not necessary
I.	Stop contraceptive method four weeks before surgery

These clinical scenarios relate to women seeking advice relating to surgery and the risks of thromboembolism. In each case you should decide on the best course of action with regard to hormonal medication and select the most appropriate advice.

Each option may be used once, more than once or not at all.

2.46 A 26-year-old woman is on the waiting list for scoliosis surgery and seeks advice about whether she should continue taking her combined oral contraceptive pill.

Answer [   ]

2.47 A 26-year-old woman is being admitted to hospital for scoliosis surgery in six weeks time and seeks advice about whether she should have her next dose of depot medroxy progesterone acetate, which is now due.

Answer [   ]

2.48 A 26-year-old woman is on the waiting list for diagnostic laparoscopy to diagnose her pelvic pain. She is currently taking Dianette® for contraception and in the hope that it will improve her acne.

Answer [   ]

2.49 A fit 50-year-old woman started on systemic HRT (sequential tablet formulation) six months ago because of severe vasomotor and vaginal dryness symptoms. She has felt much better on it but is now on the waiting list for a posterior vaginal repair for prolapse. Apart from the surgery, you do not identify any risk factors for thromboembolism in her medical notes.

Answer [   ]

2.50 A 45-year-old woman is taking tibolone (Livial®) hormone replacement therapy having had a complete pelvic clearance for endometriosis six months previously. She is about to undergo carpal tunnel surgery and seeks advice about her tibolone medication.

Answer [   ]

Curriculum module 3

Antenatal care

Syllabus

- You will be expected to understand and demonstrate appropriate knowledge and attitudes in relation to periconceptional care, antenatal care and maternal complications of pregnancy.
- An awareness of substance misuse, psychiatric illness, problems of pregnancy at extremes of reproductive age and of domestic violence in relation to pregnancy is expected. An appreciation of emotional and cultural issues is needed too.
- You will be expected to have a good understanding of common medical disorders and the effect that pregnancy may have on them, and also their effect, in turn, upon the pregnancy. You will be expected to demonstrate your ability to assess and manage these conditions.
- Knowledge of therapeutics in antenatal care is expected.
- You will need to show understanding of the roles of other professionals, the importance of liaison and empathic teamwork.
- You will be expected to understand the principles of antenatal screening including screening for structural defects, chromosomal abnormalities and haemoglobinopathies and the effects of relevant infections during pregnancy on the fetus and neonate.

Learning outcomes

In the past GPs were more involved in provision of antenatal care than they are now. Although few run antenatal clinics now, having delegated this responsibility to midwives, it is not uncommon for midwives to consult the GP for advice when they are dealing with a difficult case or if the patient needs a prescription. When deciding whether to refer a pregnant woman for hospital care, midwives will work to protocols and national guidelines but may consult the GP if they are unsure. Some patients may seek a second opinion if they are unhappy about or need more information about advice given to them by the midwife or the obstetricians.

The Confidential Enquiry into Maternal and Child Health Report has highlighted the important role of the GP where women have pre-existing medical disorders. For these reasons the DRCOG exam continues to test knowledge about the antenatal care of pregnant women.

MULTIPLE CHOICE QUESTIONS

3.1 Referring a pregnant woman for an antenatal glucose tolerance test is indicated in the following situations:

A. Obesity [T] [F]
B. Previous pregnancy ending in stillbirth [T] [F]
C. Polyhydramnios in this pregnancy [T] [F]
D. One episode of glycosuria [T] [F]
E. Recurrent urinary tract infections during pregnancy [T] [F]

3.2 The community midwife asks you to see a 23-year-old woman who has presented for antenatal care late in her first pregnancy. She has needle tracks on her arms and on questioning admits to injecting heroin and often smokes cannabis.

With regard to the effect of her drug habit on her pregnancy:

A. Drug users commonly suffer from iron and vitamin deficiency [T] [F]
B. Methadone substitution is contraindicated while she is pregnant [T] [F]
C. Premature labour is likely [T] [F]
D. She is at increased risk of thromboembolism [T] [F]
E. Cannabis is linked with low birthweight [T] [F]

3.3 Screening tests for Down syndrome:

A. Carry a risk of miscarriage [T] [F]
B. Are mandatory [T] [F]
C. Rarely miss an affected pregnancy [T] [F]
D. Should only be offered to high-risk mothers [T] [F]
E. The result indicates the chance of the pregnancy being affected [T] [F]

3.4 The following are maternal risk factors for intrauterine growth restriction:

A. Antiphospholipid syndrome [T] [F]
B. Maternal diabetes mellitus [T] [F]
C. Cocaine use during pregnancy [T] [F]
D. Being 'small for gestational age' herself at birth [T] [F]
E. Continuing to work until term [T] [F]

3.5 Symphysis pubis dysfunction in pregnancy:

A. Will give the woman more pain the wider the gap in the symphysis [T] [F]
B. Is made worse by maternal obesity [T] [F]
C. Caesarean section is of proven benefit to the patient [T] [F]
D. Can happen in the first trimester [T] [F]
E. Has been shown to be improved by physiotherapy [T] [F]

3.6 **Concerning the dental health of pregnant women:**

A. The immune response to plaque bacteria is altered in pregnancy   [T]   [F]
B. Pregnant women are entitled to free dental care only until the baby [T]   [F]
    is born
C. Hyperemesis can result in damage to maternal teeth   [T]   [F]
D. Periodontitis is a risk factor for low birthweight   [T]   [F]
E. There is an association between pregnancy and gingival   [T]   [F]
    hyperplasia

3.7 **In a pregnancy affected by obstetric cholestasis:**

A. The condition is characterized by intense pruritus without a   [T]   [F]
    skin rash
B. The serum bilirubin is usually markedly raised   [T]   [F]
C. The itching particularly affects the palms and soles of the feet   [T]   [F]
D. Postnatal resolution of symptoms and biochemical abnormalities [T]   [F]
    are required to confirm the diagnosis
E. Ursodeoxycholic acid therapy has been shown to reduce the   [T]   [F]
    incidence of stillbirth

3.8 **If you are looking after a pregnant woman with a personal history of venous thromboembolism:**

A. She should be referred to a consultant clinic early for risk   [T]   [F]
    assessment
B. Low molecular weight heparin is contraindicated if she wishes to [T]   [F]
    breastfeed
C. If the previous DVT was associated with a causative factor she   [T]   [F]
    may not need anticoagulation during pregnancy
D. Anticoagulation with warfarin is preferable to heparin in   [T]   [F]
    pregnancy
E. She is likely to be offered induction of labour if she is on heparin   [T]   [F]

3.9 **Concerning the management of a woman with epilepsy in pregnancy:**

A. Antiepileptic drugs are associated with an increased risk of   [T]   [F]
    congenital abnormalities
B. Monotherapy with one drug is the preferred option in pregnancy [T]   [F]
C. Epileptic women intending pregnancy should be advised to take [T]   [F]
    0.5 mg folic acid daily
D. Sodium valproate is associated with the least risk of abnormality [T]   [F]
E. Pregnant women are more at risk of seizure-related death than   [T]   [F]
    non-pregnant women

3.10 **Screening for the following infections is routinely offered during antenatal care of pregnant women in the UK**

A. Parvovirus B19   [T]   [F]
B. Hepatitis B   [T]   [F]
C. Gonorrhoea   [T]   [F]
D. Human immunodeficiency virus   [T]   [F]
E. Syphilis   [T]   [F]

SINGLE BEST ANSWER QUESTIONS

3.11 Intrahepatic cholestasis of pregnancy is an uncommon but serious complication. Which of the following statements about this condition is not correct?

A. The baby is at risk of intrauterine death

B. Antenatal administration of vitamin K to the mother reduces the risk of postpartum haemorrhage

C. Meconium in the liquor during labour can be ignored as it is to be expected

D. The condition can run in families

E. The recurrence risk in a subsequent pregnancy is over 50%

Answer [　]

3.12 Which of the following statements concerning HIV in pregnancy is true:

A. In HIV positive mothers on antiretroviral treatment breastfeeding is safe

B. Interventions reduce the risk of vertical HIV transmission from 30% to zero

C. All infants born to women who are HIV positive should be treated with antiretroviral therapy from birth

D. Women who do not require treatment for their own health do not need to take antiretroviral therapy during pregnancy

E. The use of short-term steroids to promote fetal lung maturation is inadvisable

Answer [　]

3.13 A refugee woman from Ethiopia books for antenatal care in her first pregnancy and discloses to the midwife that she has undergone female genital mutilation (FGM) in the past. Which of these statements about FGM is true?

A. UK law states that the suturing can legally be restored after delivery

B. She must be delivered by elective caesarean section

C. The FGM can be surgically 'undone' before delivery

D. A female baby may be at risk of FGM as a teenager in the future

E. It usually involves complete closure of the vaginal introitus except for a tiny hole

Answer [　]

3.14 You see a pregnant woman in your surgery who has just been to the hospital for a dating scan at 11 weeks gestation which reveals that she has monochorionic twins in separate sacs. Which of the following statements is true about this type of twin pregnancy?

A. Monochorionic twins are at lower risk of twin–twin transfusion syndrome than dichorionic twins

B. She will be having regular growth scans from 32 weeks gestation

C. She should be delivered by caesarean section as there is a risk of cord entanglement

D. Delivery should be planned for 37 weeks if she has not laboured

E. She will not be able to have any sort of non-invasive screening for Down syndrome

Answer [　]

3.15 You are consulted by a primigravid woman at 24 weeks gestation who has an unbearable headache. She has a history of severe migraine about which she has consulted you before several times. You do a thorough examination and find epigastric tenderness. Testing her urine reveals proteinuria +++. Which one of the following statements about her situation is correct?

A. The diagnosis cannot be pre-eclampsia because of the early gestation

B. If her blood pressure is 125/80 mmHg the diagnosis cannot be pre-eclampsia

C. Fundal height is irrelevant as IUGR will not be apparent at this early gestation

D. She needs assessment by an obstetrician urgently

E. Prescribing antibiotics without awaiting the results of an MSU is not advisable

Answer [ ]

3.16 Consultant referral is necessary so that antenatal serial growth scans can be arranged to check on fetal growth if the pregnancy is affected by which one of the following conditions in the mother:

A. 'Slapped cheek' syndrome

B. Recurrent unexplained antepartum haemorrhage

C. Previous delivery by caesarean section

D. History of polycystic ovarian syndrome

E. Maternal vitamin B12 deficiency

Answer [ ]

3.17 A 14-year-old schoolgirl is brought to your surgery by her angry mother having been sent home with a note from the school nurse suggesting that she might be pregnant. On examination it is obvious that her abdominal swelling is due to a pregnancy of about 36 weeks gestation; fetal movements can be clearly seen and the fetal heart auscultated. Which one of the following statements is true with regard to this teenage pregnancy?

A. She is no more likely to deliver a small-for-dates infant than mothers ten years older

B. You should involve the police because her pregnancy must be the result of rape

C. There is no point in discussing contraception

D. There is a higher incidence of sexually transmitted infections in teenage mothers

E. Her due date can be accurately predicted when she has her first scan at the hospital

Answer [ ]

3.18 A 34-year-old woman who has had two uncomplicated pregnancies before expresses a wish to have a home birth this time. At her 28-week check-up with the midwife she mentions that she has had a couple of minor episodes of vaginal bleeding following intercourse during the previous few weeks. Her blood group is A Rhesus negative. Which one of the following statements about her situation is correct?

A. If she had a normal anomaly scan the diagnosis cannot be placenta praevia

B. The bleeding will not be due to cervical cancer if her prepregnancy smear was normal

C. Kleihauer testing will help diagnose placental abruption

D. This woman could still have a home birth as requested if the placenta is not low

E. She should be referred to consultant-led antenatal care for growth scans

Answer [   ]

3.19 You see a primigravid woman in clinic who has just had a 20-week detailed (anomaly) scan which reveals a low-lying placenta. Which of these is the most appropriate advice for her?

A. Take folic acid 5 mg daily

B. Avoid sexual intercourse

C. Take an increased dose of oral iron three times daily

D. Admission to hospital will be necessary later in the pregnancy

E. Delivery will be by caesarean section at 37 weeks

Answer [   ]

3.20 You are looking after a 'grand multip', pregnant with her fifth baby, who has had four normal births before. She is particularly at risk of which pregnancy complication?

A. Anaemia

B. Hypertension

C. Low-lying placenta

D. Postpartum haemorrhage

E. Placenta accreta

Answer [   ]

EXTENDED MATCHING QUESTIONS

A.	Alpha fetoprotein level
B.	Amniocentesis
C.	Chorionic villus sampling
D.	Combined nuchal translucency scan and serum screening
E.	Cordocentesis
F.	Detailed ultrasound scan
G.	Karyotype both parents for balanced (Robertsonian) translocation
H.	Nuchal translucency scan
I.	Serum screening with hCG/alpha fetoprotein/estriol levels
J.	Third-trimester growth scan
K.	3-D ultrasound scan

The clinical scenarios below relate to prenatal screening and diagnostic tests. For each woman select the most appropriate investigation.

Each option may be used once, more than once or not at all.

3.21 The wife of a prominent politician is referred to a private obstetric clinic at ten weeks gestation because she has conceived unexpectedly many years after the birth of her last child and is now aged 42. She wishes to be absolutely reassured that the baby does not have Down syndrome as soon as possible because she feels that it would hamper her contribution to her husband's career.

Answer [　]

3.22 A patient with a history of a previous pregnancy affected by neural tube defect wishes to have the most sensitive test in this current pregnancy.

Answer [　]

3.23 A 36-year-old woman has conceived after many years of infertility. She wishes to have a screening test for Down syndrome with the least false positive rate.

Answer [　]

3.24 A couple who know that they are both carriers of cystic fibrosis present at nine weeks gestation requesting prenatal diagnosis.

Answer [　]

3.25 A 40-year-old woman who has reached 15 weeks gestation having had three previous first-trimester miscarriages wishes to have a diagnostic test for Down syndrome because her partner has a balanced Robertsonian translocation.

Answer [　]

A.	Abruptio placentae
B.	Appendicitis
C.	Constipation
D.	Pancreatitis
E.	Pre-eclampsia
F.	Red degeneration of a uterine fibroid
G.	Torsion of an ovarian cyst
H.	Ureteric calculus
I.	Urinary tract infection
J.	Uterine rupture

The clinical scenarios below relate to the emergency presentation of a pregnant woman with abdominal pain. For each woman select the most likely diagnosis for her pain.

Each option may be used once, more than once or not at all.

3.26 Two years after a myomectomy operation, a 42-year-old woman has conceived following IVF treatment. At 32 weeks gestation she is admitted to the obstetric unit with increasing pain in her abdomen for three days, which only responds to opiate analgesia. Apart from nausea she has no systemic symptoms. On examination she is apyrexial and normotensive but has a tachycardia. There is localized tenderness only at the fundus of the uterus.

Answer [ ]

3.27 An 18-year-old primigravid woman presents in A&E at 16 weeks gestation with lower abdominal pain and vomiting. She has fetor oris and a temperature of 37.8 °C.

Answer [ ]

3.28 At 32 weeks gestation a woman pregnant with her second baby is admitted in an ambulance having collapsed in a supermarket due to sudden onset of severe abdominal pain. Her observations are stable apart from a maternal tachycardia. The uterus is tender and unfortunately no fetal heart beat is detectable.

Answer [ ]

3.29 At 17 weeks gestation a 38-year-old primigravid woman is rushed in to A&E with severe unilateral colicky loin pain. She was writhing about on the bed but the pain has now subsided following a dose of morphine. Urinalysis reveals haematuria and her temperature is normal.

Answer [ ]

3.30 A primigravid woman on holiday in London attends an NHS 'walk-in' centre with severe epigastric pain and headache. Her pregnancy has been uncomplicated so far and she is now 30 weeks gestation. On admission, urinalysis reveals that there is a lot of protein in her urine.

Answer [   ]

A.	Aim for vaginal delivery but with a shortened second stage
B.	Await spontaneous labour and aim for vaginal delivery
C.	Classical caesarean section
D.	Elective caesarean section at 39 weeks gestation
E.	Elective caesarean section at 39 weeks gestation and sterilization
F.	Elective caesarean section at 40 weeks gestation
G.	Emergency caesarean section
H.	Induction of labour at 38 weeks gestation and aim for vaginal delivery
I.	Offer external cephalic version and await spontaneous labour
J.	Offer external cephalic version and if successful induce labour

The following scenarios relate to a woman with a complicated pregnancy or underlying medical condition. How would you counsel her with regard to delivery?

Each option may be used once, more than once or not at all.

3.31 Having been delivered by caesarean section in both previous pregnancies a 30-year-old woman books for antenatal care at 17 weeks gestation in her third pregnancy.

Answer [   ]

3.32 Having had a myomectomy operation a few years ago, a 39-year-old woman is followed up carefully in antenatal clinic because she has several more fibroids in the uterus. Serial growth scans show that the baby is OK but at 37 weeks the ultrasonographer notes that the fibroid in the lower segment has grown to 8 cm diameter and the baby is lying transversely above it.

Answer [   ]

3.33 A woman with HIV attends antenatal clinic at 36 weeks gestation. She is on antiretroviral medication and her viral load is extremely low < 50 copies per ml.

Answer [   ]

3.34 A primigravid woman is referred to hospital antenatal clinic at 37 weeks gestation because the presentation is found to be breech. Scan confirms that the baby is of average size and the presentation is flexed breech.

Answer [   ]

3.35 Just prior to conceiving, a 34-year-old woman was treated for a cerebral aneurysm, which was successfully clipped leaving no neurological deficit. Her craniotomy wound has healed well and she is now 36 weeks gestation in her first pregnancy.

Answer [   ]

A.	Admit immediately to a psychiatric 'mother and baby' unit
B.	Advise that depression is common and resolves after delivery
C.	Advise that she should stop medication as it can harm the baby
D.	Arrange specialist counselling
E.	Ask a psychiatric liaison worker to visit at home
F.	Continue medication and seek psychiatric advice
G.	Recommence psychiatric medication immediately
H.	Refer her back to her previous psychiatrist
I.	Refer for a routine opinion from a specialist obstetric psychiatric clinic
J.	Refer for an urgent opinion from a specialist obstetric psychiatric clinic
K.	Suggest that she considers short-term use of sleeping tablets
L.	Suggest that she takes an antidepressant

The following scenarios relate to psychiatric problems in pregnant women. In each case decide the most appropriate course of action.

Each option may be used once, more than once or not at all.

3.36 Having been diagnosed with schizophrenia at university many years ago, a 34-year-old woman books for antenatal care very late at 36 weeks gestation as she had not realized that she was pregnant until the third trimester. She has been off medication for many years and has been psychiatrically well since.

Answer [   ]

3.37 A primigravid woman at 28 weeks gestation consults you in surgery about feeling very low in mood and having trouble sleeping following the death of her mother. She denies thoughts of self harm.

Answer [   ]

3.38 A young woman with bipolar disorder has been well controlled on lithium for a few years and seeks preconceptual counselling. She is planning pregnancy in the near future and has no other medical problems.

Answer [   ]

3.39 The midwife caring for one of your patients contacts you with concerns about a 42-year-old first time mother who has refused to allow her access to the house for the previous three days. The husband reveals on the telephone that his wife has not slept since the baby was born and is making bizarre comments about the health of the baby. Her psychiatric liaison worker has left a written care plan in her obstetric notes.

Answer [   ]

3.40 A woman books for antenatal care at ten weeks in her second pregnancy. She gives a history of postnatal depression which involved several months of inpatient care following her previous delivery. She is currently well and not on any medication.

Answer [   ]

A.	Abdominal ultrasound scan
B.	Computed tomogram scan
C.	Doppler measurement
D.	Electronic cardiotocograph fetal monitoring
E.	Fetal growth scan in two weeks
F.	Speculum examination of the cervix with fibronectin swab
G.	Speculum examination of the cervix with microbiology swabs
H.	Transvaginal scan
I.	Ultrasound scan with umbilical artery doppler
J.	Vaginal examination in theatre with the operating team standing by

These clinical scenarios relate to women in the third trimester of pregnancy, presenting with vaginal bleeding. In each case, choose the most appropriate initial investigation.

Each option may be used once, more than once or not at all.

3.41 A woman attends the labour ward at 35 weeks gestation on account of a small amount of vaginal bleeding which has now stopped. Initially there was some minor abdominal pain but this has settled and there is no uterine activity. There have been reduced fetal movements since the episode of bleeding. On examination the size of the uterus is compatible with dates.

Answer [   ]

3.42 A primigravid 37-year-old woman presents with a heavy vaginal bleed at 39 weeks gestation. The uterus is non-tender and the baby is well grown but appears to be lying transversely. There are no contractions and the condition of both the mother and the baby is stable.

Answer [   ]

3.43 A primigravid patient is seen in the antenatal assessment unit because of recurrent episodes of antepartum haemorrhage over the previous few weeks. The uterine fundus measures 'small for dates' at 37 weeks gestation. An ultrasound scan confirms that the baby's abdominal circumference is on the tenth centile of the growth chart and the liquor volume is less than expected.

Answer [   ]

3.44 Having booked late for antenatal care because she tried to conceal her pregnancy, a 15-year-old primigravid woman comes in to labour ward late one evening with a small amount of postcoital bleeding at term. The baby is moving normally and the uterus is non-tender.

Answer [   ]

3.45 The emergency ambulance brings a 23-year-old woman to hospital at 34 weeks in her second pregnancy because she experienced sudden onset of abdominal pain and vaginal bleeding an hour ago. On examination the uterus is very tender and feels hard.

Answer [   ]

A.	Candida albicans
B.	Chlamydia trachomatis
C.	Escherichia coli
D.	Gardnerella vaginalis
E.	Gonococcus
F.	Group B streptococcus
G.	Listeria monocytogenes
H.	Parvovirus B19
I.	Rubella
J.	Streptococcus faecalis
K.	Toxoplasma gondii

The clinical scenarios below relate to women with infectious diseases in pregnancy. For each case select the single most likely infecting organism.

Each option may be used once, more than once or not at all.

3.46 A woman presents in the surgery at 22 weeks gestation complaining of increasing abdominal discomfort and on examination the uterus is tense and large for dates. She gives a history of a mild flu-like illness two weeks previously. The community midwife refers her to hospital for an ultrasound scan which shows polyhydramnios and fetal hydrops.

Answer [   ]

3.47 A primigravid woman presents at 34 weeks gestation with a history of feeling increasingly unwell, rigors, and right upper quadrant pain. On examination she is flushed, has a tachycardia of 100 bpm and has a temperature of 38 °C. She is tender in the right renal angle.

Answer [   ]

3.48 A 17-year-old woman presents at 30 weeks gestation in her first pregnancy with a history of recurrent postcoital bleeding. Her booking scan at 20 weeks showed a normally sited placenta. Speculum examination reveals a florid ectropion with contact bleeding on taking swabs.

Answer [   ]

3.49 In antenatal clinic at 17 weeks gestation a primigravid woman complains of vaginal discharge and soreness. On speculum examination there is a thick white discharge adherent to the vaginal walls.

Answer [   ]

3.50 A 28-year-old primary school teacher is pregnant for the first time. Several children in her class have 'slapped cheek syndrome' at the start of term and when she comes to hospital for her routine anomaly scan her baby is found to be hydropic.

Answer [   ]

Curriculum module 4

Management of labour and delivery

Syllabus

- You will be expected to have the knowledge, understanding and judgement to be capable of initial management of intrapartum problems in a hospital and in a community setting.
- This will include: knowledge and understanding of normal and abnormal labour, data and investigation interpretation, induction and augmentation of labour, assessment of fetal wellbeing and compromise.
- An understanding of the management of all obstetric emergencies is expected. You will need to demonstrate appropriate knowledge of regional anaesthesia, analgesia and operative delivery including caesarean section.
- You will need to be able to demonstrate respect for cultural and religious differences in attitudes to childbirth.

Learning outcomes

Times have changed from the days of the family doctor when GPs came into hospital to look after some of their patients in labour and few GPs are involved in intrapartum care these days. You might think that there is not much point in acquiring knowledge about what happens on the labour ward and some trainees in O&G posts on the GP training scheme don't enjoy being on duty for labour ward. Nevertheless, patients expect their GP to be aware of what can go wrong during delivery and many seek the opinion of their GP if they are worried about issues around delivery or after the event if they have had a complication.

This part of the exam will be much easier if you have worked on a labour ward since you were a medical student. However, you will find some useful information on the RCOG website in terms of advice for consent for obstetric procedures, which detail complications and potential problems. In addition there are several RCOG 'Green-top' guidelines and NICE guidelines relevant to obstetric care which are a good source of information for this part of the syllabus.

MULTIPLE CHOICE QUESTIONS

4.1 Considering vaginal birth in women who have previously been delivered by caesarean section (VBAC):

A. The chance of a successful vaginal birth occurring next time is about 70% [T] [F]

B. They should never consider vaginal delivery if they have had two previous caesarean sections [T] [F]

C. If the mother is obese the chance of a successful VBAC is reduced [T] [F]

D. The risk of uterine rupture is increased if the previous section was complicated by infection [T] [F]

E. Can have a 'water birth' as long as it is in hospital [T] [F]

4.2 A woman who has developed severe pre-eclampsia in pregnancy is at risk of the following problems:

A. Fetal distress in labour [T] [F]

B. Reduced uterine response to synthetic oxytocin [T] [F]

C. Cerebrovascular accident (stroke) [T] [F]

D. Excess bleeding due to disseminated intravascular coagulation [T] [F]

E. Renal failure [T] [F]

4.3 The following obstetric conditions predispose to cord prolapse during labour:

A. Unstable lie [T] [F]

B. Breech presentation [T] [F]

C. Maternal diabetes [T] [F]

D. Placenta praevia [T] [F]

E. Polyhydramnios [T] [F]

4.4 Induction of labour is indicated in the following conditions:

A. Maternal urinary tract infection [T] [F]

B. Symphysis pubis dysfunction [T] [F]

C. Pregnancy-induced hypertension [T] [F]

D. Pathological CTG tracing [T] [F]

E. Undiagnosed antepartum haemorrhage [T] [F]

4.5 The following are contraindications to a home delivery:

A. Twin pregnancy [T] [F]

B. A woman with a BMI of 37 who has had two normal births before [T] [F]

C. Grand multiparity [T] [F]

D. Second labour after previous forceps delivery [T] [F]

E. Poor rapport with community midwife [T] [F]

4.6 Planning to labour in a birthing pool of water in hospital is safe for the following pregnant women:

A. A primigravid woman whose baby is in the occipito-posterior [T] [F] position at the start of labour

B. A pregnant woman with a BMI of 45 [T] [F]

C. A multiparous woman whose pregnancy is complicated by mild [T] [F] Rhesus disease

D. A woman with an uncomplicated postmature pregnancy being [T] [F] induced

E. A woman with an otherwise uncomplicated pregnancy who has [T] [F] had a successful external cephalic version

4.7 Concerning certification of stillbirth:

A. If a child is born dead, the doctor or midwife will issue a medical [T] [F] certificate of stillbirth

B. Any child born in the 20th week of pregnancy that did not breathe [T] [F] or show any other signs of life should be registered as a stillbirth

C. The Stillbirth Register is separate from the standard Register of Births [T] [F]

D. A fetus papyraceus (usually one of a twin pregnancy which died in [T] [F] utero many weeks previously) should not be registered as a stillbirth

E. Hospitals may provide certification for a fetus lost too early in [T] [F] pregnancy to be classified as a stillbirth if the parents request it

4.8 The indications for assisted vaginal delivery (shortening the second stage of labour with forceps or ventouse) include:

A. Maternal cardiac disease [T] [F]

B. Fetal prematurity [T] [F]

C. Suspected fetal compromise [T] [F]

D. Maternal hypertensive disease [T] [F]

E. Previous third-degree tear [T] [F]

4.9 Placental abruption:

A. Is associated with pre-eclampsia [T] [F]

B. Can cause fetal death [T] [F]

C. May occur in the absence of vaginal bleeding [T] [F]

D. Makes it difficult to feel fetal parts on examination of the woman's [T] [F] abdomen

E. Can cause disseminated intravascular coagulation in the mother [T] [F]

4.10 An obstetric anaesthetist will be unwilling to site an epidural until they have seen a recent normal platelet count and clotting screen for a woman whose pregnancy is complicated by:

A. Pre-eclampsia [T] [F]

B. Maternal diabetes [T] [F]

C. Twin pregnancy [T] [F]

D. Placental abruption [T] [F]

E. Intrauterine fetal death [T] [F]

SINGLE BEST ANSWER QUESTIONS

4.11 An ambulance is summoned by a community midwife who is conducting a home delivery for a multiparous woman who has had two normal deliveries before. Half way through the first stage of labour the patient has become increasingly distressed and is complaining of severe abdominal pain. The pain continues between contractions, which are occurring every three minutes and the midwife has noticed that the uterus is tender and hard on palpation. Which of the following is the most likely complication?

A. Obstructed labour
B. Concealed placental abruption
C. Hyperstimulated labour
D. Chorioamnionitis
E. Uterine rupture

Answer [　]

4.12 You are in a labour room trying to cope with a severe postpartum haemorrhage while waiting for the registrar to arrive. The inexperienced student midwife hands you a selection of drugs to choose from to try and stop the uterine bleeding. Which of these drugs has she picked up in error?

A. Atosiban
B. Carboprost
C. Ergometrine
D. Misoprostol
E. Oxytocin

Answer [　]

4.13 A woman books for antenatal care in her fourth pregnancy. Her obstetric history includes three previous deliveries by caesarean section. She is predisposed to which obstetric complication?

A. Cord prolapse
B. Haemorrhage
C. Placenta accreta
D. Pre-eclampsia
E. Unstable lie

Answer [　]

4.14 The most important reason that administration of ergometrine to control postpartum haemorrhage is contraindicated in a woman with pre-eclampsia is:

A. It is likely to make her vomit profusely
B. It does not work as well as oxytocin
C. It gives a sustained effect rather than a quick onset of action
D. It is likely to increase her blood pressure
E. It could decrease her intracranial pressure

Answer [　]

4.15 As a junior doctor on the labour ward, it often feels as though you are being asked to insert an intravenous line on every woman in labour. Which of the following pregnant women does not need a cannula when she is admitted?

A. A woman with an uncomplicated pregnancy delivering her sixth baby
B. A primigravid woman whose haemoglobin was 95 g/l two weeks ago
C. A woman who had a postpartum haemorrhage in her last delivery
D. A woman who had a forceps delivery for fetal distress in her previous pregnancy
E. A woman who had an emergency caesarean for fetal distress in her last pregnancy

Answer [ ]

4.16 Having had a massive postpartum haemorrhage following the delivery of her first baby a 34-year-old woman has received eight units of blood, two units of cryoprecipitate and fresh frozen plasma during the previous couple of hours. She has developed pulmonary oedema with an oxygen saturation of 55%. Currently her temperature is 37.5 °C, her pulse is 110 beats per minute, her blood pressure 90/40 mmHg and her urine output is reduced to only 5 ml per hour. The clotting screen is normal and her haemoglobin is currently 95 g/l. What is likely to be the cause of this clinical situation?

A. Bacterial contamination of the blood transfused
B. Adult respiratory distress syndrome
C. Blood borne viral infection
D. Delayed transfusion reaction
E. Inadequate transfusion

Answer [ ]

4.17 You are looking after a woman in labour who has had two fetal blood samples done already because of an abnormal cardiotocograph trace, the results of which are normal so far. The obstetric anaesthetist is keen for her to have an epidural inserted, thereby avoiding a general anaesthetic if emergency delivery becomes necessary later. The most important reason for avoiding general anaesthetic in labour is:

A. The mother does not have to be kept 'nil by mouth' in labour
B. General anaesthetic in an emergency takes longer than topping up an epidural
C. Ventouse delivery is more difficult under GA because the mother cannot push
D. The mother is at risk of Mendelssohn's syndrome (aspiration pneumonitis)
E. Epidural can lower her blood pressure and improve placental perfusion

Answer [ ]

4.18 When performing a fetal blood sample in the first stage of labour it is preferable to place the mother in the left lateral position for the following reason:

A. The midwife is more easily able to support the mother's legs
B. Placental perfusion is improved by relieving pressure on maternal vena cava
C. The cervical os is easier to access with the amnioscope
D. Necessary equipment for the procedure can be placed on the bed within reach
E. The baby may be lying on the placenta, thereby compressing the umbilical cord

Answer [ ]

4.19 While on labour ward you notice a commotion in one of the delivery rooms and hear someone shouting for help with shoulder dystocia. Which of the following procedures may help the birth attendants deliver the baby in this life-threatening situation?

A. McRobert's manoeuvre to hyper-flex the maternal hips
B. Løvset manoeuvre to rotate the baby
C. Delivering the anterior arm of the baby
D. Mauriceau–Smellie–Veit manoeuvre to flex the baby's neck
E. Fundal pressure on the uterus

Answer [ ]

4.20 A primigravid woman has been in labour for nearly 20 hours and actively pushing for 90 minutes so a decision is made to perform an assisted vaginal delivery on account of delay in the second stage. The woman is at increased risk of which complication?

A. Fetal distress
B. Inverted uterus
C. Postpartum haemorrhage
D. Cervical dystocia
E. Paravaginal haematoma

Answer [ ]

EXTENDED MATCHING QUESTIONS

A.	Amniotomy
B.	Elective caesarean section
C.	Electronic fetal monitoring
D.	Emergency caesarean section
E.	Intermittent auscultation
F.	Request a clotting screen
G.	Routine elective episiotomy
H.	Titrated synthetic oxytocin infusion
I.	Vaginal examination in theatre with the operating team standing by
J.	Ventouse delivery

The following clinical scenarios apply to women delivering in a hospital obstetric unit. In each case, select the most appropriate management plan.

Each option may be used once, more than once or not at all.

4.21 A primigravid 32-year-old woman presents early in the first stage of spontaneous labour at 38 weeks gestation, contracting once every ten minutes. Her membranes have just ruptured spontaneously and fresh meconium is seen in the liquor.

Answer [   ]

4.22 During vaginal examination in a woman's third labour, the midwife finds the cervix to be 8 cm dilated and feels a pulsatile cord alongside the fetal head. The head is below the ischial spines and in the occipito-anterior position.

Answer [   ]

4.23 A primigravid woman had had an uncomplicated pregnancy so far under midwifery care and presents with a heavy vaginal bleed at 39 weeks gestation. The uterus is non-tender and the baby is well grown with a cephalic presentation, five-fifths palpable. The condition of both mother and baby is stable but she is contracting strongly every three minutes and the blood continues to trickle from the vagina.

Answer [   ]

4.24 Having been admitted to labour ward four hours previously experiencing three contractions every ten minutes, a low-risk primigravid patient is examined and her cervix is found to be 6 cm dilated with intact membranes. She mobilizes in her labour room using nitrous oxide for analgesia and four hours later the cervix is 7 cm dilated.

Answer [   ]

4.25 A midwife calls you in to a delivery room because of a small vaginal bleed in a low-risk primigravid woman whose labour has been progressing normally. The midwife is auscultating the baby's heartbeat which has been 70 beats per minute for five minutes. The mother's pulse is 90, her blood pressure is stable and the cervix is 8 cm dilated.

Answer [   ]

A.	Arrange emergency caesarean section
B.	Check airway and administer oxygen by facial mask
C.	Check plasma glucose level
D.	Commence electronic fetal monitoring
E.	Contact the consultant haematologist on-call
F.	Cross-match blood
G.	Counsel about postpartum sterilization
H.	Perform a vaginal examination to exclude cord prolapse
I.	Rapid IV administration of 1 litre crystalloid
J.	Request urgent ultrasound scan
K.	Site IV cannula and check haemoglobin

These clinical scenarios relate to an emergency situation involving a woman on the labour ward in the third trimester of pregnancy. In each case, choose the most appropriate initial management plan.

Each option may be used once, more than once or not at all.

4.26 A 28-year-old woman with type 1 diabetes at 30 weeks gestation attends triage on labour ward early one morning because of an antepartum haemorrhage. She collapses in the waiting room and when you attend to sort out the situation she appears confused and is asking where she is.

Answer [   ]

4.27 A 34-year-old woman is admitted to delivery suite at term in her eighth pregnancy. She has delivered six live children previously. On examination the cervix is 7 cm dilated and she is involuntarily pushing.

Answer [   ]

4.28 The labour ward is very busy when a young primigravid woman is admitted at 38 weeks gestation in labour. Yesterday in the midwifery antenatal clinic she was found to have a breech presentation and is awaiting a consultant outpatient appointment arranged for tomorrow. On admission she experiences spontaneous rupture of membranes and the student midwife in triage tells you that 'the fetal heart is dropping intermittently to 80 beats per minute'.

Answer [   ]

4.29 A woman who has just delivered twin boys collapses in the delivery room at the end of the second stage. The placenta is still *in situ* and the registrar is trying to deliver it. The midwife who pushed the emergency call button tells you that she has just noticed a large amount of blood in the bed. The patient is unresponsive and has a tachycardia of 120 beats per minute.

Answer [   ]

4.30 Having been admitted with a fresh antepartum haemorrhage, a primiparous patient is diagnosed with a placental abruption at 34 weeks gestation. Both mother and baby are stable at the moment, but the haematology technician has just bleeped you to say that the clotting screen you sent to the lab an hour ago is not normal.

Answer [   ]

A.	Cryoprecipitate
B.	Iron infusion
C.	Iron injections weekly
D.	Oral iron
E.	Platelet transfusion
F.	Recombinant Factor VIIa
G.	Transfuse 'O negative' blood
H.	Transfuse type-specific blood
I.	Transfuse cross-matched blood
J.	Transfuse blood from cell saver

Each of these clinical scenarios describes a pregnant woman whose clinical condition is or could be compromised by haemorrhage; for each patient pick the best management option given the information that you are presented with.

Each option may be used once, more than once or not at all.

4.31 During a routine caesarean section under spinal anaesthetic the consultant you are assisting unexpectedly comes across a low-lying placenta and the woman loses 2500 ml blood before the baby is delivered and the placenta is removed from the uterus. Her haemoglobin done the previous day is 105 g/l. Her blood pressure has dropped to 70/40 mmHg and she has become unresponsive to questions.

Answer [　]

4.32 A primigravid woman has a blood test at 36 weeks gestation and is found to have a haemoglobin level of 69 gm/l. She has not been taking the iron tablets prescribed by her GP because of severe nausea, and has tried three different preparations.

Answer [　]

4.33 A 31-year-old primigravid woman is known to have beta-thalassaemia and has a haemoglobin level of 80 g/l by the time she reaches 38 weeks gestation. She is symptomatic, feeling very tired and slightly breathless.

Answer [　]

4.34 You are the junior doctor on labour ward assisting the registrar dealing with a manual removal of placenta under general anaesthetic. During the last 15 minutes the woman started having a major haemorrhage and so far has lost 3 litres of blood. The consultant obstetrician has been called and the two units of blood stored on the labour ward have already been transfused. Her heart rate is 120 bpm and her blood pressure is 90/50 mmHg.

Answer [　]

4.35 A 35-year-old woman pregnant with twins attends antenatal clinic at 28 weeks gestation for a growth scan. She has a routine blood test done and her haemoglobin is 90 g/l.

Answer [   ]

A.	Attempt to turn the baby (version) for vaginal delivery
B.	Arrange an emergency caesarean section
C.	Arrange an elective caesarean section
D.	Ask the anaesthetist to site an epidural
E.	Conduct an assisted vaginal delivery with ventouse or forceps
F.	Conduct a breech extraction
G.	Obtain a fetal blood sample from the scalp
H.	Obtain a fetal blood sample from the cord
I.	Obtain maternal serum for cross-matching blood
J.	Obtain maternal serum for a clotting screen
K.	Perform a vaginal examination to exclude cord prolapse
L.	Put up a syntocinon drip to increase the contractions
M.	Rupture the membranes with an amnihook

As the junior doctor on the labour ward you have been called to assist the midwives with the management of labouring women experiencing a complication.

In each scenario, choose the most appropriate immediate action that you think the obstetric team (not necessarily you personally) should take.

Each option may be used once, more than once or not at all.

4.36 One hour after administration of a prostaglandin pessary to induce labour for postmaturity, a primigravid woman is found to be having more than six contractions in ten minutes. You are asked to site an intravenous cannula while the midwife removes the pessary. Although the contractions lessen in frequency to three in ten the baby becomes bradycardic and you can hear that the fetal heart rate has been at 90 beats per minute for four minutes so far.

Answer [   ]

4.37 A 21-year-old primigravid woman was admitted in spontaneous labour six hours previously when the cervix was 7 cm dilated and has been relaxing in the birthing pool, coping without formal analgesia. The liquor is clear and intermittent auscultation of the fetal heart is reassuring. The cervix is now 8 cm dilated and the baby appears to be lying in the occipito-posterior position.

Answer [   ]

4.38 A multiparous woman has delivered her first twin vaginally 15 minutes ago and there is no sign of the second twin appearing although the contractions are continuing every two minutes. On examination it is apparent that the second twin is lying transversely in the uterus.

Answer [   ]

4.39 A rather frightened 17-year-old primigravid woman is in spontaneous labour and the cervix is 6 cm dilated. The midwife has noted meconium in the liquor and there are late decelerations on the cardiotocograph. The woman has asked for more analgesia and the midwife says that she is becoming more and more uncooperative.

Answer [   ]

4.40 A multiparous woman who has had three previous uncomplicated vaginal births is admitted in advanced labour at term and to everyone's surprise the presentation of the baby is found to be breech, station at the ischial spines and the cervix 9 cm dilated. The membranes rupture just after the vaginal examination and the liquor is clear. The midwife commences a cardiotocograph trace, which shows occasional early decelerations.

Answer [   ]

A.	Abruption of the placenta
B.	Cervical laceration
C.	Disseminated intravascular coagulation
D.	Placenta accreta
E.	Placenta praevia
F.	Retained succenturiate lobe of placenta
G.	Rupture of the uterus
H.	Uterine atony
I.	Vasa praevia
J.	Velamentous insertion of the cord

Given the clinical information provided, select the most likely diagnosis for each of these obstetric patients experiencing vaginal bleeding.

Each option may be used once, more than once or not at all.

4.41 A woman has just delivered her first baby and while the midwife is inspecting the placenta the patient has a brisk vaginal bleed of about 600 ml. Maternal observations are stable and the uterus feels well contracted. The midwife points out to you that there are blood vessels running through the membranes.

Answer [   ]

4.42 A primigravid woman aged 21 presents to labour ward at 39 weeks gestation because of a brisk painless vaginal bleed of about 100 ml following intercourse. The uterus is non-tender with a transverse fetal lie. The fetal heart is steady at 140 beats per minute.

Answer [　]

4.43 You are called to see a primigravid woman who has started bleeding half way through the first stage of labour, losing 200 ml in a couple of minutes. In spite of her epidural she seems to be in a lot of pain and there are unmistakeable signs of severe fetal distress on the cardiotocograph.

Answer [　]

4.44 During her second labour a 35-year-old woman starts to lose fresh blood per vaginam. Her first baby was delivered by caesarean section because of fetal distress related to chorioamnionitis at 6 cm dilatation in the first stage. This time the cervix has reached 7 cm dilatation but the contractions have stopped.

Answer [　]

4.45 The midwife looking after a primigravid woman in labour at term ruptured the membranes five minutes ago with an amnihook to speed up the progress of the first stage of labour, as cervical dilatation has been stuck at 5 cm for the last four hours. You are called because the midwife is concerned that the liquor is very heavily bloodstained. The uterus is non-tender, contracting four in ten minutes and the fetal heart rate has risen from a baseline of 120 before amniotomy to 180 beats per minute with late decelerations.

Answer [　]

A.	Administer oral benzylpenicillin
B.	High vaginal swab on admission
C.	Induction of labour and intrapartum IV benzylpenicillin
D.	Prescribe intrapartum IV benzylpenicillin
E.	Prescribe intrapartum IV erythromycin
F.	Prescribe intrapartum IV clindamycin
G.	Prescribe intrapartum IV metronidazole
H.	Reassure the patient that no action is necessary
I.	Vaginal cleansing with chlorhexidine on admission in labour

Each of these pregnant women has been found to be carrying group B streptococcus on vaginal swabs at some stage in this or a previous pregnancy. For each patient select the most appropriate management plan to prevent early-onset neonatal group B streptococcal disease.

Each option may be used once, more than once or not at all.

4.46 A primigravid woman has been admitted to labour ward for elective caesarean delivery for persistent breech presentation. She had a swab taken last week by her GP which has grown group B streptococcus.

Answer [   ]

4.47 A woman is admitted in established labour at term. A swab done at 12 weeks gestation when she had a threatened miscarriage grew group B streptococcus.

Answer [   ]

4.48 At 37 weeks gestation a multiparous woman is admitted with prelabour rupture of the membranes. She was found to have group B streptococcus on a high vaginal swab done a few weeks previously when she was seen in another maternity unit in Skegness on holiday.

Answer [   ]

4.49 A woman presents in spontaneous labour at term with her second baby. In her previous pregnancy she had a swab done in the first trimester which grew group B streptococcus; then she delivered at term and the baby was fine. She has not had any swabs done in this pregnancy.

Answer [   ]

4.50 A woman is admitted in established labour at 38 weeks with ruptured membranes. Her previous baby developed meningitis after delivery, which was subsequently found to be due to group B streptococcus. Following that delivery she developed a rash when she was given penicillin in the puerperium to prevent her from developing endometritis.

Answer [   ]

Curriculum module 5

Postpartum problems (the puerperium) including neonatal problems

Syllabus

- You will be expected to understand and demonstrate appropriate knowledge, management skills and attitudes in relation to postpartum maternal problems including: the normal and abnormal postpartum period, postpartum haemorrhage, therapeutics, perineal care, psychological disorders, infant feeding and breast problems.
- You will be expected to demonstrate an understanding of the investigation and management of immediate neonatal problems including neonatal resuscitation.

Learning outcomes

Even in the past when women stayed in hospital for days 'lying-in' (and acquiring venous thrombosis!) it has been the remit of the GP to diagnose problems in the puerperium. The management of patients recovering from traumatic deliveries is now an increasing part of the GP's workload as cost and social pressures result in patients spending very little time in hospital after delivery. Some patients are even leaving hospital the following day when they have been delivered by caesarean section. For this reason obstetricians feel that the problems that can occur in the puerperium are core knowledge for a GP working in the UK and the RCOG continues to expand the bank of questions on this topic.

MULTIPLE CHOICE QUESTIONS

5.1 Concerning maternal mental health in the puerperium:

A. The incidence of puerperal psychosis is 0.02 per 1000 births   [T]   [F]

B. Women who suffer from depression in pregnancy are less likely   [T]   [F]
to breastfeed

C. Psychosis typically presents within the first 90 days postnatally   [T]   [F]

D. Suicide is an important preventable cause of maternal death in the UK [T]   [F]

E. Less than 1% of recently delivered women will develop a   [T]   [F]
depressive illness

5.2 A primigravid woman sustains a fourth-degree tear during a normal delivery, which is repaired by the registrar on duty. With regard to her perineal trauma:

A. The tear should be repaired as soon as possible in the delivery room [T] [F]
B. There is likely to be damage to the anorectal mucosa [T] [F]
C. Laxatives will be needed postpartum [T] [F]
D. She should be followed up in secondary care [T] [F]
E. She may experience deep dyspareunia as a result [T] [F]

5.3 Potentially fatal causes of maternal pyrexia in the puerperium include:

A. Endometritis [T] [F]
B. Mastitis [T] [F]
C. Deep vein thrombosis [T] [F]
D. Streptococcal sore throat [T] [F]
E. Breast abscess [T] [F]

5.4 A woman who delivered her first baby two days ago is having problems breastfeeding because of sore nipples. She is considering bottle feeding instead and the midwife asks you to discuss breastfeeding with the woman. Which of the following statements are true or relevant to her situation?

A. She should stop breastfeeding until the soreness has resolved [T] [F]
B. Sore nipples mean that she is already developing mastitis [T] [F]
C. She will need antibiotics in order to continue breastfeeding [T] [F]
D. She is not likely to resume menstruation while she is breastfeeding [T] [F]
E. She does not need to use contraception while she is breastfeeding [T] [F]

5.5 Babies born to mothers who have used cocaine in pregnancy are at increased risk of the following:

A. Low birthweight [T] [F]
B. Placental abruption [T] [F]
C. Neonatal abstinence (withdrawal) syndrome [T] [F]
D. Nasal septum defect [T] [F]
E. Abnormal brain development [T] [F]

5.6 You are asked to review a woman who had a forceps delivery of her first baby 12 hours ago after a long labour, because she is keen to go home. The midwives are unhappy to let her leave the hospital because she has not yet passed urine.

With regard to the management of her bladder and urine output:

A. Dehydration is the most likely cause [T] [F]
B. She should be catheterized [T] [F]
C. A referral to urology is indicated [T] [F]
D. The problem is likely to be related to damage to her bladder from the forceps [T] [F]
E. She is at risk of long-term voiding problems [T] [F]

5.7 A woman who had just been delivered by caesarean section weighs 130 kg. She runs an excess risk of the following complications compared with mothers who have a normal BMI:

A. Pulmonary embolus [T] [F]

B. Wound infection [T] [F]

C. Pressure sore [T] [F]

D. Urinary tract infection [T] [F]

E. Postpartum haemorrhage [T] [F]

5.8 A woman who is HIV positive has just been delivered of her first baby by caesarean section. With regard to the postnatal care of the neonate:

A. She should be advised against breastfeeding the baby [T] [F]

B. The baby should not have any invasive tests such as [T] [F] blood tests

C. Cord blood should be sent for viral load [T] [F]

D. The baby should receive antiretroviral therapy [T] [F]

E. The baby should be isolated from the mother until she has stopped [T] [F] bleeding

5.9 You are asked to review a woman on the postnatal ward because the midwives suspect that she has had a pulmonary embolus 48 hours after an emergency caesarean section for slow progress in labour.

Regarding her clinical situation:

A. A renal and liver function test should be requested before [T] [F] commencing anticoagulation treatment

B. She should be fully anticoagulated while awaiting the results [T] [F] of tests

C. Breathlessness may be the only symptom [T] [F]

D. She cannot breastfeed while on heparin [T] [F]

E. Anticoagulation should be delayed as it may cause her section [T] [F] wound to bleed

5.10 You are reviewing a woman on the postnatal ward whose first pregnancy was complicated by intrahepatic cholestasis of pregnancy (obstetric cholestasis). Her labour was induced because of it and her baby was born without complications eight hours ago. With regard to her condition:

A. She is likely to have a persistent skin rash as well as severe [T] [F] itching

B. The pruritus will have mainly affected her hands and feet [T] [F]

C. She should have another liver function test done ten days [T] [F] postpartum

D. There is a high recurrence rate of over 50% in subsequent [T] [F] pregnancies

E. She should not use a contraceptive method containing estrogen [T] [F]

SINGLE BEST ANSWER QUESTIONS

5.11 A woman has just delivered her second baby yesterday and requests sterilization before she goes home. Her partner is not keen for her to have this done as he is having trouble coping with their toddler and wants her to go home immediately. While you are counselling her about puerperal sterilization, which one of the following statements is correct about this situation?

A. Clip sterilization is more likely to fail as the fallopian tubes are thicker
B. If she is sterilized now it will take longer for the uterus to involute
C. Laparoscopic sterilization is feasible immediately postpartum
D. Puerperal sterilization requires the written consent of both partners
E. She should defer the decision 24 hours for further discussion to avoid regret

Answer [ ]

5.12 A woman is recovering on the postnatal ward following an emergency caesarean section. On the third day she complains of discomfort and swelling in her right leg, which is clearly larger than the left leg, with a tender calf. The most appropriate medication while awaiting the results of further investigation is:

A. Enoxaparin 20 mg daily
B. Enoxaparin 40 mg daily
C. Enoxaparin 1 mg per kg twice daily
D. TED stockings
E. Loading dose of warfarin

Answer [ ]

5.13 You are called to the obstetric postnatal ward to see a recently delivered patient with a swelling on her vulva. The delivery was normal and she had an episiotomy sutured by the midwife four hours ago. She seems to be in severe discomfort and cannot pass urine. The most likely diagnosis is:

A. Acute herpes infection of the vulva
B. Paravaginal haematoma
C. Bartholin's abscess
D. Thrombosed haemorrhoid
E. An infection in the episiotomy wound

Answer [ ]

5.14 A community midwife asks you to attend a home delivery because she cannot determine the sex of the baby. On examination the newborn infant is well but the genitalia are ambiguous with a small phallus and some scrotal-like development of the skin. Bilateral swellings palpable in the inguinal canals might be gonads. Which is the most appropriate course of action?

A. Advise the parents to choose a name that could be either male or female
B. Reassure the parents that the child is male with undescended testes
C. Send a referral letter to paediatric clinic so karyotyping can be arranged
D. Send the baby into hospital for urgent paediatric review
E. Take the baby's blood for 17-hydroxyprogesterone levels

Answer [ ]

5.15 A woman consults you in surgery about feeling very low in mood for the last four weeks. She is experiencing bouts of crying, is off her food and having trouble sleeping. She delivered her first baby six weeks ago and is very upset that she has had to give up breastfeeding as she felt unable to cope.

What is the most appropriate course of action to deal with her symptoms?

A.   Suggest that she takes an antidepressant and monitor her progress
B.   Inform her that her symptoms are very common and will resolve shortly
C.   Inform her that she has a mental illness and should see a psychiatrist
D.   Admit her urgently to a 'mother and baby unit'
E.   Refer to a breastfeeding counsellor

Answer [   ]

5.16 You have just finished assisting at a difficult caesarean section during which the woman sustained a massive haemorrhage. She is at present on the High Dependency Unit having a blood transfusion but her condition seems to have stabilized and her husband is at her bedside looking after the newborn baby. His mother came into hospital with them but only one person was allowed into the operating theatre with her. In the hospital coffee bar you meet the mother-in-law who is anxiously waiting for news and asks you why the delivery is taking so long.

You have to deal with her enquiry but what should you tell her?

A.   That the mother and baby are both fine
B.   That she is not on labour ward but you are not allowed to tell her why
C.   That you will send the husband to give her information
D.   The delivery has been complicated but everything is all right now
E.   To go to the High Dependency Unit to see the new mother and baby

Answer [   ]

5.17 The highest risk factor for the occurrence of puerperal psychosis is:

A.   A history of postnatal depression in a previous pregnancy
B.   A previous history of bipolar disorder
C.   Eating disorder as a teenager
D.   Family history of puerperal psychosis
E.   Personality disorder

Answer [   ]

5.18 On the evening shift you go to the postnatal ward and find that the midwives have been waiting for you to complete a list of prescribing tasks they have been saving up. Which one takes priority?

A. A woman who delivered a stillborn baby this morning is waiting for a prescription for cabergoline to suppress lactation.

B. A woman who had a caesarean section three days ago is ready to be discharged and is awaiting a prescription for analgesic drugs to take home.

C. A woman who has just been readmitted with puerperal sepsis is waiting for antibiotics. Her temperature is 35.8 °C, BP 90/60 mmHg and pulse 120 bpm.

D. A woman who suffered a major postpartum haemorrhage yesterday is waiting for you to prescribe a blood transfusion. Her haemoglobin is 60 g/l.

E. A woman who had an emergency caesarean section two hours ago is waiting for a prescription of low molecular weight heparin prophylaxis.

Answer [ ]

5.19 A 34-year-old primigravid Jehovah's Witness signed an advance directive refusing any type of blood transfusion or blood products when she first booked for antenatal care. She has just been readmitted a week postpartum with a massive haemorrhage and is on the operating table where the consultant is having difficulty stopping the bleeding. Her haemoglobin is currently 30 g/l and her life hangs in the balance. Which of the following statements is correct with regard to the management of this situation?

A. Her husband can give consent for her to have a blood transfusion

B. Transfuse her without consent because it is in her best interests

C. Get an emergency court order to transfuse

D. Respect her advance directive and withhold transfusion

E. Transfuse her own blood from the cell saver

Answer [ ]

5.20 This morning a woman was delivered of her first baby using forceps because of fetal distress in the second stage of labour. The baby is doing fine but the mother sustained a third-degree tear, which has been repaired by your consultant. When debriefing her about the third-degree tear, which of the following statements is true?

A. The tear will have involved the anal mucosa as well as the sphincter muscle

B. She will be given antibiotics and laxatives postpartum

C. She is very likely to be incontinent of flatus in the future

D. If she has another baby she will need a caesarean section

E. Third-degree tears do not occur with normal deliveries

Answer [ ]

EXTENDED MATCHING QUESTIONS

A.	Combined oral contraceptive pill
B.	Condoms
C.	Copper intrauterine device
D.	Depot medroxy progesterone acetate
E.	Diaphragm
F.	Female sterilization
G.	Levonorgestrel intrauterine system
H.	Progesterone only pill
I.	Spermicide gel
J.	Vasectomy

The clinical scenarios below describe mothers requesting contraceptive advice in the postpartum period. Select the most appropriate method of contraception for each woman.

Each option may be used once, more than once or not at all.

5.21 Having just delivered her first baby a 15-year-old schoolgirl is very keen to avoid getting pregnant again.

Answer [ ]

5.22 A 40-year-old woman who was delivered by caesarean section yesterday has now had two children. She wishes to start secure contraception immediately before she leaves hospital but does not want to rule out having another child in the future.

Answer [ ]

5.23 An overweight 35-year-old woman with a BMI of 45 attends for her postnatal check-up with her first baby. She conceived after IVF treatment because of infertility due to polycystic ovarian syndrome. She still has some frozen embryos in storage but does not want to conceive again just yet as she has been advised to lose a lot of weight first.

Answer [ ]

5.24 Having used the pill with no problems in the past, a 25-year-old wishes to restart contraception after delivering her first baby a week ago. She had a normal delivery, her lochia is normal and she is successfully breastfeeding.

Answer [ ]

5.25 A woman who used to suffer from premenstrual syndrome wishes to have a secure form of contraception after delivering her first baby. She has decided that she is very sensitive to hormones and requests a method that does not involve using hormones.

Answer [ ]

A.	Arrange a district nurse to supervise dressings
B.	Arrange a visit from a breastfeeding peer support group
C.	Arrange readmission to the obstetric unit for review
D.	Arrange urgent admission to the emergency medical ward
E.	Ask the community midwife to visit at home
F.	Prescribe broad-spectrum antibiotics
G.	Send her in to A&E
H.	Take the sutures out and allow the wound to drain

These clinical scenarios describe recently delivered women who have developed complications. In each case, select the most appropriate management plan.

Each option may be used once, more than once or not at all.

5.26 A woman who had a caesarean section two days ago was discharged home yesterday. She has asked for a home visit this morning because there is copious sero-sanguinous fluid discharging from the wound.

Answer [ ]

5.27 Two days after a normal delivery, a primiparous women telephones the surgery to report heavy vaginal bleeding with clots.

Answer [ ]

5.28 You are asked to do a home visit to look at the caesarean wound of a patient who has been out of hospital for four days. She has an absorbable subcuticular suture *in situ* in the skin and there is a spreading cellulitis around the scar.

Answer [ ]

5.29 A primiparous patient who delivered four days ago is having problems with breastfeeding due to pain. On examination her nipples are cracked and sore but there is no unusual swelling of the breasts.

Answer [ ]

5.30 The community midwife is doing a home visit for a woman who has been discharged from hospital two days after a forceps delivery. She is struggling with breastfeeding and has asked for help. The midwife telephones you because she has noticed that the woman's left leg is swollen.

Answer [ ]

A.	Blood transfusion
B.	Evacuation of retained products of conception
C.	Examination under anaesthetic
D.	Full blood count
E.	Intravenous antibiotics
F.	Norethisterone 5 mg tds
G.	Oral antibiotics
H.	Pelvic ultrasound scan
I.	Reassure the patient
J.	Resuture the perineum

The clinical scenarios below relate to women in the puerperium following a vaginal delivery. For each scenario select the most appropriate course of action from the list above.

Each option may be used once, more than once or not at all.

5.31 You are seeing a 24-year-old woman in your GP surgery for her postnatal check. She had a normal vaginal delivery six weeks ago with a small second-degree perineal tear. She is breastfeeding and is feeling well. She tells you that she still has a pink loss vaginally but there have been no clots and the loss is not offensive.

Answer [　]

5.32 You are the junior obstetric doctor on-call overnight and at midnight you are asked to see a woman who has been readmitted three days after the delivery of her third child. Over the last few hours her lochia has become heavier and she is passing clots vaginally. Her observations are: pulse 90 bpm, blood pressure 125/85, temperature 37.5 °C, respiratory rate 14. The midwife has already taken a high vaginal swab.

Answer [　]

5.33 The midwives ask you to review a woman on the postnatal ward one day after delivery. She had a right mediolateral episiotomy which was repaired by the registrar and now she is complaining of severe perineal pain so she can't sit comfortably. On examination her temperature is 36.5 °C, pulse 75 bpm, blood pressure 110/65. The perineal sutures are intact and the perineum is bruised with a 3 cm swelling underlying the sutures. The vaginal sutures are also intact and there is no swelling in the vagina.

Answer [　]

5.34 Eight hours after delivery a woman who has just arrived on the postnatal ward suddenly starts to bleed heavily per vaginam, losing another 200 ml on top of the 300 ml estimated blood loss at delivery. Her predelivery haemoglobin done on admission in labour was 115 g/l. The notes indicate that the placenta was removed in pieces after the cord came off during controlled cord traction.

Answer [　]

5.35 A woman is readmitted by her community midwife because she is worried about the appearance of the perineal wound a week after delivery. On examination you find that the wound has broken down and the tissues are covered in a sloughy yellow-green exudate, which smells offensive.

Answer [ ]

A.	Bimanual pressure to compress the uterus
B.	Controlled cord traction (Brandt–Andrews method)
C.	Ergometrine 500 mg IM
D.	Evacuation of uterus
E.	Inject carboprost (Hemabate®) into the uterus
F.	IV infusion of 40 units of oxytocin over four hours
G.	IV dose of 40 units of oxytocin stat
H.	Manual removal of placenta
I.	Place a Bakri balloon into the uterine cavity

Each of these obstetric patients has either bled heavily after delivery or is at risk of doing so and this question refers to the prevention or treatment of postpartum haemorrhage. Choose the most appropriate management plan for each woman.

Each option may be used once, more than once or not at all.

5.36 A 35-year-old woman has just had an emergency caesarean section for failure to progress in labour and the baby weighed 4.8 kg. During the delivery the blood loss was estimated at nearly a litre but she is no longer bleeding actively. As they are suturing the skin at the end of the operation, the registrar asks you to prescribe something in order to keep the uterus contracted.

Answer [ ]

5.37 A woman has delivered her third baby at home two hours ago but the community midwife has transferred her in to hospital because she has not been able to deliver the placenta in spite of active management of the third stage. There is quite a big blood clot in the bed, which amounts to about 600 ml.

Answer [ ]

5.38 A woman is urgently brought back to labour ward six hours after a normal delivery because she suddenly bleeds heavily vaginally, losing 500 ml in a couple of minutes. Looking through her previous notes you see that a succenturiate lobe was mentioned on her anomaly scan at 21 weeks gestation.

Answer [ ]

5.39 You are the only doctor on labour ward when a woman who was being induced for pre-eclampsia unexpectedly starts pushing and rapidly delivers the baby and placenta. She has a brisk postpartum haemorrhage of 500 ml. She has already had ten units of oxytocin given as the baby was delivering and you have put up an oxytocin infusion with another 40 units so she is now nearing the maximum dose. The registrar is in the gynaecology emergency theatre dealing with a woman in extremis due to a ruptured ectopic pregnancy and you are waiting for the obstetric consultant to arrive from home. She continues to bleed heavily, so you must select the best course of action to save her life.

Answer [　]

5.40 The midwives ask you to put up an intravenous infusion on a woman who is bleeding heavily after delivery of her placenta. You are sure the bleeding is coming from the uterus but every time the senior midwife stops massaging the uterus the bleeding starts again. You are having trouble getting a cannula into a vein so you send for the anaesthetist and ask the midwife to continue rubbing the fundus. The registrar is on the way but you need to give something quickly to make the uterus contract.

Answer [　]

A.	Arterial blood gas
B.	Blood cultures
C.	CT pulmonary angiogram
D.	CT brain
E.	Chest x-ray
F.	D-dimer
G.	Electrophoresis
H.	Haemoglobin
I.	Liver function test daily until results are normal
J.	Liver function test ten days after delivery
K.	Liver ultrasound
L.	Lumbar puncture
M.	Pelvic x-ray
N.	Pulmonary V/Q scan

These clinical scenarios relate to postpartum women with complicated pregnancies experiencing problems or seeking advice after delivery. For each woman, select the most appropriate initial investigation that will help you make a diagnosis.

Each option may be used once, more than once or not at all.

5.41 You are asked to see an unwell 27-year-old woman on the postnatal ward who delivered yesterday. She is complaining of a fronto-occipital headache which is so severe that she can hardly move and is associated with nausea. She had an epidural in labour which was initially ineffective and while it was being resited the dura was inadvertently punctured. Her temperature is 38 °C.

Answer [   ]

5.42 A woman whose labour was induced for obstetric cholestasis has returned home from hospital and you are asked to review her by the community midwife. She asks you what tests she needs now that the baby is safely delivered.

Answer [   ]

5.43 A woman with sickle cell disease is on the postnatal ward after a caesarean section for the delivery of her first baby. She complains of pain at the top of her right leg near the hip joint and cannot stand up comfortably. There is no swelling of either leg on examination.

Answer [   ]

5.44 Following an unsuccessful attempt at induction of labour over three days, a primigravid woman has an emergency caesarean section at 42 weeks gestation. The baby has been admitted to the Special Care Baby Unit (SCBU) with meconium aspiration and you are asked by the SCBU staff to review the mother there the following day because she has become increasingly short of breath.

Answer [   ]

5.45 A primigravid woman has a rather prolonged second stage but achieves a normal delivery of a 4 kg baby after pushing really hard for two hours. Shortly after delivery she becomes progressively short of breath and complains of mild left-sided chest pain on inspiration. On examination there is decreased air entry on the left side of her chest. Her midwife brings the saturation probe from theatre and tells you that her oxygen levels are normal.

Answer [   ]

A.	Elective caesarean section at 37 weeks
B.	Elective caesarean section at 39 weeks
C.	External cephalic version
D.	Induce labour before term
E.	Vaginal birth and consider episiotomy
F.	Vaginal birth with CTG monitoring
G.	Vaginal birth with oxytocin drip
H.	Take low-dose aspirin 75 mg in pregnancy
I.	Terminate the pregnancy

These clinical scenarios relate to women who have recently delivered and have returned to the hospital postnatal clinic for debriefing. In each case, select the most appropriate advice with regard to her next pregnancy.

Each option may be used once, more than once or not at all.

5.46 After being induced for severe pre-eclampsia at 34 weeks gestation, a primigravid woman is delivered by emergency caesarean section for fetal distress at 8 cm dilatation. She is thinking of embarking on another pregnancy in about a year's time as her husband is keen to have another baby soon.

Answer [ ]

5.47 After a very prolonged first stage of labour, the registrar unsuccessfully attempted a forceps delivery in theatre for a primigravid woman who has been pushing for two hours. The position of the baby's head was occipito-anterior at the ischial spines with moulding ++. A caesarean section was performed after three strong pulls, during which there was no descent of the fetal head. The baby weighed 3.8 kg and was two weeks overdue.

Answer [ ]

5.48 Half way through her labour, when the membranes ruptured at 5 cm dilatation, a primigravid woman was found to have a breech presentation and therefore had her first baby delivered by caesarean section. You note from the operation notes that there was a bicornuate uterus which might lead to another breech presentation next pregnancy. Choose the best course of action if the next baby is breech too.

Answer [ ]

5.49 During a forceps delivery performed for fetal distress, a primigravid woman sustains a third-degree tear. At her follow-up appointment it has healed well and she has made a full recovery with no symptoms related to the anal sphincter. She wishes to discuss plans for her next birth.

Answer [ ]

5.50 Having reached 8 cm cervical dilation in her first labour, a primigravid woman was delivered by emergency caesarean section because of a fetal bradycardia associated with fresh vaginal bleeding. The labour was progressing well up to that point but unfortunately the bradycardia turned out to be due to placental abruption and the baby did not survive. She does not feel strong enough to contemplate another pregnancy just yet, but is wondering about the mode of delivery next time.

Answer [ ]

Curriculum module 6
Gynaecological problems

Syllabus

- You will be expected to demonstrate appropriate knowledge, management skills and attitudes in relation to benign gynaecological problems including: urogynaecology, paediatric and adolescent gynaecology, endocrine problems, pelvic pain and abnormal vaginal bleeding. This will include knowledge of early pregnancy loss, including clinical features, investigation and management of disorders leading to early pregnancy loss: miscarriage (including recurrent), ectopic pregnancy and molar pregnancy.
- You will be expected to demonstrate an ability to assess and manage common sexually transmitted infections including HIV/AIDS and be familiar with their modes of transmission and clinical features. You will be expected to understand the principles of contact tracing. You will also be expected to know the basis of national screening programmes and their local implementation through local care pathways.
- You will be expected to demonstrate appropriate knowledge of clinical features, investigation and management of premalignant and malignant conditions of the female genital tract. You will be expected to have an understanding of the indications and limitations of screening for premalignant and malignant disease. An understanding of the options available for palliative and terminal care including relief of symptoms and community support will be expected.
- The examiners will expect you to demonstrate appropriate knowledge and attitudes in relation to subfertility. This includes an understanding of the epidemiology, aetiology, management and prognosis of male and female fertility problems. You will be expected to have a broad-based knowledge of investigation and management of the infertile couple in a primary care setting and appropriate knowledge of assisted reproductive techniques including the legal and ethical implications of these procedures.

Learning outcomes

This represents a large part of the workload of a GP with an interest in women's health and consequently there are a large number of these questions on the examination bank.

In 'benign gynaecology' areas of knowledge covered (many of which overlap) are menstrual problems, endocrinology, e.g. polycystic ovarian syndrome and the menopause, pelvic pain, pelvic inflammatory disease and vaginal discharge and paediatric/adolescent issues such as delayed puberty.

There is also an area mysteriously called 'issues relevant to a migrant population' which involves subjects such as female genital mutilation, infectious diseases and ethical problems.

This module of the curriculum also covers sexually transmitted infections, subfertility, early pregnancy loss, urogynaecology including prolapse and gynaecological oncology. Patients with problems in any of these areas are likely to present initially to the GP so this part of the curriculum features heavily in the actual examination. Questions are likely to concentrate on making a diagnosis and knowing when to refer rather than detailed knowledge of the specialized management once she reaches hospital, although the contents of national guidelines should be referred to in revision as they are likely to be relevant.

MULTIPLE CHOICE QUESTIONS

6.1 The following gynaecological problems can present with intermenstrual bleeding:

A.	Genital chlamydia infection	[T]	[F]
B.	Nabothian follicle on the cervix	[T]	[F]
C.	Subserous fibroids	[T]	[F]
D.	Granulosa cell tumour of the ovary	[T]	[F]
E.	Endometrial polyp	[T]	[F]

6.2 An asymptomatic nulliparous 39-year-old woman attends for a routine cervical smear and the practice nurse discovers a large pelvic mass, making the cervix difficult to access. The following are possible differential diagnoses for this mass:

A.	Uterine fibroid	[T]	[F]
B.	Diverticular abscess	[T]	[F]
C.	Ovarian cyst	[T]	[F]
D.	Urethral diverticulum	[T]	[F]
E.	Haematocolpos	[T]	[F]

6.3 Bacterial vaginosis:

A.	Causes vaginal discharge with a characteristic fishy smell	[T]	[F]
B.	Is associated with pruritus and vulvovaginitis	[T]	[F]
C.	Is associated with a lowered vaginal pH	[T]	[F]
D.	May be treated with metronidazole	[T]	[F]
E.	Should be treated if detected during pregnancy	[T]	[F]

6.4 Women with polycystic ovarian syndrome:

A.	Have a raised body mass index	[T]	[F]
B.	May develop gestational diabetes	[T]	[F]
C.	Cannot conceive without ovulation induction	[T]	[F]
D.	Are more likely to miscarry than women without the syndrome	[T]	[F]
E.	During an IVF cycle are more likely to develop hyperstimulation syndrome	[T]	[F]

6.5 Regarding hormone replacement therapy (HRT):

A. It should be offered to patients with premature ovarian failure [T] [F]
B. It protects against unwanted pregnancy in perimenopausal [T] [F]
women
C. The incidence of cardiovascular disease is reduced in the first year [T] [F]
of use
D. It is first-line management in a patient at risk of osteoporosis [T] [F]
E. The risk of breast cancer returns to baseline five years after [T] [F]
stopping HRT

6.6 A 29-year-old woman attends surgery complaining of urinary leakage on coughing since the birth of her first son 14 months ago. On examination there is demonstrable stress incontinence but no vaginal wall prolapse and urodynamic study shows a stable bladder. The following are appropriate treatments to consider in her case:

A. Duloxetine tablets [T] [F]
B. Oxybutynin tablets [T] [F]
C. Bladder drill (retraining) [T] [F]
D. Pelvic floor muscle training [T] [F]
E. Pelvic floor repair operation [T] [F]

6.7 Features of premenstrual syndrome include:

A. Occurrence in anovulatory cycles [T] [F]
B. Relief of symptoms at menstruation [T] [F]
C. An association with dysmenorrhoea [T] [F]
D. Abnormally high progesterone levels [T] [F]
E. Cyclical pelvic pain [T] [F]

6.8 A woman from Somalia brings her four-year-old daughter to paediatric A&E as she has become acutely unwell on return from a holiday to visit family back home. The child seems to be unable to talk and is sweaty, shivering and incontinent of urine. You can see that there is blood on her pyjamas.

The following conditions should be considered in the differential diagnosis:

A. Genital mutilation [T] [F]
B. Malaria [T] [F]
C. Sexual abuse [T] [F]
D. Tetanus [T] [F]
E. Urinary tract infection [T] [F]

6.9 The following are features of human papilloma virus infection:

A. Koilocytes on a cervical biopsy [T] [F]
B. Genital warts [T] [F]
C. Intermenstrual bleeding [T] [F]
D. Painful ulcers on the vulva [T] [F]
E. Cervical stenosis [T] [F]

6.10 In your GP surgery you see a woman aged 32 with severe premenstrual syndrome (premenstrual dysphoric syndrome). She has regular periods which are not heavy and does not need contraception because her husband has had a vasectomy. She is hoping for a solution for her mood changes.

The following treatments have been shown to be effective in PMS:

A. Transdermal estradiol   [T]   [F]
B. Progesterone given in the luteal phase of the menstrual cycle   [T]   [F]
C. Psychological treatment in the form of cognitive behavioural   [T]   [F]
    therapy (CBT)
D. Combined oral contraceptive pill   [T]   [F]
E. Selective serotonin reuptake inhibitors (SSRIs) given in the   [T]   [F]
    luteal phase

SINGLE BEST ANSWER QUESTIONS

6.11 A 68-year-old woman with a BMI of 30 presents to her GP with a history of urinary urgency and frequency almost every hour with urge incontinence. She has to wear a pad all the time and rarely leaves the house as a result. Vaginal examination reveals no prolapse and urinalysis is negative. Which one of the following management options is most likely to ameliorate her symptoms?

A. Colposuspension operation
B. Electrical stimulation of pelvic floor muscle
C. Weight loss
D. Prescription of duloxetine
E. Bladder drill (retraining)

Answer [   ]

6.12 A 38-year-old woman attended for a routine cervical smear during which an asymptomatic polyp is noted on the surface of the cervix. The result of the smear was normal. In counselling her about the polyp, which one of the following statements is true?

A. It could be caused by chlamydia
B. It is unlikely to be associated with endometrial pathology
C. It is most likely to be a nabothian follicle
D. It is associated with human papilloma virus infection
E. It should be removed because it is likely to be malignant

Answer [   ]

6.13 When you are on-call for gynaecological emergencies in your hospital, you are frequently asked to organize management for women attending the Early Pregnancy Clinic. Which one of these statements is correct with regard to the management of miscarriage?

A. Medical management is associated with an increased incidence of pelvic infection

B. Women having a surgical evacuation should be screened for chlamydia

C. Expectant management is the treatment of choice if the uterus is septic

D. Histological proof that the uterus contained trophoblastic tissue excludes ectopic pregnancy

E. Perforation of the uterus during surgical evacuation is more likely in incomplete rather than missed miscarriage

Answer [   ]

6.14 You see a woman in clinic with urinary frequency and urgency who you suspect might have overactive bladder (detrusor instability) and counsel her about it. Which of these statements is not correct in this context with regard to detrusor instability?

A. It can be confidently diagnosed from the history without further investigation

B. Bladder drill (retraining) is recommended treatment

C. It may be a symptom of multiple sclerosis

D. It will respond to oral anticholinergics

E. It can be improved by pelvic floor exercises

Answer [   ]

6.15 A routine 'dating' scan arranged by the midwife shows that a primigravid woman has suffered a missed miscarriage. The sac contains a fetus about 9 weeks size but there is no fetal heart pulsation seen. She was not expecting this as she has not had any bleeding at all during the pregnancy, so is extremely upset and would like to deal with the problem as quickly as possible. Which would be the best management plan in her case?

A. Admit to hospital for medical management with methotrexate

B. Evacuate the uterus with cervical preparation

C. Expectant management with another scan in two weeks to see if she has miscarried

D. Give 800 micrograms of misoprostol

E. Prescribe mifepristone orally and follow up after two weeks

Answer [   ]

6.16 A 24-year-old woman whose scan reveals polycystic ovarian syndrome (PCO) consults you about management of her facial hirsutism. Her serum testosterone is within normal limits and she does not wish to conceive. Which of these treatments for PCO is the most appropriate management option?

A. Clomifene citrate

B. Co-cyprindiol combined oral contraceptive pill

C. Cyproterone acetate

D. Metformin

E. Ovarian drilling

Answer [   ]

6.17 In your GP surgery you see a diabetic woman aged 49 years who seeks treatment for irregular heavy menstrual bleeding. Her pelvis feels normal on examination and speculum reveals a healthy cervix. Which of the following statements about her management is correct?

A. LH/FSH levels are a useful investigation

B. Serum ferritin should be measured as well as haemoglobin at the first visit

C. She should be referred to gynaecology clinic

D. Testing for coagulation disorders should be done prior to commencing treatment

E. Tranexamic acid can be prescribed as first-line therapy without referral

Answer [ ]

6.18 You are seeing a 48-year-old woman for a preoperative check-up. She is due to have a hysterectomy for fibroids next week and is thinking of having her normal ovaries removed at the same time as the uterus. She wishes to discuss the possible benefits and problems associated with a surgical menopause. Which one of her ideas about the bilateral oophorectomy operation is actually correct?

A. Oophorectomy will not affect her libido

B. She will need sequential HRT to get rid of her menopausal symptoms

C. It will completely prevent her from getting any gynaecological cancer in later life

D. She should consider oophorectomy if her mother had ovarian cancer

E. Oophorectomy will increase the operating time substantially

Answer [ ]

6.19 A 23-year-old woman with a BMI of 50 attends your GP surgery to discuss her fertility problems because she and her husband have been trying to conceive for 18 months. She has irregular periods with a cycle varying from 35 to 42 days and the ovulation predictor kits she has purchased from the chemist indicate that she is not ovulating. Her husband has two children from his previous marriage. Which of the following is the most appropriate piece of advice?

A. Continue trying for six more months then you will refer her to infertility clinic

B. Commence taking folic acid 10 mcg daily

C. Make an appointment for her husband to arrange a semen analysis

D. Prescribe clomifene citrate to be taken on days two to six of the cycle

E. To avoid pregnancy until she has lost weight

Answer [ ]

6.20 A young woman attends her GP's surgery with a positive pregnancy test after seven weeks of amenorrhoea. She is anxious because has suffered two previous early pregnancy losses; a miscarriage at ten weeks followed by an ectopic pregnancy which was managed surgically. Which course of action is most appropriate?

A. Admit to gynaecology ward
B. Arrange midwifery booking
C. Refer for early scan
D. Refer to antenatal clinic
E. Take blood for serum hCG in the surgery

Answer [ ]

EXTENDED MATCHING QUESTIONS

A.	Ascorbic acid
B.	Clomifene citrate
C.	Danazol
D.	Depot medroxy progesterone acetate
E.	Dianette®
F.	LHRH analogues
G.	Medroxyprogesterone acetate
H.	Mefenamic acid
I.	Tamoxifen
J.	Tibolone
K.	Tranexamic acid

Each of these clinical scenarios describes a woman presenting to her GP requesting help with menstrual problems; for each patient pick the most appropriate treatment option given the information that you are presented with.

Each option may be used once, more than once or not at all.

6.21 A 22-year-old nulliparous woman who is not currently sexually active seeking treatment for menorrhagia and primary dysmenorrhoea.

Answer [ ]

6.22 An obese teenager with acne and frequent heavy periods seeking contraception.

Answer [ ]

6.23 A 34-year-old overweight woman with irregular heavy bleeding whose endometrial biopsy reveals cystic hyperplasia with no atypia.

Answer [ ]

6.24 A 30-year-old woman with three children has just undergone a third termination of pregnancy without complications. She has attended the surgery twice in the past for help with her menorrhagia and dysmenorrhoea.

Answer [   ]

6.25 A sterilized 32-year-old woman whose menorrhagia has not responded to treatment with non-steroidal anti-inflammatory drugs.

Answer [   ]

A.	Anterior colporrhaphy operation
B.	Antibiotics
C.	Biofeedback
D.	Bladder drill (retraining)
E.	Helmstein bladder distension
F.	Injection of phenol into the bladder trigone
G.	Sacrocolpopexy operation
H.	Supervised pelvic floor physiotherapy
I.	Tension-free vaginal tape (TVT) operation

Each of these scenarios describes a woman presenting to gynaecology clinic with urinary incontinence; for each patient pick the most appropriate treatment option given the clinical information that you are presented with.

Each option may be used once, more than once or not at all.

6.26 Eighteen months after a colposuspension operation for stress incontinence, a 60-year-old woman presents with a recurrence of her incontinence. She brings with her the results of a private urodynamic study that she had done after surfing the internet. This shows that she has a compliant bladder on filling in a sitting position, but when she stands up there is demonstrable leakage of urine associated with spikes of high detrusor pressure measurements > 30 cm water.

Answer [   ]

6.27 Less than a week after her bladder pressure study where she was diagnosed as having detrusor instability, a 51-year-old postmenopausal woman comes to the surgery seeking treatment on account of a marked deterioration in her symptoms of dysuria, urinary frequency and urgency with urge incontinence.

Answer [   ]

6.28 Six months after the normal vaginal birth of her first child, a 37-year-old teacher complains of urinary incontinence when doing her aerobic classes. On examination she does have a moderate cystocoele and minor rectocoele but no uterine descent.

Answer [   ]

6.29 A bladder pressure study excludes detrusor instability in a 55-year-old woman with a mixed picture of stress and urge urinary incontinence. Her symptoms are getting worse with frequent leakage in spite of intensive supervised pelvic floor physiotherapy.

Answer [   ]

6.30 A fit 62-year-old woman has had a vaginal hysterectomy done years ago for menorrhagia. She presents with 'something coming down' and on examination of the external genitalia you can see the vaginal vault protruding.

Answer [   ]

A.	Appendicitis
B.	Ectopic pregnancy
C.	Haemorrhage into an ovarian cyst
D.	Incomplete miscarriage
E.	Missed miscarriage
F.	Normal intrauterine pregnancy
G.	Partial hydatidiform mole
H.	Threatened miscarriage
I.	Urinary tract infection

The clinical scenarios below describe women presenting with pain in early pregnancy. For each case select the most likely diagnosis.

Each option may be used once, more than once or not at all.

6.31 A 23-year-old woman comes in to the Gynaecological Admission Unit complaining of left iliac fossa pain. She is very tender on the left side of her abdomen and on pelvic examination you find cervical excitation. She has had seven weeks of amenorrhoea and her serum βhCG is 5000 IU/ml. The transvaginal ultrasound scan shows a small empty rounded structure (thought to be a gestational sac) in the uterus.

Answer [   ]

6.32 A week after her 12-week dating scan, a 24-year-old woman presents to A&E with an acute onset of central abdominal pain and nausea. On examination you find severe lower abdominal tenderness with generalized guarding and rebound. Her white cell count is 14×10^6/l, and urinalysis is negative.

Answer [   ]

6.33 An obese 35-year-old woman who had her Mirena® intrauterine system removed five months ago on account of breast tenderness attends her GP to complain of lower abdominal discomfort and that her breast tenderness persists. She remains amenorrhoeic. On examination you can feel a mass in her lower abdomen above the symphysis pubis.

Answer [   ]

6.34 A 21-year-old woman is admitted to A&E by ambulance having collapsed while out shopping. On arrival at hospital she is complaining of shoulder tip pain, and examination shows a tender abdomen with guarding. She had a coil fitted a month after the delivery of her two-year-old son, and thinks her last menstrual period was two weeks ago, although it was lighter than usual.

Answer [   ]

6.35 A primigravid woman presents to the Early Pregnancy Unit with a history of 11 weeks amenorrhoea, minor lower abdominal discomfort and a small amount of vaginal bleeding. A urine pregnancy test is positive. Pelvic examination reveals no tenderness and the uterus is the correct size for dates with a closed cervical os.

Answer [   ]

A.	Adenomyosis
B.	Appendicitis
C.	Chronic pelvic inflammatory disease
D.	Endometriosis
E.	Interstitial cystitis
F.	Irritable bowel syndrome
G.	Ovarian cyst
H.	Polycystic ovarian syndrome
I.	Urinary tract infection
J.	Uterine fibroids

The clinical scenarios below describe non-pregnant women presenting in the gynaecology clinic with lower abdominal or pelvic pain. For each case select the most likely diagnosis.

Each option may be used once, more than once or not at all.

6.36 A 22-year-old student with an 18-month history of non-cyclical intermittent lower abdominal pain and deep dyspareunia. She is tender in both adnexae and the uterus is retroverted.

Answer [   ]

6.37 As well as experiencing deep dyspareunia for six months, a 48-year-old woman has pain when her bladder is full, which is associated with urinary frequency and nocturia.

Answer [   ]

6.38 After years of being on the pill, a 35-year-old woman has developed gradually increasing severe dysmenorrhoea, intermittent pelvic pain and dyspareunia in her first pill-free year. On examination her uterus is normal size but both adnexae are tender.

Answer [   ]

6.39 A woman who has had five normal deliveries complains of increasingly severe secondary dysmenorrhoea. Her periods are regular but becoming heavier. The uterus is bulky and very tender on pelvic examination.

Answer [   ]

6.40 A 24-year-old woman has been using the pill since her teenage years to control her heavy periods as well as for contraception. She seeks help on account of intermittent pain in both iliac fossae associated with abdominal bloating and deep dyspareunia.

Answer [   ]

A.	Reassurance only
B.	Repeat pelvic ultrasound at beginning of next cycle
C.	Repeat pelvic ultrasound in three months
D.	Repeat serum CA125
E.	Routine referral to a gynaecological oncologist
F.	Routine referral to a gynaecologist
G.	Serum CA125 and repeat pelvic ultrasound scan
H.	Serum CA125 and urgent (two-week wait) referral to gynaecologist
I.	Urgent (two-week wait) referral to gynaecological oncologist
J.	Urgent (two-week wait) referral to gynaecologist

Each of these clinical scenarios relates to a woman presenting in a general practice surgery with an ovarian cyst. In each case select the most appropriate management plan for that patient.

Each option may be used once, more than once or not at all

6.41 A 54-year-old postmenopausal woman presents to your surgery with irregular vaginal bleeding over the last six months. An ultrasound scan shows an endometrial thickness of 8 mm and large bilateral multiloculated ovarian cysts. There are no other abnormal features on the scan.

Answer [   ]

6.42 A 27-year-old woman gives a history of longstanding dysmenorrhoea and deep dyspareunia. A pelvic ultrasound shows a unilocular 4 cm diameter cyst on the left ovary consistent with a 'chocolate cyst'.

Answer [   ]

6.43 A 19-year-old woman attends surgery with right iliac fossa pain, nausea and vomiting. Her last menstrual period was three weeks before and an ultrasound scan shows a 3 cm diameter right ovarian cyst with internal echoes consistent with haemorrhage. Her pain settles with simple analgesia.

Answer [   ]

6.44 A 39-year-old woman complains of left iliac fossa pain radiating down her left leg. The ultrasound shows a 9 cm diameter complex cyst on her left ovary and her CA125 level is 470.

Answer [ ]

6.45 A 65-year-old woman presents to the surgery with loss of appetite and abdominal distension, 12 years after her menopause. It started with a bout of 'gastroenteritis' which has just settled. You organize a CA125 level, which is slightly raised at 55 and an ultrasound scan of the pelvis, which is normal.

Answer [ ]

A.	Ergometrine infusion over four hours
B.	Evacuation of uterus on routine consultant list tomorrow
C.	Evacuation of uterus immediately on emergency list
D.	Evacuation of uterus after cervical priming
E.	Gemeprost pessaries
F.	Intravenous antibiotics
G.	Methotrexate injection
H.	Mifepristone and misoprostol
I.	Oxytocin infusion over four hours
J.	Repeat βhCG level in 48 hours

These clinical scenarios describe women experiencing complications in the first trimester of pregnancy. For each case, select the most appropriate management plan for that patient.

Each option may be used once, more than once or not at all.

6.46 Having developed hyperemesis, a 39-year-old primigravid patient has an ultrasound scan during her hospital admission which shows a 'snowstorm appearance'. You are asked to review the scan and plan management when you take over the night shift at 8 pm.

Answer [ ]

6.47 A 20-year-old shop assistant presents to Early Pregnancy Unit at seven weeks gestation in her second pregnancy complaining of left-sided abdominal pain. She had an ectopic pregnancy a year ago which was treated by laparoscopic right salpingectomy. Her BP and pulse are normal and scan shows an empty uterus with a mixed echo mass in the left adnexa which is 2 cm in diameter. The βhCG level is 2150 IU/ml and haemoglobin is 117 g/l.

Answer [ ]

6.48 A routine 'dating' ultrasound scan shows that a 21-year-old woman who had a ventouse delivery for her previous child nine months ago, has suffered a missed miscarriage.

Answer [ ]

6.49 On admission to the gynaecology ward, you note that a young woman admitted with bleeding at ten weeks gestation has a temperature of 38.5 °C and a tender uterus. There is a small amount of bleeding on speculum examination but the cervical os is open and you can see what looks like a gestation sac protruding through.

Answer [ ]

6.50 At 2 am you are summoned to A&E urgently to see a 23-year-old woman who is having a miscarriage. There is a lot of blood all over the bed and someone has initiated an intravenous infusion as she is hypotensive. On speculum examination you have to remove clots from the vagina to visualize the cervix and find that the cervical os is wide open.

Answer [ ]

Curriculum module 7

Fertility control (contraception and termination of pregnancy)

Syllabus

- You will be expected to demonstrate appropriate knowledge, management skills and attitudes in relation to fertility control and termination of pregnancy.
- You will be expected to understand the indications, contraindications, complications, mode of action and efficacy of all reversible and irreversible contraceptive methods.
- You will be expected to demonstrate appropriate knowledge of abortion and should be familiar with the accompanying laws related to abortion, consent, child protection and the Sexual Offences Act(s).
- There may be conscientious objection to the acquisition of certain skills in areas of sexual and reproductive health but knowledge and appropriate attitudes as described above will be expected.

Learning outcomes

This module covers contraception including emergency contraception (EC) and termination of pregnancy (TOP). Questions on this part of the syllabus test clinical knowledge and understanding of the law relating to termination of pregnancy and assessing Lord Fraser competency for girls under the age of 16 years requesting contraception or TOP. The questions in the exam may also test attitudes and behaviours in terms of medical ethics as applied to fertility control. The RCOG recognizes the relevance of fertility control to everyday general practice, hence it is part of the DRCOG curriculum in addition to the option of studying for the Diploma of Sexual and Reproductive Health.

MULTIPLE CHOICE QUESTIONS

7.1   If a 15-year-old schoolgirl consults you for contraception provision:

A.   You must inform her parents or legal guardians before prescribing [T]   [F]

B.   There are unlikely to be child protection issues if she is deemed   [T]   [F]
competent to give consent for treatment

C.   She should be advised to have a cervical smear as she has become [T]   [F]
sexually active

D.   She cannot attend a family planning clinic until she reaches the age [T]   [F]
of 16 years

E.   You must enquire about her sexual history regarding partners   [T]   [F]

7.2 In women who are thinking of using the combined pill for contraception:

A. The risk of thromboembolism is the same as in pregnancy [T] [F]
B. The risk of mortality from large bowel cancer is reduced [T] [F]
C. A family history of breast cancer is an absolute [T] [F]
   contraindication
D. An alternative method should be sought if they are [T] [F]
   planning a long high-altitude trek
E. The failure rate in typical use rather than in ideal use is 9% [T] [F]

7.3 A woman comes to see you in your GP surgery requesting female sterilization as she has had trouble with various other forms of contraception. She is not in a stable relationship currently but has had six pregnancies; five children and one ectopic pregnancy. You agree to write a referral letter to the hospital but should counsel her regarding:

A. A lifetime failure rate of 1 in 2000 [T] [F]
B. Future risk of ectopic pregnancy [T] [F]
C. Mirena® IUS has a much lower Pearl index [T] [F]
D. A history of previous ectopic pregnancy is a contraindication [T] [F]
E. If she regrets her decision, reversal involves laparoscopic clip [T] [F]
   removal

7.4 Regarding non-oral hormonal contraception:

A. The combined transdermal patch (Evra®) works primarily by [T] [F]
   inhibiting ovulation
B. With the progesterone implant the release of hormone is highest [T] [F]
   just after insertion
C. The levonorgestrel intrauterine system (Mirena®) should [T] [F]
   normally be changed every five years to maintain contraceptive
   efficiency
D. The effectiveness of Mirena® is reduced by liver enzyme-inducing [T] [F]
   drugs
E. The vaginal contraceptive ring (NuvaRing®) is inserted at [T] [F]
   the beginning of the cycle and removed on day 22

7.5 Possible complications of vasectomy include:

A. Scrotal haematoma [T] [F]
B. Recanalization of the vasa [T] [F]
C. Loss of libido [T] [F]
D. Formation of antisperm antibodies [T] [F]
E. High testosterone levels [T] [F]

7.6 In combined oral contraceptive formulations, the following may be found as the estrogen component:

A. Mestranol [T] [F]
B. Estriol [T] [F]
C. Estradiol valerate [T] [F]
D. Conjugated equine estrogen [T] [F]
E. Ethinylestradiol [T] [F]

7.7 A woman who has had two children has a copper IUCD fitted in the Family Planning Clinic. She turns up in the surgery for a check-up six weeks later but on speculum examination you cannot find the coil strings. Which of the following statements are true with regard to her situation?

A. She could be pregnant with the coil in the uterus [T] [F]

B. The coil could have been extruded per vaginam without her noticing [T] [F]

C. The next step is to try and retrieve the coil strings with a thread retriever [T] [F]

D. An ultrasound scan is indicated [T] [F]

E. She is not covered for contraception [T] [F]

7.8 When advising women about copper intrauterine devices:

A. They are considered unsuitable for nulliparous teenage girls [T] [F]

B. Additional contraceptive measures are required when they are first fitted [T] [F]

C. Women should be screened preinsertion for sexually transmitted infections [T] [F]

D. Most IUDs are impregnated with barium so they can be located on x-ray [T] [F]

E. All copper IUDs are licensed for five years use [T] [F]

7.9 In women using progesterone-only pill (POP) oral contraception:

A. There is no need to stop taking POP prior to major surgery [T] [F]

B. The window for missed pill taking is only three hours for all formulations [T] [F]

C. There is a link between POP use and breast cancer [T] [F]

D. Additional measures are not required if the method is initiated on days 1 to 5 of the menstrual cycle [T] [F]

E. There is no proven evidence of weight gain associated with POP use [T] [F]

7.10 When advising women about postcoital emergency contraception:

A. The levonorgestrel pill (Levonelle®) can be used more than once in a cycle [T] [F]

B. The copper device should be fitted within five days of unprotected intercourse [T] [F]

C. Ulipristal (EllaOne®) works primarily by altering the endometrium to prevent implantation [T] [F]

D. Women experiencing pain having used any method of emergency contraception within the previous few weeks should seek medical advice [T] [F]

E. Women with poorly controlled asthma should avoid ulipristal (EllaOne®) [T] [F]

SINGLE BEST ANSWER QUESTIONS

7.11 Which is the single best course of action if a woman presents to your surgery at 12 weeks gestation having conceived with an IUCD *in situ*?

A. Repeat the pregnancy test to check for miscarriage
B. Remove the coil if the strings can be visualized
C. Request an x-ray to localize the coil
D. Take triple swabs as infection is likely in this situation
E. Do serial βhCG estimations to exclude ectopic pregnancy

Answer [ ]

7.12 A woman whose pelvic ultrasound scan indicates that she has polycystic ovarian syndrome consults you because she does not wish to conceive for a couple of years. She has sought help previously for management of her facial hirsutism and her serum testosterone is within normal limits.

Select the most appropriate management option in her case from the list below:

A. Clomifene citrate
B. Cyproterone acetate
C. Co-cyprindiol (cyproterone acetate and 35 mcg ethinylestradiol)
D. Levonorgestrel-releasing intrauterine system
E. Metformin

Answer [ ]

7.13 Which one of the following statements about laparoscopic female sterilization is correct?

A. The patient should regard it as an irreversible method of contraception
B. The operation is usually done under local anaesthetic
C. The clips are made of nickel so can't be used if a woman is allergic to base metal
D. Diathermy sterilization increases the chances of successful reversal
E. Applying two clips to each tube is advisable to improve efficacy

Answer [ ]

7.14 A 28-year-old woman who is virgo intacta wishes to start contraception in advance of her marriage which is arranged for a few months' time. She has polycystic ovarian syndrome which was diagnosed when she saw a gynaecologist with oligomenorrhoea and she is worried that she will develop hirsutism, which would spoil her wedding photographs.

From the list given below, select the most appropriate form of contraception for her in these unusual circumstances:

A. Cerazette®
B. Dianette®
C. Marvelon®
D. Nexplanon®
E. NuvaRing®

Answer [ ]

7.15 A woman has unprotected intercourse with a stranger at a party two days before she consults you for emergency contraception. She has since heard that he is HIV positive and she has made herself an appointment with the local GUM clinic this afternoon.

Choose the best option for emergency contraception in her case:

A. Levonelle 1500®
B. Mirena®
C. EllaOne®
D. Marvelon®
E. Multiload Cu375®

Answer [   ]

7.16 A 26-year-old woman had her first smear three weeks ago. She is using a copper IUD for contraception and asks you to check on the smear result when she attends your surgery for her family planning check-up. She is asymptomatic and pelvic examination is normal. Her LMP was two weeks ago and she had intercourse yesterday. Her smear result shows no cytological abnormality but mentions the presence of actinomycosis-like organisms. What is the correct course of action?

A. Remove the IUD immediately and admit to gynaecology ward
B. Remove the IUD and prescribe emergency contraception
C. Remove the IUD, prescribe emergency contraception and penicillin
D. Leave the IUD in place and reassure her as she is asymptomatic
E. Leave the IUD in place and arrange ultrasound to exclude pelvic abscess

Answer [   ]

7.17 A neurology consultant colleague has written to you about an epileptic patient on your surgery list whose compliance with her phenytoin medication is poor so that she is having frequent fits. She attends surgery asking for contraceptive advice, having found a new partner. What is the best method of contraception for her?

A. Cerazette®
B. Evra®
C. Marvelon®
D. Mirena®
E. NuvaRing®

Answer [   ]

7.18 Which of the following statements is true of abortions performed in the UK?

A. Patients are routinely scanned to check gestational age of the pregnancy
B. Patients are not usually screened for STIs if undergoing medical rather than surgical termination
C. Over 90% of terminations are performed in the first trimester below 13 weeks gestation
D. Subsequent subfertility can be reliably prevented by administering routine antibiotic prophylaxis effective against chlamydia
E. Simultaneous sterilization should be carried out on request if the patient is having a general anaesthetic

Answer [   ]

7.19 A 40-year-old woman with mild learning difficulties needs contraception because she is having a sexual relationship with another patient in the same residential accommodation. An ultrasound scan is requested because her periods are known to be heavy and this reveals multiple small submucosal fibroids distorting her uterine cavity.

Select the most appropriate form of contraception in her case:

A. Copper IUD
B. Hysterectomy
C. Mercilon®
D. Mirena®
E. Nexplanon®

Answer [ ]

7.20 Which of the following statements is not true about the use of the combined oral contraceptive pill?

A. It will reduce primary dysmenorrhoea
B. It ameliorates the symptoms of premenstrual syndrome
C. It is associated with an increased risk of pelvic inflammatory disease
D. It reduces the incidence of benign breast disease
E. It reduces the risk of ovarian cancer in later life

Answer [ ]

EXTENDED MATCHING QUESTIONS

A.	Combined oral contraceptive pill
B.	depot medroxy progesterone acetate
C.	Etonogestrel subdermal implant
D.	Female sterilization
E.	Intrauterine contraceptive device
F.	Levonelle®
G.	Levonorgestrel intrauterine system
H.	Male condom
I.	Progesterone only pill
J.	Vasectomy

These clinical scenarios relate to women attending your surgery for contraceptive provision. In each case select the most appropriate method for her.

Each option may be used once, more than once or not at all.

7.21 An 18-year-old student is about to go abroad on a 'gap year' and wishes to organize effective contraception while she is away. She has regular periods and no relevant medical or family history.

Answer [ ]

7.22 The development of a latex-allergy rash on the vulva results in a 38-year-old woman requesting a change in her contraceptive plans. She has four children and has consulted you recently for heavy periods.

Answer [ ]

7.23 A 17-year-old hairdresser has just had her second termination of pregnancy. Both pregnancies occurred as a result of running out of supplies of the pill.

Answer [ ]

7.24 At her postnatal appointment, a 38-year-old mother of three children seeks advice about a reliable method of contraception. She experienced severe breast tenderness on the progesterone-only pill and is therefore not keen on taking any hormones.

Answer [ ]

7.25 A 32-year-old woman attends gynaecology clinic, having been referred by her GP for sterilization. She reveals that her husband and father of her two children has just found out about her extramarital affair and left the family home. Her lifestyle is rather chaotic and she needs a very secure method of contraception.

Answer [ ]

A.	Three months
B.	Six months
C.	12 months
D.	24 months
E.	Five years
F.	Seven years
G.	Ten years
H.	15 years
I.	20 years

These statements refer to a 47-year-old woman seeking contraceptive advice. Choose the most appropriate time option given the clinical information in each scenario.

Each option may be used once, more than once or not at all.

7.26 If the 47-year-old woman chooses the Mirena® how long will it be effective as a contraceptive in her particular case?

Answer [ ]

7.27 If the 47-year-old woman chooses a non-hormonal method, how long should she continue to use the method if she has her menopause (last ever period) next year?

Answer [ ]

7.28 The 47-year-old woman makes an informed decision to choose the combined pill as she has no cardiovascular risk factors. When she eventually stops taking the pill, for how long after cessation could she expect a protective effect against ovarian cancer?

Answer [   ]

7.29 If the 47-year-old woman makes an informed decision to choose the combined pill, how soon should you check her blood pressure after initiating the prescription?

Answer [   ]

7.30 If the 47-year-old woman makes an informed decision to choose the combined pill, how often should she attend for blood pressure checks?

Answer [   ]

A.	Administer a GnRH analogue
B.	Commence antibiotics
C.	Commence the combined oral contraceptive pill (COC)
D.	Commence oral progestogens for 25 days
E.	Continue with the next pack of the COC without a pill-free period
F.	Insert an intrauterine contraceptive device (IUCD)
G.	No intervention is required
H.	Remove the IUD
I.	Use condoms as an additional form of contraception

These clinical scenarios relate to women seeking advice in the family planning clinic in your surgery. For each case, select the most appropriate management plan.

Each option may be used once, more than once or not at all.

7.31 A 26-year-old woman using depot medroxy progesterone acetate who has a BMI of 27 kg/m^2 is suffering from breakthrough bleeding. This is now causing relationship difficulties as she does not want to have intercourse when she is bleeding and she is annoyed that she needs to carry pads around with her all the time. She wishes to control the bleeding if possible.

Answer [   ]

7.32 A 32-year-old woman attends surgery because she is feeling unwell and on examination she has a large boil in her left armpit after shaving. You prescribe flucloxacillin 500 mg qds for seven days. She is using Microgynon® for contraception and has five pills left in her pack.

Answer [   ]

7.33 A 29-year-old woman attends surgery. She has a BMI of 34 kg/m². She has bought the antiobesity drug orlistat over the counter at a chemist and is worried as she has developed severe diarrhoea since taking it. You discover that she is using Mercilon® for contraception but she has not had sexual intercourse since the commencement of orlistat.

Answer [   ]

7.34 A 27-year-old woman attends surgery having discovered that she is eight weeks pregnant via a scan organized by the local Accident and Emergency Department where she went complaining of severe nausea. This has confirmed an intrauterine pregnancy and she has a Multiload Cu375® in place. She is shocked to find herself pregnant but wishes to continue with the pregnancy.

Answer [   ]

7.35 A 34-year-old woman attends your surgery. She has a Nova T380® copper intrauterine device *in situ* for contraceptive purposes. She had a casual sexual encounter with a stranger four days ago and now she is suffering from abdominal pain. On examination she is apyrexial, a yellow discharge is noted and the uterus is tender to palpate.

Answer [   ]

A.	At any time in the menstrual cycle
B.	After three weeks
C.	After six weeks
D.	After eight weeks
E.	After 12 weeks
F.	After three months
G.	After three years
H.	After five years
I.	After seven years
J.	Day 1–5 of cycle
K.	Day 19 of cycle
L.	Day 21 of cycle

Each of the clinical scenarios below relate to women requesting contraceptive advice. For each patient select the single most appropriate advice to give from the list above.

Each option may be used once, more than once or not at all.

7.36 An 18-year-old woman attends for repeat emergency contraception having had a second episode of unprotected intercourse in this menstrual cycle. You offer her levonorgestrel 1.5 mg orally and counsel her about the need for contraception. She is keen to have the etonogestrel implant (Nexplanon®) inserted and asks you when is the most appropriate time that this can be done.

Answer [   ]

7.37 A 23-year-old woman has opted to use injection depot medroxy progesterone acetate for contraception. She enquires when she will need her second injection.

Answer [   ]

7.38 A 45-year-old woman attends for replacement of her levonorgestrel intrauterine system (Mirena IUS®), which she uses both for contraception and for control of her heavy menstrual bleeding. She is currently amenorrhoeic with the IUS in place. She asks you when she will need the next IUS if she hasn't gone through the menopause.

Answer [   ]

7.39 A 25-year-old woman is requesting the combined oral contraceptive pill (COC) for contraception postnatally. She had a normal vaginal delivery and is bottle feeding her baby. When should she commence the COC?

Answer [   ]

7.40 A 25-year-old woman attends your surgery requesting to commence the combined oral contraceptive pill for the first time. She has been amenorrhoeic for some time but her pregnancy test is negative. When can she commence her pill?

Answer [   ]

A.	Copper IUCD delayed until chlamydia swab results available
B.	Copper IUCD with chlamydia antibiotic prophylaxis
C.	depot medroxy progesterone acetate injection
D.	Levonorgestrel (Levonelle®) 1.5 mg oral dose
E.	Levonorgestrel intrauterine system (Mirena®)
F.	Nexplanon® etonogestrel implant
G.	No prescription needed; reassure
H.	Ulipristal acetate (EllaOne®) 30 mg oral dose
I.	Repeat ulipristal acetate (EllaOne®) 30 mg oral dose

These clinical scenarios relate to women seeking emergency contraception. For each case, select the most appropriate method.

Each option may be used once, more than once or not at all.

7.41 A shy 35-year-old woman presents to her local police station the morning after an alleged rape and is seen at the Sexual Assault Referral Centre (SARC). She has had a full infection screen done and thinks that her last period was about 12 days ago. She does not usually use contraception as she has never been sexually active and is very distressed at the thought of possible pregnancy as a result of the attack.

Answer [   ]

7.42 The same shy 35-year-old woman returns to the SARC three hours later having just vomited in the car on the way home.

Answer [   ]

7.43 Three months after her first delivery, a woman is still fully breastfeeding her baby. She has not had a period yet and thought that she didn't need to use contraception at all so had unprotected intercourse two days ago. It took her a long time to get pregnant and you suspect that her subfertility might have been due to previous episodes of pelvic inflammatory disease related to proven chlamydia infection.

Answer [   ]

7.44 A 24-year-old woman normally uses depot medroxy progesterone acetate for contraception but has forgotten to return for her usual injection, which is now over a month overdue. She has been amenorrhoeic since she started on depot medroxy progesterone acetate three years ago and she is keen to continue using it because her periods had been heavy previously. She had unprotected intercourse three days ago.

Answer [   ]

7.45 On return from her holidays, a teenage woman seeks help four days after a condom failure abroad. She is now on day 18 of an irregular cycle and uses a Ventolin inhaler several times a day for her asthma (which has been severe enough to necessitate hospital admission in the past).

Answer [   ]

A.	24 hours
B.	72 hours
C.	120 hours
D.	Anytime in the cycle
E.	Day 1–5 of the menstrual cycle
F.	Day 1–7 of the menstrual cycle
G.	Five days after expected ovulation
H.	Immediately
I.	Next expected menses
J.	Two weeks
K.	Three to four weeks

The following clinical scenarios relate to timing of commencement of contraceptive methods. For each scenario select the most appropriate option.

Each option may be used once, more than once or not at all.

7.46 A 19-year-old drug user had a vaginal delivery yesterday and the baby has been taken into care. She has a chaotic lifestyle and this was her third unplanned pregnancy. She is happy to have an etonogestrel implant but is keen to leave hospital and asks you when is the soonest that the device can be inserted.

Answer [   ]

7.47 A 19-year-old woman has just completed the second part of a medical abortion. Following counselling she has requested the etonogestrel subdermal implant (Nexplanon®) for ongoing contraception. When should she have this inserted?

Answer [   ]

7.48 A woman using depot medroxy progesterone acetate for contraception has forgotten to attend her appointment for her next injection. She telephones the surgery to make another appointment and asks how much time she has got before she cannot rely on the injection for effective contraception.

Answer [   ]

7.49 A 32-year-old woman has been using a Progesterone only pill (POP) for a year following the birth of her second child. She has stopped breastfeeding now and is unhappy with the intermenstrual bleeding that she has with the POP. She is keen to switch to the combined oral contraceptive (COC) and asks how long after finishing her POP packet she should start the COC.

Answer [   ]

7.50 A 16-year-old woman requests emergency contraception for her first episode of unprotected intercourse due to condom failure. She is in a steady relationship and is keen to start the combined oral contraceptive pill (COC). When would you advise her to start taking the COC?

Answer [   ]

Curriculum module 1: Answers

MULTIPLE CHOICE QUESTIONS

1.1 Concerning symptoms caused by endometriosis:

A. Patients often complain of deep dyspareunia   T

Other causes of pain on intercourse are chronic pelvic inflammatory disease, adenomyosis and irritable bowel syndrome.

B. There is a correlation between the severity of pain symptoms and the extent of the endometriotic lesions found at laparoscopy   F

This is one of the great conundrums about endometriosis. We do not know why some patients with minimal disease experience severe pain whereas we have all come across patients with such awful disease that they have a 'frozen pelvis' but they have very little pain.

C. Dyschezia is caused by endometriosis in the rectovaginal septum   T

Dyschezia is pain on defecation which may be caused by deposits of endometriosis in the rectovaginal septum or in the Pouch of Douglas.

D. Patients with endometriosis may suffer from chronic fatigue   T

The mechanism is unclear but this makes endometriosis difficult to separate from chronic pelvic inflammatory disease on symptomatology; the cyclical nature of the pain may help.

E. Primary dysmenorrhoea is a common symptom of endometriosis   F

Secondary dysmenorrhoea may be due to endometriosis. Classically secondary dysmenorrhoea lasts throughout the period and may even get worse towards the end of the period. Primary dysmenorrhoea is classically spasmodic pain just before or during the first one or two days of a period and is functional pain in the absence of pelvic pathology.

Source: RCOG Green-top guideline number 24. *The Investigation and Management of Endometriosis.*

1.2 Regarding early pregnancy complications:

A. Diarrhoea may be due to intra-abdominal bleeding   T

An important learning point: blood or pus in the Pouch of Douglas irritates the rectum and may cause the patient to have diarrhoea. Consequently each 'Confidential Enquiries into Maternal Death' report describes cases where ectopic pregnancy was misdiagnosed as gastroenteritis and the patient died as a result of delayed intervention.

B. Hyperemesis is a recognized presentation of hydatidiform mole   T

One of the reasons for scanning patients admitted with hyperemesis is to rule out molar pregnancy (the other is to diagnose multiple pregnancy).

C. Missed abortion usually presents with light bleeding   F

Missed abortion means that the patient has had no bleeding and therefore is unaware that her pregnancy has miscarried. The diagnosis is usually made when

she presents for a dating scan at the end of the first trimester, thinking that the pregnancy is OK.

D. Pain in the shoulder indicates that the patient may have an ectopic pregnancy   T

Referred pain caused by blood irritating the peritoneum underneath the diaphragm is felt over the C3,4,5 dermatomes (remember your undergraduate anatomy: 'C3,4,5 keeps the diaphragm alive').

E. A patient with an ectopic pregnancy may not have missed a period   T

When an ectopic pregnancy implants in the tube the decidualized endometrium lining the uterus sometimes sheds at the time a period would have occurred. The bleeding is often not as heavy as a period, so the next question is 'Was that a normal period?'

1.3 Considering domestic abuse in an O&G setting:

A. Pregnancy is known to provoke episodes of domestic violence   T

Several studies have highlighted this association, which underlines the importance of staff in antenatal clinics feeling that it is their responsibility to ask the right questions. One would assume that pregnancy would be protective but it appears to provoke attacks rather than prevent them.

B. Community midwives are required to ask about domestic violence during routine antenatal care even if it seems unlikely (e.g. the patient works as a doctor)   T

Domestic violence knows no boundaries of social class or race. It could be happening to a colleague in a hospital residence near you.

C. Female relatives can be used to translate when asking about domestic violence to ensure a non-English speaker has understood the question   F

A victim of domestic violence may be reluctant to disclose the problem in the presence of a relative because of the likely repercussions within the family. It is good practice for a midwife to see a woman alone at some stage during the pregnancy to ask about this and it may involve the use of an independent translator.

D. There is a recognized association between domestic violence and repeated requests for termination of unwanted pregnancy   T

'Repeated termination' is recognized as a marker for domestic violence and some victims of abuse may be coerced into requesting termination of pregnancy against their will. Others may view the child as tying them into an abusive relationship; the psychology is complex.

E. Domestic abuse may involve control of a woman's finances   T

Domestic abuse is intentional abuse inflicted on one partner by another while in an intimate relationship. It includes physical, sexual, emotional, psychological or financial abuse.

1.4 These conditions may cause amenorrhoea:

A. Polycystic ovarian syndrome   T

PCO causes anovulation in some women, which may result in irregular or absent periods.

B. Endometrial hyperplasia   F

This causes heavy irregular bleeding.

C. Mullerian agenesis   T

This results in congenital absence of the uterus (and sometimes vagina too) which presents with primary amenorrhoea.

D. Asherman syndrome — T

This syndrome is a result of over-enthusiastic curettage of the uterus at evacuation or termination of pregnancy, which causes failure of the endometrium to regenerate and the formation of intrauterine adhesions.

E. Anorexia nervosa — T

Drastic weight loss results in the hypothalamic–pituitary axis switching off. Cessation of periods is usually a sign that the eating disorder condition is becoming serious.

1.5 A 37-year-old woman attends your surgery to inform you that she is six weeks pregnant. She has a BMI of 38 and has had four previous caesarean sections, delivering babies of over 4 kg each time.

She is at increased risk of the following pregnancy complications:

A. Placenta accreta — T

With every successive caesarean section the chance of having placenta praevia increases and the risk of the low-lying placenta also being accreta increases exponentially. This situation could result in torrential haemorrhage necessitating emergency hysterectomy and is one of the reasons obstetricians like to limit caesarean sections to three.

B. Postpartum haemorrhage — T

On the fifth and subsequent babies, we label a mother as being a 'grand multip' whatever the mode of delivery for her previous babies. The significance of this is that she is more at risk of postpartum haemorrhage.

C. Intrauterine growth retardation — F

D. Gestational diabetes — T

Her BMI earns her a glucose tolerance test.

E. Pre-eclampsia — F

This usually occurs in women on their first pregnancy and rarely in multiparous women.

1.6 The following factors contribute to the 'Risk of malignancy index' (RMI) when evaluating the likelihood of an ovarian cyst being malignant in nature:

A. Solid areas in the cyst on ultrasound scan — T

B. The age of the woman — F

C. The CA125 tumour marker level — T

D. The menopausal status of the woman — T

E. A family history of ovarian cancer — F

The RMI is worked out using the woman's menopausal status, the CA125 level and the ultrasound findings. The score predicts the likelihood of malignancy (which guides subsequent investigations, identifies those patients that should be referred to the gynae-oncology MDT and helps to plan treatment).

1.7 A 42-year-old nulliparous woman consults you in the surgery about her urinary problems. She has been suffering with urinary frequency and urge incontinence for over a year. The following should be considered as a possible cause of her symptoms:

A. Uterine fibroid — T

Pressure in the pelvis from a large fibroid near the bladder can present with urinary frequency or incontinence.

B. Multiple sclerosis   T
Sometimes urinary difficulties are the first presenting symptom of MS.

C. Urinary tract infection   F
The length of duration of symptoms means that UTI is not a likely cause.

D. Detrusor instability   T
This fits the bill and could be diagnosed on urodynamic study.

E. Interstitial cystitis (IC)   T
This is a chronic inflammatory condition of the bladder wall which can be diagnosed at cystoscopy. The cardinal features of IC are pain at the end of micturition as the bladder empties.

1.8 When assessing a gynaecological patient with pelvic pain, these examination findings are recognized signs of endometriosis:

A. Fixed retroversion of the uterus   T
B. Palpable nodules in the rectovaginal septum   T
C. A tender swelling situated within the umbilicus   T
D. Adnexal tenderness   T
E. Contact bleeding of the cervix   F
Endometriosis may cause severe adhesions in the pelvis, which can fix the uterus down in retroversion. Tender nodules are typical of endometriosis, which can be found in odd places even the umbilicus. It is possible to get endometriosis on the cervix too, but it will look like a tiny chocolate cyst that does not bleed when you touch it.

1.9 Non-sensitized, Rhesus-negative women should receive anti-D immunoglobulin in the following situations:

A. Miscarriage below 12 weeks when the uterus is evacuated surgically   T
B. Ectopic pregnancy   T
C. Incomplete miscarriage over 12 weeks   T
D. Complete miscarriage under 12 weeks when bleeding is heavy   T
E. Threatened miscarriage below 12 weeks when the fetus is viable   F
The rules for administration of anti-D have changed recently to avoid giving it to women who are under 12 weeks gestation and have had a spontaneous miscarriage with conservative management or a threatened miscarriage, as the risk of sensitization is very low.
Source: RCOG Green-top guideline number 22. *The Use of Anti-D Immunoglobulin for Rhesus D Prophylaxis.*

1.10 Concerning maternal death:

A. The maternal mortality rate is lower in the UK than in the USA   T
B. Reducing the number of maternal deaths worldwide by the year 2050 is a 'millennium development goal'   F
C. The maternal mortality ratio is defined as the number of maternal deaths per 100 000 pregnancies   F
D. The details of every maternal death in the UK are scrutinized to look for elements of substandard care   T
E. There has been an increase in maternal deaths from sepsis related to sore throats   T

Surprisingly the chance of dying in pregnancy is much higher in the USA and the rate is increasing. Perhaps this reflects access to health care but the reasons remain obscure. Millennium development goal number 5 is to achieve a 75% reduction in the worldwide maternal mortality ratio by 2015 and it is very unlikely that this will be realized. The maternal mortality ratio is the number of deaths per 100 000 maternities, which is the number of pregnancies which result in either a live birth or stillbirth occurring from 24 weeks gestation onwards. Stillbirths at or after 24 weeks have to be reported by law and the number of pregnancy losses before this time is unknown: therefore using maternities rather than pregnancies as a denominator is more accurate and allows comparison between time periods.

SINGLE BEST ANSWER QUESTIONS

1.11 Taking over the gynaecology on-call duties one evening, you are given this list of tasks to be done. Which one would you do first?

A.   Site an intravenous infusion for a severely dehydrated patient with hyperemesis

B.   Sign a death certificate as a patient's husband is waiting on the ward for it

C.   Review the scan report of a woman with a suspected ectopic pregnancy

D.   Review a woman who has just miscarried an 18-week fetus but not delivered the placenta

E.   Clerk a new patient that a GP has sent in to hospital with a suspected torted ovarian cyst

The reason for choosing the 18-week miscarriage patient first is that she is likely to bleed heavily as she has a retained placenta. If you cannot remove the placenta easily on the ward she needs to go to theatre. The later on in pregnancy the miscarriage happens, the greater the bulk of the placenta and the more bleeding you get. With a second-trimester miscarriage it is likely to be very heavy indeed. In addition there could well be an element of infection here which puts her at increased risk of haemorrhage.

The patient with a possible torted ovarian cyst is likely to be in severe pain, but a potential haemorrhage takes precedence over that.

The patient with a possible ectopic has already been clerked and is likely to have established IV access; she only goes to the top of the list if she drops her blood pressure.

1.12 You are trying to persuade a postoperative woman with a haemoglobin of 55 g/l that she would not be so breathless if she had a blood transfusion, but she is concerned about the risk of acquiring HIV. The chance of acquiring HIV infection as a result of blood transfusion in the UK is approximately:

A.   1 in 6000

B.   1 in 60 000

C.   1 in 600 000

D.   1 in 6 million

E.   1 in 60 million

This is useful information to have at your fingertips if you are counselling a woman who needs a blood transfusion.

Source: RCOG Green-top guideline number 47: *Blood Transfusion in Obstetrics.*

1.13 The community midwife doing an antenatal clinic in your GP surgery asks you to see a 37-year-old obese woman who has come for a routine check-up at 32 weeks gestation in her first pregnancy. Her booking blood pressure in the first trimester was 130/88 but it is now 160/95 and the midwife has checked the blood pressure twice. The woman is asymptomatic. Which is the most appropriate course of action?

A. Urinalysis and prescribe antihypertensives if no proteinuria
B. Send urgent full blood count, urate and liver function test
C. **Refer her urgently to hospital for further investigation and treatment**
D. Urinalysis and request urgent antenatal appointment if no proteinuria
E. Twenty-four hour urine collection for protein analysis

This woman probably has underlying essential hypertension. However it is irrelevant to your immediate decision whether she has proteinuria or not (and therefore superimposed pre-eclampsia) because her blood pressure is at a level where cerebrovascular accident is a real possibility. The maternal mortality reports stress that a systolic of 160 mmHg is a critical level where treatment must be instituted to prevent this complication. There is also a need for fetal assessment to check for placental insufficiency, so referral to hospital is a sensible solution rather than treating the hypertension in primary care.

1.14 A 52-year-old woman presents to your surgery with a very sore vulva. On examination you find thickening of both labia minora with a couple of shallow ulcers on both sides and a split area at the fourchette. What is the most likely diagnosis in her case?

A. Eczema
B. Genital herpes
C. Lichen planus
D. **Lichen sclerosus**
E. Vulval intraepithelial neoplasia (VIN)

Lichen sclerosus is the most common cause of these findings on the vulva. Women of this age do not usually get genital herpes and lichen planus and VIN are rare.

1.15 The clinical scenarios detailed below describe gynaecological patients admitted as an emergency. Which patient is most likely to have a diagnosis of ectopic pregnancy?

A. Acute onset of central abdominal pain and nausea at 12 weeks gestation. On examination severe lower abdominal tenderness with generalized guarding and rebound, also fetor oris. White cell count is $18 \times 10^9/l$ and urinalysis is negative
B. History of 11 weeks amenorrhoea and brown vaginal discharge but no pain. Pelvic examination reveals no tenderness but uterus is small for dates and the cervical os is closed. Serum βhCG is 2010 IU/ml and scan is awaited
C. Seven weeks amenorrhoea and vaginal bleeding. Pelvic examination reveals no tenderness. Uterus is soft and slightly enlarged with an open cervical os
D. Admitted with bleeding and lower abdominal pain at eight weeks gestation. Transvaginal ultrasound scan shows an intrauterine sac with a fetal pole but no heart pulsation detected. Serum βhCG is 150 000 IU/ml
E. **Patient with lower abdominal and shoulder tip pain who has a copper coil fitted. Last menstrual period was two weeks ago and on examination has a tender abdomen with guarding. Urinary hCG test positive in A&E**

Patient A probably has appendicitis and ectopic pregnancies usually present before 12 weeks gestation. Patient B probably has a missed miscarriage as the uterus is small for dates. Patient C either has an inevitable or incomplete miscarriage as the os is open. Patient D's pregnancy has come to grief and it may be a partial hydatidiform mole as the hCG is so high. Patient E is most likely to have an ectopic because of the shoulder tip pain and the coil. Many patients presenting with ectopic pregnancies do not have a history of amenorrhoea (although the bleeding a couple of weeks before is not a normal 'period' but uterine decidua being shed).

1.16 A 46-year-old woman presents to her GP seeking help with her period problems which date back almost a year. Her cycles are still regular with a cycle of 26 days but the bleeding is now very heavy with clots. She complains of severe secondary dysmenorrhoea but no other pelvic pain. On examination there are no masses palpable in the pelvis. The uterus is enlarged to the size of an orange, smooth and very tender but mobile with no adnexal tenderness.

Select the most likely gynaecological cause of this clinical picture:

A. **Adenomyosis**
B. Chronic pelvic inflammatory disease
C. Endometriosis
D. Endometrial hyperplasia
E. Fibroids

The enlargement of the uterus combined with tenderness suggests the diagnosis of adenomyosis. Fibroids are not usually tender and you would not suspect endometriosis without some other pelvic pain and/or tenderness. If she had chronic pelvic inflammatory disease it would have presented before the age of 46 and endometrial pathology causes irregular bleeding.

1.17 A 39-year-old woman asks for a hospital referral so that she can be investigated for recurrent miscarriage, having suffered three first-trimester pregnancy losses. She believes that her miscarriages are due to stress. She works long hours as a computer programmer and smokes 15 cigarettes a day. Which of the following factors is the most likely cause of her recurrent miscarriages?

A. Working with visual display units
B. Smoking
C. **Advanced maternal age**
D. Natural killer cells
E. Bacterial vaginosis

Maternal age over 35 is associated with a 25% risk of miscarriage.

Source: RCOG Green-top guideline number 17. *The Investigation and Treatment of Couples with Recurrent Miscarriage.*

1.18 In your GP surgery the practice nurse asks you to see a 25-year-old woman who is unable to tolerate speculum examination for her first smear test. The patient tells you that she has experienced severe dyspareunia since her marriage two years ago and discloses that she was sexually abused as a child. Which of the following statements about child abuse is untrue?

A. **Abuse in childhood predisposes to depressive illness in later life which does not respond to treatment**
B. Child abuse encompasses neglect as well as physical and sexual abuse

C. Somatization as an adult can be a result of child abuse

D. Women who have been abused as children rarely disclose such a history

E. Abuse in childhood is known to be associated with illicit drug use as an adult

Childhood sexual abuse is known to result in sexual problems in later life such as vaginismus but could also lead to behaviour such as promiscuity, early pregnancy and STIs. There is also an association with psychiatric problems but they can be treated.

1.19 The mother of a 13-year-old girl attends the surgery for advice. Her daughter has been offered human papilloma virus (HPV) vaccine at school but did not bring an information leaflet home, so she wants to know more about it. Which of these statements about the bivalent vaccine (Cervarix®) is correct?

A. She will require two doses of the vaccine over six months

B. The vaccine will reduce the chance of her developing genital warts as well as cervical intraepithelial neoplasia

C. If she completes the course of vaccinations she will not need cervical smears in the future

D. The duration of protection offered by the vaccine is unknown

E. The vaccine is made from live attenuated human papilloma virus

The bivalent vaccine contains particles of HPV viruses 16 and 18, which are associated with over 70% of cases of cervical cancer. As it does not prevent all cases of CIN and cancer women do need to stay on the smear programme, although this is likely to develop into HPV typing in the future rather than just cytology. The vaccine is given as a course of three doses but we are still not sure how long the antibody levels will persist in vivo.

The quadrivalent vaccine (Gardasil®) also contains HPV 6 and 11, which are associated with CIN and genital warts too.

1.20 Which of the following statements is true in relation to women with Turner syndrome?

A. They have no problems with learning difficulties

B. Estrogen therapy may result in spontaneous fertility

C. There is a high prevalence of left-sided congenital heart malformation

D. Administration of growth hormone at puberty will not produce any extra height

E. They all have karyotype 46XO

The prevalence of bicuspid aortic valve is up to 17% and aortic coarctation is up to 10%. When the diagnosis of Turner syndrome is made, the woman should have investigations as cardiovascular malformations are responsible for much of the reduced life expectancy in these women.

If they are given growth hormone and estrogen at puberty, they can achieve normal height. The HRT treatment will prevent osteoporosis but does not make Turner syndrome patients ovulate.

Turner syndrome does not cause mental retardation but they can have difficulties with non-verbal learning disorders (problems with spatial relationships and mathematics, problems with motor control).

The karyotype is 45XO, although it is also possible to have a mosaic karyotype.

EXTENDED MATCHING QUESTIONS

A.	CT scan of the pelvis
B.	Cystoscopy
C.	Diagnostic laparoscopy
D.	Dye laparoscopy
E.	High vaginal swab for chlamydia
F.	Hysterosalpingogram
G.	MRI scan of the pelvis
H.	Serum CA125 level
I.	Transvaginal ultrasound scan
J.	Urodynamic study

Each of these clinical scenarios describes a woman presenting with symptoms of pelvic pain; for each case pick the most appropriate initial investigation given the information that you are presented with.

Each option may be used once, more than once or not at all.

1.21 Secondary dysmenorrhoea in a 40-year-old nulliparous woman with a BMI of 48. Over the last year her periods have become heavier and she is not currently sexually active.

I. Transvaginal ultrasound scan

Possible causes of secondary dysmenorrhoea in this woman include fibroids, adenomyosis and endometriosis. Chronic PID is less likely in a woman of this age, especially as she is not sexually active. The choice is between laparoscopy and scan to investigate this. Laparoscopy might be difficult in view of her BMI and an ultrasound is an easier option initially, although it will not diagnose non-ovarian endometriosis.

1.22 A 38-year-old woman complains of premenstrual pain, severe secondary dysmenorrhoea and dyschezia

C. Diagnostic laparoscopy

Dyschezia means pain on opening bowels and this lady is likely to have endometriosis with this collection of symptoms. Ultrasound will show endometriomas on her ovaries but may be normal if the ovaries are unaffected.

1.23 A 24-year-old secretary with non-cyclical pain and deep dyspareunia, who has been trying to get pregnant for two years

D. Dye laparoscopy

The most likely diagnosis here is pelvic inflammatory disease and an ultrasound scan, while it will show hydrosalpinges and ovarian cysts, will not help much with the diagnosis as much as a laparoscopy – and the dye to investigate the fertility aspect, instead of just doing a diagnostic laparoscopy. Although chlamydia swabs are indicated, especially prior to flushing dye through the fallopian tubes, you take cervical swabs for chlamydia not a high vaginal swab.

1.24 A perimenopausal woman with left iliac fossa pain radiating down her leg, whose abdominal ultrasound shows a 9 cm septated cyst adjacent to the uterus on the left side with free fluid around it

H. Serum CA125 level

There are a couple of worrying features about this cyst – the free fluid and the fact that it is not simple. Also it is quite large and she is perimenopausal so it is not likely to be an ovulatory cyst. The CA125 level will help to calculate the Risk of Malignancy Index (RMI), which will aid the management decision regarding surgery, i.e. to remove the cyst only or to perform a hysterectomy and bilateral salpingo-oophorectomy in case it is malignant on histology. Serum CA125 is raised in over 80% of ovarian cancer cases and, if a cut-off of 30 U/ml is used, the test has a sensitivity of 81% and specificity of 75%.

Although she might have a CT scan done later if the Risk of Malignancy Index is high and she is referred to gynae-oncology, this would not be an initial investigation.

Source: RCOG Green-top guideline number 34. *Ovarian Cysts in Postmenopausal Women.*

1.25 A 62-year-old woman with severe urinary frequency for eight weeks associated with dyspareunia

B. Cystoscopy

This woman is in the right age group for a transitional cell carcinoma of the bladder and her symptoms have persisted for many weeks. We have not given you an MSU option and it is important not to miss a cancer. If the bladder is normal at cystoscopy, urodynamics may help you establish a diagnosis eventually.

A.	Bleeding corpus luteum cyst
B.	Ectopic pregnancy
C.	Gastroenteritis
D.	Heterotopic pregnancy
E.	Ovarian hyperstimulation syndrome
F.	Ovarian torsion
G.	Pelvic sepsis
H.	Pulmonary embolism
I.	Threatened miscarriage

These women have all undergone assisted conception treatment with IVF and have developed complications. For each clinical scenario select the most likely diagnosis.

Each option may be used once, more than once or not at all.

1.26 Following a cycle of IVF six weeks ago, a young woman is pregnant for the first time. She presents to A&E with increasing lower abdominal pain and diarrhoea. She has had brown vaginal loss for a couple of days. On examination she is pale with a tachycardia of 100 beats per minute but her blood pressure is normal. An urgent ultrasound scan shows an endometrial thickness of 12 mm but no gestation sac seen.

B. Ectopic pregnancy

The diarrhoea might lead you to think that she has gastroenteritis but diarrhoea can also be caused by blood in the pelvis irritating the bowel. Her tachycardia may be due to sepsis but the overall picture suggests ectopic pregnancy with intra-abdominal bleeding.

1.27 A slightly obese woman with polycystic ovarian syndrome is admitted a week after an IVF cycle during which 12 oocytes were collected. She had an embryo transfer five days previously and now has shortness of breath, nausea and abdominal pain. Her abdomen is distended on examination.

E. Ovarian hyperstimulation syndrome

The combination of her breathlessness and abdominal distension are the key to the diagnosis of hyperstimulation syndrome. Pulmonary embolus will also cause breathlessness and several of the other diagnoses will cause abdominal pain (gastroenteritis, heterotopic pregnancy, bleeding corpus luteum, torsion, sepsis, ectopic, miscarriage and perforation) but they should not cause breathlessness.
Polycystic ovary (PCO) patients are more at risk of hyperstimulation during IVF treatment.

1.28 A 27-year-old woman is admitted to the gynaecology ward as an emergency with severe abdominal pain and vomiting. She is unable to lie still and scores her pain 9 out of 10. On examination she is apyrexial, tachycardic and normotensive. She has a tender mass on the left side of the pelvis. She had a cycle of IVF recently with oocyte recovery ten days previously, followed by embryo transfer two days later.

F. Ovarian torsion

The severe pain in combination with vomiting suggests torsion and it is too early in the process for it to be an ectopic pregnancy. Sepsis is unlikely because she is apyrexial and gastroenteritis should not produce a tender mass in the pelvis.

1.29 Three weeks after a cycle of IVF a 34-year-old woman presents to her GP with increasing pain in the lower abdomen and rigors. She only had one embryo replaced in the uterus because only one of the oocytes that were retrieved actually fertilized.

G. Pelvic sepsis

Pain and rigors suggest infection and pelvic sepsis is a possible consequence of oocyte retrieval as it is usually done by inserting a catheter into the ovarian follicles individually, transvaginally under ultrasound control.

1.30 A pregnant woman is rushed to A&E in the UK having collapsed at the airport. She had a cycle of IVF in another country seven weeks ago, during which three embryos were replaced in the uterus. She has a scan picture with her showing an intrauterine pregnancy with a viable six-week fetus. Her blood pressure is 85/45 mmHg, her pulse is 120 bpm, her temperature is 36.5 °C and on abdominal examination she has rigidity, rebound tenderness and guarding. Pelvic examination reveals tenderness in the left adnexa and she has cervical excitation. Her haemoglobin is 95 g/l and her white cell count is 8×10^9/l.

D. Heterotopic pregnancy

The abdominal and pelvic examinations suggest a diagnosis of ectopic, sepsis or ovarian cyst accident. An ovarian cyst would have been noted on her scan and her normal temperature and white cell count rule out sepsis. Although there is an intrauterine pregnancy on the scan, it is possible that there is another one in her left fallopian tube, especially as more than one embryo was replaced.

A.	Bacterial vaginosis
B.	Beta-haemolytic streptococcus
C.	Candida
D.	Chlamydia
E.	Gonorrhoea
F.	Herpes genitalis
G.	Primary syphilis
H.	Streptococcus A (streptococcus pyogenes)
I.	Trichomonas vaginalis

These clinical scenarios relate to women presenting to a hospital clinic or general practice surgery. Select the most likely infecting organism given the clinical information for each woman.

Each option may be used once, more than once or not at all.

1.31 A 23-year-old woman admitted two days postpartum with severe sepsis. Her temperature is 38 °C, pulse 110 bpm, her respiratory rate is raised and her uterus is enlarged and tender. She has a sore throat with a red pharynx and white spots on her tonsils on examination.

H. Streptococcus A

In the 2006–2008 Maternal Mortality Report, the leading cause of maternal death was sepsis with Group A strep mentioned as the causative organism for the first time. Women seem to become very sick very quickly and every hospital has since introduced a sepsis protocol as timely antibiotics save lives. It is also possible to acquire chlamydial pharyngitis through sexual activity.

1.32 A 55-year-old diabetic woman presents to her GP with a six-week history of a sore vulva. On examination her vulva is red and excoriated.

C. Candida

These sort of changes on the vulva are sometimes described as 'diabetic vulva' and often thrush infection is underlying the problem, although diabetic women can look like this with negative swabs if their control is poor.

1.33 A 19-year-old presents to the practice nurse with postcoital bleeding and on speculum examination her cervix bleeds on contact.

D. Chlamydia

The most likely cause of postcoital bleeding in teenagers is cervical infection, with chlamydia being the likely organism (although most chlamydial infections are asymptomatic).

1.34 A primigravid woman is admitted in labour at term. Her uterus is tender and a diagnosis of chorioamnionitis is made. Postnatally the baby develops meningitis.

B. Beta-haemolytic streptococcus

The chorioamnionitis is likely to have resulted from ascending infection from the vagina and in combination with the neonatal meningitis, group B strep is the most likely organism on this list.

1.35 A 22-year-old woman is admitted to the gynaecology ward with acute retention of urine. On examination she has a sore vulva.

F. Herpes genitalis

Very few conditions cause urinary retention especially in young women but a primary attack of genital herpes will do this. The key to the diagnosis is finding herpetic ulcers on the vulva, which are often secondarily infected too.

A.	Colposcopy
B.	Colposcopy and cervical biopsy
C.	Dilatation and curettage
D.	Endometrial biopsy using sampling device
E.	Hysteroscopy and endometrial biopsy
F.	Human papilloma virus typing
G.	Liquid-based cervical cytology
H.	MRI scan of abdomen and pelvis
I.	Transvaginal ultrasound scan

The scenarios described below relate to women whose GP suspects that they might have cancer so they have been referred to gynaecology clinic with an urgent 'two-week wait' appointment. For each patient select the most appropriate investigation given the clinical information described in each case.

Each option may be used once, more than once or not at all.

1.36 A 48-year-old diabetic woman with a BMI of 48 presents with a history of irregular periods and intermenstrual bleeding. She is nulliparous.

E. Hysteroscopy and endometrial biopsy

There is a good chance that this woman will have endometrial cancer because of her obesity and diabetes. Although you might be able to get a diagnosis from sampling the endometrium in clinic, this may not be easy as she is nulliparous and the gold standard is hysteroscopy because you can be sure that you are taking the biopsy from the correct part of the uterus. Ultrasound would be a useful investigation especially in relation to her ovaries (which will be difficult to feel because of her size) but a tissue diagnosis is needed here.

1.37 A 26-year-old woman attends for her first smear at the GP's surgery and mentions that she has experienced postcoital bleeding for the last six months. While taking the smear, a friable 3 mm diameter red lesion is noted on her cervix, which bleeds profusely.

B. Colposcopy and cervical biopsy

As there is clinical suspicion of cancer in this case, a cervical biopsy is necessary, whatever the result of the smear.

1.38 A 57-year-old woman goes to see her GP complaining of indigestion and abdominal distension. She has had a CA125 blood test done privately and the result is 60 IU/l.

I. Transvaginal ultrasound scan

The CA125 level is higher than normal and this suggests a closer look at the ovaries. Ultrasound is the cheapest and easiest method.

1.39 A worried 31-year-old refugee woman presents to the surgery a few weeks after arrival in the country saying that her younger sister has just died of cervical cancer back home. She wishes to be reassured that she does not have it too.

G. Liquid-based cervical cytology

Cervical cancer is not inherited or genetic in any way but the patient's anxiety is understandable. A smear should be adequate and she should commence on the screening programme anyway.

1.40 A 32-year-old nulliparous woman presents with lower abdominal pain and severe dysmenorrhoea three years after radiotherapy treatment for cancer of the cervix. On examination her cervix looks normal but atrophic with radiotherapy changes and an ultrasound scan shows that the cavity of the uterus is distended with blood.

C. Dilatation and curettage

This patient has a haematometria which is probably the result of radiotherapy. Although it is important to rule out recurrence of her original cancer, the situation needs treatment to let the blood out of the uterus and get rid of her pain. We do not do dilatation and curettage as a diagnostic procedure anymore (now that hysteroscopy is available and is more accurate) but in this case it is actually the correct procedure.

A.	Discuss with on-call consultant
B.	Discuss with on-call registrar (Specialty Trainee year 4)
C.	Leave for consultant to deal with on his return
D.	No action required
E.	Phone GP
F.	Phone patient

G.	Post a prescription to patient
H.	Recall urgently to gynaecology clinic next week
I.	Refer to gynae-oncology multidisciplinary team (MDT) meeting
J.	Routine gynaecology clinic follow-up
K.	Write to GP
L.	Write to patient

The rest of your clinical team are away and your consultant's secretary has asked you to go through some messages and results in her in-tray. For each of the scenarios below select the most appropriate course of action to ensure the best use of NHS time and resources, as well as considering the most safe and convenient solution for the patient.

Each option may be used once, more than once or not at all.

1.41 A 28-year-old woman attended the antenatal clinic a few days ago for a growth scan at 28 weeks gestation and gave a history of an offensive vaginal discharge for the last week. The result of the high vaginal swab is reported as showing clue cells on microscopy and profuse anaerobes on culture.

G. Post a prescription to patient

The results of the HVS suggest bacterial vaginosis (BV) and since she is symptomatic she needs antibiotic treatment. In addition, we always treat BV in pregnancy as it can cause miscarriage and premature labour. The most efficient way of organising this is to provide a prescription directly to the patient. An alternative would be to write to her asking her to see her GP for a prescription but that would mean an extra visit to the GP and possibly a delay in starting treatment.

1.42 An 18-year-old woman attended the emergency gynaecology clinic two days ago with pelvic pain, discharge and postcoital bleeding for the preceding fortnight. The endocervical swab result shows *Chlamydia trachomatis* detected by PCR.

L. Write to patient

The reason for writing to the patient rather than just issuing a prescription is that she needs to be informed of the result and referred to the GUM clinic for treatment, screening for other STIs including HIV and contact tracing. Your letter would be able to explain all this. You would copy this to the GP but you wouldn't write to the GP asking them to do the referral to GUM as it is the gynaecology team's responsibility to action results on investigations they have done.

1.43 A GP has written a letter about a 30-year-old woman with a two-year history of pelvic pain. She has been previously seen in the gynaecology clinic by your consultant and was advised to start the combined oral contraceptive pill. She is getting headaches so has discontinued the pill but is still getting pelvic pain.

J. Routine gynaecology clinic follow-up

Since this woman is unable to tolerate the suggested management plan, she should be seen again in clinic to explore other options and possibly consider laparoscopy but it is not an urgent situation.

1.44 A 23-year-old woman was seen in the gynaecology clinic two weeks ago with a three-month history of pelvic pain throughout the cycle. Examination showed no abnormality, in particular no tenderness on vaginal examination and the high vaginal and endocervical swabs were negative. In clinic, you gave her an advice leaflet about irritable bowel syndrome and organized an ultrasound scan. The scan result shows a normal-sized anteverted uterus, both ovaries are clearly seen and are normal. There is no free fluid and there are no adnexal masses.

L. Write to patient

It is a more efficient use of time and resources to write to the patient directly with results rather than bring them back to a gynaecology clinic just to tell them that everything is normal. There is good evidence that functional bowel pain is a significant cause of pelvic pain. If she continues to have pain it would be more appropriate for her to see her GP and have a trial of treatment with laxatives and antispasmodics before considering referral back to the gynaecology clinic for laparoscopy.

1.45 A 22-year-old woman was admitted as an emergency one week ago. She was found to have a torted ovarian cyst and had a laparoscopic oophorectomy. The rest of her pelvis was normal and she was given that information before discharge. The histology report on the cyst shows a mature cystic teratoma (dermoid cyst).

L. Write to patient

The patient needs to know the result and writing to her is the most efficient use of time and resources. Since this was laparoscopic surgery she doesn't need to be seen back in clinic for review of wound healing; this would only be necessary if she'd had a laparotomy. Since this is a mature dermoid cyst it is benign so there is no need to involve the gynae-oncology MDT.

A.	Appendicitis
B.	Complete mole
C.	Ectopic pregnancy
D.	Hyperemesis gravidarum
E.	Incomplete miscarriage
F.	Missed miscarriage
G.	Partial hydatidiform mole
H.	Threatened miscarriage
I.	Urinary tract infection

The clinical scenarios below describe pregnant women presenting with acute problems. In each case select the most likely diagnosis.

Each option may be used once, more than once or not at all.

1.46 Having had a positive pregnancy test two weeks after her missed period, a 29-year-old primigravid woman is referred to have a scan because of vaginal bleeding. On arrival in the Early Pregnancy Unit the bleeding is noted to be heavy and when you insert a speculum you find that the cervical os is open.

E. Incomplete miscarriage

The cervical os being open gives this diagnosis. It could also be an inevitable or complete miscarriage – a scan would differentiate – but we have not given you these options.

1.47 A 28-year-old woman has a transvaginal ultrasound scan on the Early Pregnancy Unit at eight weeks gestation because of vaginal bleeding. The uterus is larger than expected with a closed os. The scan shows an abnormal looking intrauterine sac with a fetal pole but no heart pulsation detected. Her serum βhCG is 150 000 IU/ml.

G. Partial hydatidiform mole

The very high hCG levels suggest this diagnosis. Partial moles often present as miscarriage (unlike complete moles which have a typical snowstorm appearance on scan).

1.48 A 28-year-old woman attends her GP's surgery asking for a pregnancy test after 14 weeks of amenorrhoea. She feels unwell and has been vomiting throughout the day. On examination she is tachycardic, sweaty and has a tremor. Her uterus is easily palpable and the fundus is just below the umbilicus.

B. Complete mole

The combination of a uterus which is large for dates and symptoms of thyrotoxicosis suggest this diagnosis (hCG has an alpha subunit in common with TSH). The diagnosis could also be hyperemesis with the pregnancy being more advanced than expected from the dates (which would account for the uterus reaching the umbilicus) but hyperemesis usually occurs in the first trimester.

1.49 Having reached 11 weeks gestation, a 22-year-old woman is relieved when her morning sickness disappears. A week later she is devastated when her booking scan shows an irregular sac which is ten weeks' size. A fetal pole is present but cardiac activity is absent.

F. Missed miscarriage

The diagnosis is missed miscarriage because she has had no bleeding. The woman is unaware that her pregnancy has failed and the diagnosis is often made in the scan department.

1.50 A GP asks you to admit a pregnant 19-year-old at 14 weeks gestation because she has been vomiting for the last week. She has no diarrhoea but is clinically very dehydrated. Urine dip is positive for ketones, nitrites and protein.

I. Urinary tract infection

The diagnosis could be hyperemesis gravidarum but the nitrites and protein as well as ketones in the urine suggest UTI instead. It is also a bit unusual to start experiencing hyperemesis in the second trimester.

Curriculum module 2: Answers

MULTIPLE CHOICE QUESTIONS

2.1 Potential complications of delivery by elective caesarean section include:

A. Placenta accreta in the next pregnancy   T

The chance of having this serious complication of pregnancy where the placenta is invading the myometrium is higher the more caesareans you have and it might even result in caesarean hysterectomy. It is one of the main reasons we want to reduce the caesarean section rate in the UK.

B. Urinary tract infection   T

This is usually due to having been catheterised for the section.

C. Arterial thromboembolism   F

Venous thromboembolism is well recognized but patients with arterial thrombosis are rare and usually have some underlying clotting disorder – it is nothing to do with the mode of delivery.

D. Subsequent subfertility   T

This is a recognized association, which is sometimes due to postoperative adhesions causing tubal damage and sometimes is unexplained.

E. Prolonged ileus   T

This is an uncommon complication and if it is prolonged should prompt a review of the electrolyte situation; also consider the possibility of intra-abdominal sepsis or urine leakage from a fistula.

2.2 An 'alert' notice should be added to the operating list to warn theatre staff in advance of patients with the following issues as they may need to change the order of the list or arrange special equipment:

A. Latex allergy   T

There should be no latex in the atmosphere when these patients are in theatre so you need to allow time (20 minutes) for air change before they come in – in practice we normally put them on first so as not to hold up the list.

B. HIV infection   T

Staff will dispose of the linen in different bags and the instruments will need special treatment in addition to the staff wearing more protective clothing, e.g. double gloves.

C. Previous abdominal surgery in a patient undergoing laparoscopy   F

This may be an issue for the surgeon (more likely to find bowel adherent to the anterior abdominal wall) but we don't usually need to warn the theatre staff as the possibility of having to get out extra equipment to open up the abdomen is extremely remote.

D. BMI over 50   T

They may need to arrange extra staff or lifting equipment to actually transfer the patient to the operating table, which must also be able to withstand the extra weight.

E. A Jehovah's Witness 'advance directive' refusing transfusion   T

If haemorrhage is likely during the operation, the patient will have told you what they would accept, e.g. autotransfusion so the 'cell saver' might be needed.

2.3 **The following operations are likely to result in primary haemorrhage needing transfusion, so cross-matched blood should be available rather than just 'group and save' being requested:**

A. Hysterectomy for dysfunctional uterine bleeding   F

It is unusual to get severe intraoperative bleeding and 'group and save' will suffice.

B. Posterior vaginal repair   F

Not usually a very bloody operation

C. Salpingectomy for ruptured ectopic pregnancy   T

If the ectopic has ruptured the abdomen is usually full of blood and women still die from this – see the maternal mortality reports. Cross-match recommended.

D. Adhesiolysis   F

Patients do not usually bleed very much during these operations.

E. Laparotomy for ovarian cancer   T

Cancer operations – whether for ovarian or uterine cancer – have a higher risk of significant intraoperative blood loss and cross-match is recommended.

2.4 **Perioperative antibiotic prophylaxis is advisable for patients undergoing:**

A. Caesarean section   T

B. Vaginal hysterectomy   T

C. Laparoscopic removal of ectopic pregnancy   F

D. Anterior vaginal repair   T

E. Oophorectomy for ovarian cyst   F

Any surgery that involves opening up the vagina or operating on the vagina leads to an increased risk of infection, so that prophylactic antibiotics are indicated.

2.5 **The following are possible causes of pyrexia on the third day following an open (laparotomy) operation to remove an adherent endometrioma of the ovary:**

A. Chest infection   T

B. Deep vein thrombosis   T

C. Ureteric injury   T

D. Urinary tract infection   T

E. Small bowel obstruction   F

All of these are complications of this sort of surgery but they do not all cause pyrexia. Ureteric injury usually involves infection of the kidney above the obstructed ureter so that the patient has a swinging pyrexia associated with loin pain. Ureteric injury is especially likely with ovarian cyst operations because the ureter runs below the ovary on the pelvic side wall and this is one of the sites that it is most vulnerable.

2.6 **The risk of ureteric injury at hysterectomy is higher if:**

A. There is heavy bleeding during the operation   T

B.	The patient has a duplex kidney	T
C.	The ovaries are being conserved	F
D.	The patient's obstetric history involves caesarean deliveries	T
E.	The operation is being done for endometriosis	T

The chance of injuring a ureter is increased if there is abnormal anatomy (the duplex kidney may have two ureters) or adhesions due to endometriosis or previous surgery (after caesarean the bladder can be stuck to the uterus) or heavy bleeding obscuring the view. If the ovaries are not being dissected off the pelvic side wall and removed, the risk of ureteric injury is less.

2.7 The following situations might render laparoscopic sterilization more difficult:

A.	A woman with a BMI less than 20	T
B.	A woman with a BMI over 40	T
C.	Previous diagnostic laparoscopy	F
D.	Previous caesarean section	T
E.	A woman with a history of endometriosis	T

Laparoscopy can be exceedingly hazardous in women who are thin because the chances of hitting a major blood vessel are increased. In a morbidly obese patient, laparoscopy can be more difficult despite the use of longer instruments to access the abdominal cavity. Endometriosis can cause adhesions in the pelvis obscuring the fallopian tubes. The same applies to previous surgery but a laparoscopy alone should not cause adhesions.

2.8 When looking after elderly women on a postoperative gynaecology ward, wound dehiscence is an important complication to look out for. Following a hysterectomy, postoperative dehiscence of an abdominal wound is more likely to occur if:

A.	The patient is being treated for cancer	T
B.	The wound becomes infected	T
C.	The patient develops a postoperative ileus	T
D.	The wound is transverse rather than vertical	F
E.	The patient develops a vault haematoma	F

Elderly, unfit patients with poor nutritional status, especially those with cancer, are at risk of wound breakdown. Poor healing can be expected if the wound gets infected or if the abdomen is distended because of ileus.

The Pfannenstiel incision we use for most gynaecological surgery is very robust and rarely comes apart, so we sew the rectus sheath up with dissolvable suture material, whereas we have to use more long-lasting stitches for vertical wounds as the rectus sheath in the midline has a relatively poor blood supply and healing takes longer than a transverse incision.

2.9 A clinically appropriate reason for advising a woman to have her ovaries removed at the time of hysterectomy is:

| A. | So she can have postoperative estrogen replacement therapy | F |

Although she might need postoperative HRT, depending on her age when she has the operation, this is not a valid reason for removing the ovaries.

| B. | The hysterectomy is treatment for carcinoma of the endometrium | T |

If the hysterectomy is for cancer, the ovaries are removed for histology in order to stage the cancer accurately.

C. Oophorectomy eliminates premenstrual syndrome T

Patients who are having a bad time with PMS might want to obliterate their ovarian cycles by having them removed. We don't often do hysterectomy and bilateral salpingo-oophorectomy for PMS unless the condition is extremely severe and resistant to any other form of treatment.

D. She has a strong family history of ovarian cancer T

Some families do carry a gene for ovarian and other gynaecological cancers, so if there is a family history, we would normally discuss removing the ovaries at the time of hysterectomy. Ovarian cancer presents at a late stage because the symptoms are so nebulous and this gives an opportunity to prevent it.

E. To prevent metabolic effects of polycystic ovarian syndrome, e.g. diabetes F

Although this sounds like a nice idea theoretically, there is no evidence that oophorectomy makes any difference to the chances of her developing diabetes or any of the other long- term effects of PCOS.

2.10 Surgery can be carried out without written consent if:

A. Permission is obtained via a court order T
B. The patient is unconscious and it is in her best interests T
C. The patient is a child who is Fraser-competent F
D. The woman's husband agrees to it F
E. The operation is a dire emergency, e.g. caesarean for fetal bradycardia T

Written consent is the norm. If it is not possible to obtain written consent because of the extreme nature of the emergency, e.g. cord prolapse, then verbal consent is acceptable. We have to record the reasons for proceeding without written consent in the notes. Where a woman's capacity to consent is in doubt legal advice is obtained if time allows in accordance with the Mental Capacity Act 2005. Relatives cannot consent on behalf of an adult patient who lacks capacity, although it is good practice to involve the next of kin in any discussions. If a child is thought to be Fraser competent, you must use a written consent form.

SINGLE BEST ANSWER QUESTIONS

2.11 You are about to sign a consent form with a patient who is having a caesarean section. After you have listed the complications for her, she asks you which is the most common:

A. Wound dehiscence
B. Subsequent subfertility
C. Pseudo-obstruction of the bowel
D. Excess blood loss during surgery
E. Fetal laceration

All of these complications of caesarean section occur relatively rarely except the excess blood loss, which is almost inevitable. We teach our Specialist Registrars (SpRs) how to minimize blood loss at caesarean but patients usually lose far more than those who have a vaginal delivery.

2.12 In the antenatal clinic you see a primigravid woman who has been referred by her community midwife at 37 weeks because the fetus is lying transversely. You organize an ultrasound scan which shows that the reason for the abnormal lie is an 8 cm diameter ovarian cyst filling her pelvis. Your consultant tells you to arrange a caesarean section and the woman asks you

about the management of the cyst. Select the most appropriate advice in this clinical situation:

A. It will be dealt with later as ovaries are not accessible during a caesarean
B. Spontaneous resolution of the cyst is likely after delivery
C. Removing the cyst at the time of caesarean will require a general anaesthetic
D. Caesarean and removal of the cyst should take place now in case the cyst torts
E. Ovarian cystectomy during a caesarean at 39 weeks is appropriate

You will have seen the surgeon checking the ovaries routinely at the end of a caesarean operation before closing the abdomen, so the ovaries are obviously accessible. Spontaneous resolution is unlikely as this cyst cannot be an ovulatory cyst; otherwise it would have disappeared months ago while she has been pregnant. It does need to come out at the time of the caesarean, which is possible after the baby is delivered and the uterine incision closed. It can be done under spinal anaesthetic as it shouldn't increase the operating time by very much so it is unlikely that the spinal will wear off before the cystectomy has been done. In terms of the timing of the caesarean, the knowledge that is being tested here is that if the baby is delivered at 37 weeks there is a risk of transient tachypnoea of the newborn and the paediatricians prefer us to delay elective deliveries until 39 weeks gestation.

2.13 You have seen a woman in preoperative assessment clinic who is due to undergo hysterectomy for prolapse in a few weeks time. Which one of these is the most important factor to warn the anaesthetist about from her case notes?

A. She lives alone and has no postoperative social arrangements for care
B. Her mother had a DVT during chemotherapy many years ago
C. She has hypertension, which is adequately treated with bendrofluazide
D. She is allergic to penicillin
E. There is a family history of suxamethonium apnoea

The anaesthetist will want her to have a test to see if she has suxamethonium apnoea too. Although all the other factors are relevant to her hospital admission they are not as important to the anaesthetic team.

2.14 You are filling out a thromboprophylaxis risk form in the preoperative assessment clinic, for a woman about to undergo a pelvic floor repair. Which of the following does not contribute to her risk score for venous thromboembolism?

A. The woman has a BMI of 44
B. The woman has inflammatory bowel disease
C. The woman has essential hypertension
D. The woman has protein S deficiency
E. The woman has a history of recent breast cancer

If you have ever filled out a thromboprophylaxis risk form in a preoperative clinic you will recognize most of these risk factors.

2.15 A 45-year-old woman has been put on the waiting list for endometrial ablation to treat her menorrhagia. She visits the surgery to ask for further information as she wasn't given adequate time to discuss the procedure in the gynaecology clinic. Which one of the following statements about endometrial ablation is correct?

A. Endometrial ablation is always done under general anaesthetic

B. Endometrial sampling is not required prior to the procedure

C. It cannot be undertaken in the presence of a caesarean scar

D. She should continue using contraception afterwards

E. The operation has a 90% chance of producing amenorrhoea

This operation is not contraceptive and there have been reported pregnancies following the procedure. The scarring in the uterine cavity means that they often miscarry but there have been some reports of pregnancies going to term. We do worry a bit about caesarean scars and may arrange a scan to look at the thickness of the myometrium in the lower part of the uterus, but it is not a contraindication. Some of the newer methods of ablation can be done under local anaesthetic.

2.16 A woman attends A&E due to heavy vaginal bleeding a week after having a large loop excision of the transformation zone (LLETZ procedure) for CIN 3. Her pulse and blood pressure are normal and her haemoglobin is 120 g/l. On speculum examination there is active bleeding from the cervix. What is the most appropriate initial management in this case?

A. Arrange the operating theatre immediately for suturing of the cervix

B. Pack the vagina and give broad-spectrum antibiotics

C. Prescribe oral norethisterone and allow home

D. Prescribe tranexamic acid and allow home

E. Take a swab and commence broad-spectrum oral antibiotics

As she is actively bleeding you have to do something about this situation and cannot just send her home. Secondary bleeding like this is usually due to infection so she needs some antibiotics. Packing the vagina is usually enough to stop the bleeding but she may need to go to theatre if that does not work.

2.17 You would have concerns about the legitimacy of one of these patients signing their consent form for surgery. Which patient?

A. A girl aged 15 years requesting termination of pregnancy

B. An elderly woman who has had a stroke

C. A woman requesting sterilization whose husband did not agree

D. A Jehovah's Witness who needs a caesarean for placenta praevia

E. A non-English speaking woman whose husband is translating for her

A teenager who seems competent to understand what she is agreeing to (so-called Gillick or Fraser-competent) is not a worry. Just because a patient has had a stroke, you cannot assume they lack competency. You need to carry out an assessment in accordance with the Mental Capacity Act 2005. The only problem here is the woman whose husband is the only way of communicating with her – he may have a vested interest and may not convey to her exactly what you tell him. In these circumstances, an independent interpreter is recommended.

2.18 An 86-year-old woman presents to the gynaecology outpatient clinic with postmenopausal bleeding. Having examined her, the consultant decides that hysteroscopy and cervical biopsy are necessary but she is currently taking warfarin on account of an artificial heart valve. Select the most appropriate option regarding her anticoagulation:

A. Continue with current dose of warfarin

B. Change to heparin and omit dose on morning of surgery

C. Omit warfarin for three days before surgery and check INR

D. Omit anticoagulation on morning of surgery

E.   Postpone surgery until anticoagulant therapy completed

This woman's anticoagulation therapy will not 'complete' because she will be on it for life, so option E is irrelevant. It is not advisable to continue with surgery while she is fully anticoagulated as she is likely to bleed excessively so a method of stopping it temporarily must be found. The best option is to switch to heparin, which can be stopped and restarted more easily, with the possibility of staying on heparin until the histology report is available and you know whether she is going to need major surgery such as a hysterectomy for cancer in the near future.

2.19 You are asked to review a woman on the Day Case Unit who had a laparoscopic sterilization yesterday. She has had four children between the ages of six months and four years, all delivered by caesarean section via a Pfannenstiel incision. The nurses are concerned because she has abdominal pain and she is still not well enough to go home, although your consultant saw her last night after the operating list had finished and discharged her. When you examine her you notice some watery discharge from her suprapubic incision, which is soaking through the dressing. Which one of the following statements applies to this case?

A.   Bowel damage is unlikely because her previous incision was suprapubic
B.   She is probably evading being discharged because the children exhaust her
C.   She should be sent home because your consultant discharged her
D.   There could be a hole in her bladder
E.   Unrecognized laparoscopic bowel injury produces peritonitis very quickly

Laparoscopy carries a risk of serious complications of about 2 in 1000 and it is important for GPs to be able to recognize them. If you have assisted in theatre, you will know that a Pfannenstiel incision involves opening up the peritoneum as far as the umbilicus, so it is possible to have bowel stuck to the back of the scar all the way up the anterior abdominal wall, even if the skin incision is suprapubic. As a caesarean incision heals, it is not unusual for the bladder to become adherent – to the front of the uterus and to the back of the abdominal incision – so it is possible that the second port for the sterilization has gone through the bladder. It could be urine leaking out of the wound. We know that bowel damage at laparoscopy is not always recognized at the time of injury and that the presentation is often delayed so that the patient has returned home by the time they develop symptoms of peritonitis.

Source: RCOG Green-top guideline number 49. *Preventing Entry-related Gynaecological Laparoscopic Injuries.*

2.20 An asthmatic woman is breathless on return to the Day Case Unit from the operating theatre recovery room and you are asked for advice. She has had an uncomplicated evacuation of uterus performed, but the hospital notes mention that she did have a coughing fit as she was being anaesthetized. Select the most appropriate immediate course of action in this situation:

A.   Send her for an urgent chest x-ray
B.   Organize a peak flow estimation
C.   Prescribe nebulized salbutamol
D.   Ask the anaesthetist to review her at the end of the list
E.   Check her airway and give her oxygen by face mask

All of these actions are appropriate but the first thing to do is ABC – check her airway and give oxygen. You are not sure at this stage whether she is having an exacerbation of her asthma, has a pneumothorax or has aspirated.

EXTENDED MATCHING QUESTIONS

A.	CA125 level
B.	Chest x-ray
C.	Clotting screen
D.	CT scan of abdomen and pelvis
E.	Electrocardiogram
F.	Endocervical chlamydia swab
G.	Ferritin
H.	Haemoglobin
I.	High vaginal swab
J.	Plain abdominal x-ray
K.	Pregnancy test
L.	Thrombophilia screen
M.	Ultrasound guided biopsy
N.	Ultrasound scan of the pelvis

The clinical scenarios below describe women who are on the waiting list for various gynaecological operations. Select the single most appropriate preoperative investigation for each case.

Each option may be used once, more than once or not at all.

2.21 A 31-year-old woman requesting fertility investigations is to be admitted to the Day Case Unit on day 8 of her next menstrual cycle for a laparoscopy and dye test to check tubal patency because she has a past history of pelvic inflammatory disease.

F. Endocervical chlamydia swab

Although most patients undergoing minor gynaecological procedures will have a haemoglobin estimation this is not really necessary unless they have heavy periods. For this patient it is more important to check that she does not have an undiagnosed chlamydia infection as dye laparoscopy may result in a further episode of acute pelvic inflammatory disease. Another distractor here is the pregnancy test but she is day 8 of the cycle so this is not really relevant.

2.22 To investigate her severe longstanding menorrhagia a 49-year-old woman is going to undergo hysteroscopy and endometrial biopsy and she has chosen to have it done under general anaesthetic.

H. Haemoglobin

This woman is likely to have iron deficiency anaemia and hopefully the GP will have already done the haemoglobin before referring her for a gynaecological opinion. The

*distractors are ferritin level (which you would do if she was anaemic) and
ultrasound scan of the pelvis.*

2.23 A woman aged 42 years has an ultrasound scan revealing a left ovarian cyst
measuring 9 cm with solid elements in it. The right ovary seems normal on the
scan and there is no ascites. Your consultant is trying to decide whether to
remove the uterus and other ovary as well as the diseased ovary.

A. CA125 level

*The main issue here is whether the cyst is likely to be malignant or not. If there is
any suspicion of malignancy the correct operation is total hysterectomy, bilateral
salpingo-oophorectomy and omentectomy for staging of the disease. A CT scan
might give some idea of omental or other abdominal spread of tumour but the
CA125 blood level is the most useful piece of information when deciding on the
extent of surgery to be performed. A normal chest x-ray would exclude stage 4
disease if there are no pleural effusions, but is not as useful as the CA125.*

2.24 A 32-year-old multiparous woman is admitted as a day case for laparoscopic
sterilization. She has been using a copper coil for contraception but you
cannot see the strings and she thinks it was extruded from the uterus during
an unusually heavy period four weeks ago.

K. Pregnancy test

*You might want to do a haemoglobin level in view of the recent heavy period but the
main worry here is that she has not had contraceptive protection for the last few
weeks, giving her a chance to conceive prior to being sterilized. Although she has not
actually missed her period yet, pregnancy tests are now sensitive enough to pick up
measurable levels of hCG by a week after implantation. If you are worried about
where the coil is you might want an ultrasound scan of the pelvis or even a plain
x-ray to locate it but the pregnancy test comes first.*

2.25 A 40-year-old woman is going to have a hysterectomy for endometriosis. The
preoperative ultrasound scan reveals bilateral chocolate cysts on the ovaries.
She has not had any surgery before but her mother had a DVT following
hysterectomy at the same age.

L. Thrombophilia screen

*If this woman has inherited a thrombophilia she may need anticoagulation to cover
the hysterectomy.*

A.	Chest x-ray
B.	CT scan of abdomen and pelvis
C.	Electrocardiogram
D.	Haemoglobin
E.	High vaginal swab
F.	Intravenous pyelogram (IVP) x-ray
G.	Plain abdominal x-ray
H.	Serum calcium
I.	Ultrasound scan of kidneys

J.	Urea and electrolytes
K.	Urine culture

These clinical scenarios describe women developing complications after gynae-cological operations. Select the most appropriate investigation for each case.

Each option may be used once, more than once or not at all.

2.26 Three days after a hysterectomy for endometrial cancer, a 60-year-old woman still has a distended abdomen with no bowel sounds. Which investigation will help you most with planning her management?

J. Urea and electrolytes

As she has no bowel sounds, the diagnosis is paralytic ileus. You do not really need an abdominal x-ray to diagnose this – just use your stethoscope – but it can be associated with a low potassium level therefore the U&E is more use than an x-ray in the management of this patient because it will help you decide which intravenous fluids to prescribe.

2.27 An obese 58-year-old woman who normally smokes 20 cigarettes a day develops severe left-sided chest pain two days after a prolapse operation. She is tachycardic and tachypnoeic. On examination you find an inspiratory wheeze but normal air entry all over the chest. Which investigation would you carry out initially?

C. Electrocardiogram

You would not want to send her down to the x-ray department for a chest x-ray until you have excluded acute myocardial infarction with an ECG.

2.28 Having undergone hysteroscopy and insertion of a levonorgestrel intrauterine system (Mirena®) for menorrhagia under general anaesthetic, a 42-year-old woman was not well enough to be discharged home and has stayed in hospital overnight because of severe lower abdominal pain. The next morning she is still in pain and has a temperature of 38 °C. You cannot locate the coil strings on speculum examination.

G. Plain abdominal x-ray

The suspicion is that the IUS has perforated the fundus of the uterus. You should be able to locate it on an abdominal film (although an ultrasound of the uterus would also be useful but we haven't given you this option).

2.29 On the fourth day following a difficult hysterectomy and bilateral salpingo-oophorectomy operation for endometriosis a 38-year-old woman has a swinging pyrexia and unilateral loin pain. She is still nauseous and seems to have a persistent ileus.

I. Ultrasound scan of kidneys

Although this clinical scenario sounds like pyelonephritis and therefore MSU would be indicated, there is possibly a much more sinister cause of her symptoms, which must not be overlooked. UTI does not usually cause ileus. The persistent ileus could be due to urine in the peritoneal cavity as a result of ureteric damage during surgery and the consequences of missing that diagnosis are potentially much more serious, with loss of renal function on the affected side. A normal ultrasound of the kidneys excludes ureteric damage and is a better investigation than IVP as it does not involve radiation.

2.30 Six days after leaving hospital following a vaginal hysterectomy operation, an anaemic woman is readmitted with further vaginal discharge and pain. She was sent home on iron tablets and analgesics. On readmission she is pyrexial and bimanual pelvic examination reveals a palpable tender mass at the vault with offensive brown blood in the vagina.

E. High vaginal swab

Although a haemoglobin level would be routine here, you already know that she is anaemic and is being treated for it. The diagnosis is vault haematoma, which is likely to be infected. You will be prescribing antibiotics for this patient anyway but the point of a high vaginal swab is to check that the treatment is correct, depending on the sensitivities. If you can feel a palpable haematoma, imaging is superfluous to the diagnosis.

A.	A guardian with Power of Attorney should sign the consent form
B.	Consent from the patient is valid
C.	Defer the operation until a court order can be obtained
D.	Defer the operation until an independent interpreter is available
E.	Defer the operation until the woman is fully recovered
F.	The consent already given is not valid
G.	The clinician could go ahead with surgery in the patient's best interests
H.	The woman has a right to refuse consent
I.	The woman should not be asked to participate in the research
J.	Verbal consent from the patient is adequate
K.	Written consent could be obtained from the patient's husband

These clinical scenarios describe women in different situations where consent may be an issue. Select the most appropriate advice for each case.

Each option may be used once, more than once or not at all.

2.31 A 51-year-old woman with severe learning difficulties is brought into A&E as an emergency with prolonged heavy bleeding. On admission her haemoglobin is 93 g/l. She needs a hysteroscopy to investigate the problem but cannot understand what is being proposed.

A. A guardian with Power of Attorney should sign the consent form

It is clearly in the best interests of this patient for her to have the investigation done especially as the bleeding has made her anaemic. The best option is for her family to be involved in the decision. In the absence of family it is likely that she will have a legal guardian who could sign the consent form for her. In fact the 'consent form' is form 4 which is a statement of why the procedure is in her best interests and ideally the legal guardian would sign in agreement to the procedure.

2.32 On the labour ward a primigravid woman has reluctantly had a fetal blood sample done at 4 cm dilatation and the result shows that the baby is hypoxic. She has a needle phobia and adamantly refuses caesarean section to deliver the baby quickly. Both the obstetric consultant and the paediatrician have explained the possible consequences to her.

H. The woman has a right to refuse consent

Although the consequences of this woman's decision could have profound effects on her baby's health, the baby has no rights in law until it is born. It is her right to refuse consent and the responsibility of the health professionals involved is to ensure that her decision is really fully informed. You might need to take into account the effects of any drugs she might have had for pain relief in labour and take care to document fully everything that is explained to her. Her husband cannot give consent on her behalf.

2.33 A Jehovah's Witness has a hysterectomy operation for endometrial cancer. She specifically states that she will not accept blood transfusion and signs a disclaimer form preoperatively. In the recovery room it becomes apparent that she has internal bleeding and the consultant decides to take her back to theatre. She has had a lot of opiates to control her pain and is very drowsy.

G. The clinician should go ahead with surgery in the patient's best interests

The blood transfusion issue is not relevant to consent in this situation but the longer the return to theatre is delayed, the more likely she is to die. The surgeon can take her back to theatre urgently to stop the bleeding without further consent especially as she will not accept blood transfusion. Her husband cannot give consent on her behalf.

2.34 On the labour ward a new research project is underway comparing two different drugs to treat postpartum haemorrhage. You are called in to put a drip up for a woman who has lost 400 ml of blood already and the blood loss seems to be ongoing. Although it has not been discussed previously with the patient, the midwife mentions the possibility of the patient being asked to participate in the research project.

I. The woman should not be asked to participate in the research

It is not appropriate to take consent for participation in a research project in an emergency situation. There is no time available for the woman to consider the options and either participate or withdraw consent if she wants to and these things are best discussed earlier in pregnancy.

2.35 A 15-year-old schoolgirl presents to clinic requesting surgical termination of pregnancy accompanied by her 15-year-old boyfriend. She will not tell her parents about the pregnancy and after much discussion she is thought to be able to understand the risks of the procedure.

B. Consent from the patient is valid

If the teenager is deemed to be competent to understand the implications of her decision (so-called 'Fraser competence'), then she can give consent for the procedure. It is always best if she does tell her parents (especially if she develops a complication) and we would always encourage her to think about doing that.

A.	Cancel the operation as it is not the correct procedure for this patient
B.	Go ahead with the operation as planned
C.	Postpone the operation and arrange counselling
D.	Postpone the operation and arrange review in genitourinary medicine clinic
E.	Postpone the operation and arrange routine gynaecology clinic review
F.	Postpone the operation and arrange urgent gynaecology clinic review
G.	Postpone the operation and organize an ultrasound scan
H.	Postpone the operation until you can arrange further tests
I.	Refer her urgently to her GP for a prescription
J.	Suggest that the patient has a spinal anaesthetic

The patients that you are seeing in the preoperative clinic are about to undergo gynaecological operations and unfortunately your consultant is not immediately available for advice. Select the most appropriate management plan for each clinical scenario.

Each option may be used once, more than once or not at all.

2.36 The waiting list clerk has arranged for a 49-year-old woman to fill a cancelled slot on the operating list at short notice. She is due to have an abdominal hysterectomy in three days' time and you are doing her preoperative check. She had a hysteroscopy done under local anaesthetic for irregular heavy bleeding recently but the histology on the endometrium from that operation is not yet available.

F. Postpone the operation and arrange urgent gynaecology clinic review

The original symptoms may be caused by endometrial cancer, so irregular perimenopausal bleeding should be dealt with urgently (in the same way as postmenopausal bleeding). You need to check the histology before she has her uterus removed as hysterectomy for endometrial cancer is a different operation from that for benign disease (for example the surgeon would take peritoneal washings and remove the ovaries as well).

2.37 A 37-year-old woman presented to clinic with left iliac fossa pain radiating down her left leg several weeks ago and ultrasound scan revealed a 7 cm simple left ovarian cyst. She was put on the waiting list for an ovarian cystectomy but her symptoms have now disappeared.

G. Postpone the operation and organize an ultrasound scan

It is possible that this was an ovulatory cyst, which may now have resolved. An ultrasound will resolve the issue.

2.38 A healthy 62-year-old woman is due to be admitted for a prolapse repair. She mentions a family history of 'difficulty waking up' after anaesthetics but is not sure of the clinical details.

H. Postpone the operation until you can arrange further tests

This patient may have inherited cholinesterase deficiency and be at risk of suxamethonium apnoea and it is possible to test for this. Even though she wants a spinal anaesthetic, this may not give enough analgesia on the day of surgery and the anaesthetist will want to know that it is safe to give her a general anaesthetic.

2.39 A 33-year-old woman is to be admitted for endometrial ablation to treat her menorrhagia. She has turned down the option of a Mirena® intrauterine system because she wishes to have another baby within the next couple of years.

A. Cancel the operation as it is not the correct procedure for this patient

This patient is obviously unaware that endometrial ablation is not a suitable operation if pregnancy is desired in the future. The operation is designed to remove the endometrial layers right down to the basal layer that regenerates each cycle. Pregnancy has been reported after this operation but it is not usually successful and we often recommend that patients considering this are sterilized concurrently.

2.40 When she was seen in the fertility clinic a couple of weeks ago, a 29-year-old woman had a speculum examination during which some routine swabs were taken. You look up the results before signing her consent form for a laparoscopy and dye test only to discover that the chlamydia swab is positive.

D. Postpone the operation and arrange review in the genitourinary medicine clinic

It is inadvisable to proceed with her surgery until the chlamydia infection has been adequately treated and contact tracing has been done – which is the main reason for involving the genitourinary medicine clinic. They are very good at taking a sexual history and following up contacts.

A.	Acute primary haemorrhage
B.	Chest infection
C.	Deep vein thrombosis
D.	Haemolysis
E.	Intestinal obstruction
F.	Pelvic haematoma
G.	Pulmonary embolus
H.	Secondary haemorrhage due to vault infection
I.	Ureteric injury
J.	Urinary tract infection
K.	Urinary retention
L.	Vault granulations
M.	Vault dehiscence

Each of these clinical scenarios describes a woman presenting with complications after a hysterectomy operation; for each patient pick the most likely diagnosis given the information that you are presented with.

Each option may be used once, more than once or not at all.

2.41 You are called to see a morbidly obese 40-year-old woman who had a hysterectomy for endometrial cancer three days ago. She has gradually become more breathless over the previous 24 hours and now seems a little confused. She is hypoxic and expresses discomfort when you ask for deep breaths to auscultate her chest but there is normal air entry. Her temperature is normal and you do not see any abnormality on her chest x-ray.

G. Pulmonary embolus

The hypoxia and chest pain on inspiration suggest either a chest infection, pulmonary embolism or pneumothorax. She has at least three risk factors for thromboembolism. The pain on deep inspiration and the normal chest x-ray are the reason the answer is PE rather than infection.

2.42 Three days after a hysterectomy for endometriosis, a 35-year-old woman is found to have a mild pyrexia and a tachycardia of 100 beats per minute. There is a moderate amount of old blood coming from the vagina and her haemoglobin has dropped from 127 g/l preoperatively to 82 g/l now. The estimated blood loss at operation was described as 250 ml.

F. Pelvic haematoma

Causes of pyrexia following a hysterectomy include wound infection, vault infection, urinary tract infection, chest infection, ureteric obstruction and thromboembolism. The drop in haemoglobin without a matching obvious massive vaginal loss suggests that this woman has a pelvic haematoma which is just starting to discharge down the vagina. The main distractor is secondary haemorrhage but that usually presents seven to ten days after the operation (and is due to infection involving the vaginal vault). Primary haemorrhage refers to blood loss during the operation.

2.43 A 30-year-old woman had a hysterectomy and left salpingo-oophorectomy for chronic pelvic inflammatory disease with hydrosalpinx. The operation notes document dense adhesions on the left side of the pelvis and there was perioperative blood loss of 900 ml. Two days later she is very unwell with swinging pyrexia, a prolonged ileus and severe left loin pain.

I. Ureteric injury

The prolonged ileus is a clue because this can occur as a result of urine leaking into the abdomen and it can't be bowel obstruction because she has no bowel sounds. Obstruction is associated with tinkling bowel sounds, whereas bowel sounds are absent in ileus.

Ureteric damage is more likely in the presence of adhesions especially if there is heavy bleeding obscuring the view of anatomical structures, and the loin pain gives it away.

2.44 A woman who had a hysterectomy ten weeks ago comes to your surgery because she has just started to bleed vaginally again. She has not seen any blood since a week after her hysterectomy but has not been examined following the operation as she did not go to the hospital for her postoperative check-up.

L. Vault granulations

It is so long since this woman's surgery that it cannot possibly be secondary haemorrhage due to vault infection as the vault will have healed up by now. Vault dehiscence is extremely rare and usually presents early as a result of a haematoma discharging down the vagina. The most likely finding on speculum examination will be granulation tissue, which can be treated by the application of silver nitrate.

As more postoperative care is moved out to primary care in the future, many GPs will be involved in doing the follow-up for hysterectomy patients. Excessive granulation tissue in association with watery discharge should alert you to the possibility of a fistula but this would have presented earlier than ten weeks. Vault dehiscence is very rare and presents within the first week or so as the tissue breaks down.

2.45 On her fluid balance chart on the first postoperative day, you notice that a woman has not passed urine since she returned from theatre in spite of having received over 2 litres of fluid intravenously. She has a pelvic drain *in situ* which contains 400 ml. The nurses report that she asked for a bedpan twice during the night.

K. Urinary retention

This woman is most likely to be in retention and the next step is to catheterise her. If there is no urine there, you need to consider whether she is dehydrated, has bled into her abdomen or (rarely) has a bilateral ureteric injury. She may have sustained a primary haemorrhage and be hypovolaemic but the most likely cause is retention. She needs a urinary catheter and a careful fluid balance chart until you have sorted out the problem.

A.	Advise alternative method of contraception four weeks before surgery
B.	Continue using current contraceptive method
C.	Prescribe full therapeutic anticoagulation therapy
D.	Prescribe local vaginal estrogen instead of systemic HRT
E.	Switch HRT to transdermal method before surgery
F.	Stop HRT four weeks before surgery
G.	Stop HRT 12 weeks before surgery
H.	Stopping HRT is not necessary
I.	Stop contraceptive method four weeks before surgery

These clinical scenarios relate to women seeking advice relating to surgery and the risks of thromboembolism. In each case you should decide on the best course of action with regard to hormonal medication and select the most appropriate advice.

Each option may be used once, more than once or not at all.

2.46 A 26-year-old woman is on the waiting list for scoliosis surgery and seeks advice about whether she should continue taking her combined oral contraceptive pill.

A. Advise alternative method of contraception four weeks before surgery

Scoliosis surgery will result in a prolonged period of immobility postoperatively. Combined hormonal contraception should be discontinued and another estrogen-free method used at least four weeks prior to surgery. You would not want to just stop the pill and not use another method as in option 1 because she may start her postoperative convalescence with an early pregnancy.

Source: RCOG Green-top guideline number 40. *Venous Thromboembolism and Hormonal Contraception.*

2.47 A 26-year-old woman is being admitted to hospital for scoliosis surgery in six weeks time and seeks advice about whether she should have her next dose of depot medroxy progesterone acetate, which is now due.

B. Continue using current contraceptive method

Progesterone only pill, injectables, implants and Mirena® do not seem to be associated with an increased risk of venous thromboembolism.

Source: RCOG Green-top guideline number 40. *Venous Thromboembolism and Hormonal Contraception.*

2.48 A 26-year-old woman is on the waiting list for diagnostic laparoscopy to diagnose her pelvic pain. She is currently taking Dianette® for contraception and in the hope that it will improve her acne.

B. Continue using current contraceptive method

Diagnostic laparoscopy is minor surgery not associated with prolonged immobility so she does not need to stop her contraceptive pill.

Source: RCOG Green-top guideline number 40. *Venous Thromboembolism and Hormonal Contraception.*

2.49 A fit 50-year-old woman started on systemic HRT (sequential tablet formulation) six months ago because of severe vasomotor and vaginal dryness symptoms. She has felt much better on it but is now on the waiting list for a posterior vaginal repair for prolapse. Apart from the surgery, you do not identify any risk factors for thromboembolism in her medical notes.

F. Stop HRT four weeks before surgery

Each woman requires an individual assessment of the risks and benefits of stopping HRT before elective surgery. Although concurrent use of HRT must increase the risk of postoperative VTE, the risk is likely to be small and in any case many women having surgery will also have thromboprophylaxis. The operation that this woman is having is relatively short in terms of operative time but may be associated with more immobilization than her normal lifestyle for a couple of weeks postoperatively. She is not likely to be prescribed thromboprophylaxis as she is otherwise low risk, so she should follow the guidance in the British National Formulary and stop her HRT four weeks prior to surgery.

Source: RCOG Green-top guideline number 19. *Venous Thromboembolism and Hormone Replacement Therapy.*

2.50 A 45-year-old woman is taking tibolone (Livial®) hormone replacement therapy having had a complete pelvic clearance for endometriosis six months previously. She is about to undergo carpal tunnel surgery and seeks advice about her tibolone medication.

H. Stopping HRT is not necessary

Carpal tunnel surgery is relatively minor, often done under local anaesthetic and does not usually involve a period of immobilization. There is no need to worry about her HRT.

Source: RCOG Green-top guideline number 19. *Venous Thromboembolism and Hormone Replacement Therapy.*

Curriculum module 3: Answers

MULTIPLE CHOICE QUESTIONS

3.1 Referring a pregnant woman for an antenatal glucose tolerance test is indicated in the following situations:

A. Obesity   T
These patients are definitely at risk of developing gestational diabetes although the cut-off BMI for requesting a GTT sometimes varies between hospitals.

B. Previous pregnancy ending in stillbirth   T
A GTT may have been done as part of the investigation for stillbirth but it is still indicated in the present pregnancy.

C. Polyhydramnios in this pregnancy   T
Gestational diabetes is a cause of polyhydramnios.

D. One episode of glycosuria   F
Not for single occasion but a second episode of glycosuria would trigger a GTT. In pregnancy the renal reabsorption threshold for glucose is lowered so a single episode of glycosuria may be a normal finding.

E. Recurrent urinary tract infections during pregnancy   F
Infections might be related to diabetes but recurrent UTIs are not a recognized symptom.

3.2 The community midwife asks you to see a 23-year-old woman who has presented for antenatal care late in her first pregnancy. She has needle tracks on her arms and on questioning admits to injecting heroin and often smokes cannabis.

With regard to the effect of her drug habit on her pregnancy:

A. Drug users commonly suffer from iron and vitamin deficiency   T
B. Methadone substitution is contraindicated while she is pregnant   F
C. Premature labour is likely   T
D. She is at increased risk of thromboembolism   T
E. Cannabis is linked with low birthweight   T
We do try and get heroin users to use methadone substitution during pregnancy. These are high risk pregnancies and should be looked after in a dedicated antenatal clinic with close links with the local drug services.

3.3 Screening tests for Down syndrome:

A. Carry a risk of miscarriage   F
Read the question carefully – it says screening tests not diagnostic tests.

B. Are mandatory   F

Although these tests are regarded by some as 'routine' they are clearly not and the patient is expected to 'opt in' and is not obliged to avail herself of the offer.

C. Rarely miss an affected pregnancy   F

All the tests available for screening have a significant false negative rate and may miss affected pregnancies.

D. Should only be offered to high-risk mothers   F

Screening tests as opposed to diagnostic tests are intended for the whole pregnant population.

E. The result indicates the chance of the pregnancy being affected   T

All the screening tests describe an odds ratio for the current pregnancy being affected.

3.4 **The following are maternal risk factors for intrauterine growth restriction:**

A. Antiphospholipid syndrome   T

B. Maternal diabetes mellitus   T

Diabetes as a risk factor is especially worrying if she already has vascular complications of her diabetes. Diabetic vasculopathy can lead to placental insufficiency due to poor uterine perfusion. Detecting placental insufficiency is one of the pitfalls of looking after diabetic mothers, whose babies may be macrosomic because of poor diabetic control or growth restricted due to underlying vasculopathy. Careful monitoring with growth scans and CTGs is necessary especially in the third trimester.

C. Cocaine use during pregnancy   T

Pregnant drug users are best managed in a dedicated clinic where facilities are available for monitoring fetal growth as well as monitoring maternal drug use. Apart from tobacco, the main 'recreational' drug implicated is cocaine.

D. Being 'small for gestational age' herself at birth   T

E. Continuing to work until term   F

There is no evidence that working causes IUGR but daily vigorous exercise is regarded as a major risk factor.

Source: RCOG Green-top guideline number 31. *The Investigation and Management of the Small-for-Gestational-Age Fetus.*

3.5 **Symphysis pubis dysfunction (SPD) in pregnancy:**

A. Will give the woman more pain the wider the gap in the symphysis   F

There is no correlation between the anatomical findings and symptoms.

B. Is made worse by maternal obesity   T

C. Caesarean section is of proven benefit to the patient   F

It is clearly better for patients with SPD to have a vaginal birth especially considering reduced mobility after a section, which could influence the incidence of thromboembolic complications.

D. Can happen in the first trimester   T

E. Has been shown to be improved by physiotherapy   T

Source: TOG article 2006. *Symphysis Pubis Dysfunction: A Practical Approach to Management.*

3.6 **Concerning the dental health of pregnant women:**

A. The immune response to plaque bacteria is altered in pregnancy   T

Pregnant women are more prone to dental caries.

B. Pregnant women are entitled to free dental care only until the baby is born F

They are entitled to free dental care and free prescriptions but this is not just during pregnancy – it continues until the baby is one year old.

C. Hyperemesis can result in damage to maternal teeth T

Frequent exposure to gastric acid erodes dental enamel.

D. Periodontitis is a risk factor for low birthweight T

This is the main reason for allowing pregnant women access to free dental care.

E. There is an association between pregnancy and gingival hyperplasia T

Gingival hyperplasia can sometimes be severe in pregnancy and there are pictures in textbooks if you don't know what this looks like.

Source: TOG article 2007. *Dental Manifestations of Pregnancy.*

3.7 In a pregnancy affected by obstetric cholestasis:

A. The condition is characterized by intense pruritus without a skin rash T

B. The serum bilirubin is usually markedly raised F

C. The itching particularly affects the palms and soles of the feet T

D. Postnatal resolution of symptoms and biochemical abnormalities is required to confirm the diagnosis T

E. Ursodeoxycholic acid therapy has been shown to reduce the incidence of stillbirth F

Ursodeoxycholic acid is used to treat itching and helps the woman's symptoms but it has not been shown to make any difference to the fetal outcome.

Source: RCOG Green-top guideline number 43. *Obstetric Cholestasis.*

3.8 If you are looking after a pregnant woman with a personal history of venous thromboembolism:

A. She should be referred to a consultant clinic early for risk assessment T

The advice is for the risk of thromboembolism to be assessed as early as possible in pregnancy and a thrombophilia screen performed (although pregnancy can affect the result of the screen).

B. Low molecular weight heparin is contraindicated if she wishes to breastfeed F

C. If the previous DVT was associated with a causative factor she may not need anticoagulation during pregnancy T

If the patient does not have a thrombophilia it is possible to defer anticoagulation until postpartum, although a careful risk assessment is necessary.

D. Anticoagulation with warfarin is preferable to heparin in pregnancy F

Warfarin is teratogenic and best avoided especially in the first trimester. It is also less easy to reverse if premature labour and delivery occurs.

E. She is likely to be offered induction of labour if she is on heparin T

As there is a risk of haemorrhage at delivery the usual management is to offer induction of labour at term, omitting the dose of heparin until after delivery.

Source: RCOG Green-top guideline number 37a. *Reducing the Risk of Thrombosis and Embolism during Pregnancy and the Puerperium.*

3.9 Concerning the management of a woman with epilepsy in pregnancy:

A. Antiepileptic drugs are associated with an increased risk of congenital abnormalities T

Antiepileptic drugs are associated with an increased risk of congenital abnormalities and neurodevelopmental delay but the outlook is worse if the woman stops taking them and has frequent fits as a consequence.

B. Monotherapy with one drug is the preferred option in pregnancy   T
Polytherapy carries the highest risk.

C. Epileptic women intending pregnancy should be advised to take 0.5 mg folic acid daily   F
Women and girls with epilepsy should be encouraged to take 5 mg folic acid daily in case pregnancy ensues.

D. Sodium valproate is associated with the least risk of abnormality   F
Sodium valproate is particularly worrying in terms of the risk of congenital abnormality.

E. Pregnant women are more at risk of seizure-related death than non-pregnant women   T
Source: TOG article 2006. *The Management of Women with Epilepsy.*
   Saving Mothers Lives: Reviewing Maternal Deaths to Make Motherhood Safer: 2006–2008. The Eighth Report of the Confidential Enquiries into Maternal Deaths in the United Kingdom. Published 2011 and accessible via the RCOG website.

3.10 Screening for the following infections is routinely offered during antenatal care of pregnant women in the UK

A. Parvovirus B19   F
This virus causes 'slapped cheek syndrome', which is common amongst young children but doesn't make them ill. In pregnancy it causes transplacental infection and fetal anaemia.

B. Hepatitis B   T
This is one of the routine screening tests and, if positive, the newborn is vaccinated after delivery. As a GP you might consider testing the rest of the family as well.

C. Gonorrhoea   F

D. Human immunodeficiency virus   T
We introduced HIV screening in pregnancy a few years ago when it was demonstrated that you could reduce the vertical transmission rate to 2% by taking special measures with the mother.

E. Syphilis   T
Although it is rare these days, we still screen for syphilis because the consequences of congenital syphilis are so devastating.

SINGLE BEST ANSWER QUESTIONS

3.11 Intrahepatic cholestasis of pregnancy is an uncommon but serious complication. Which of the following statements about this condition is not correct?

A. The baby is at risk of intrauterine death

B. Antenatal administration of vitamin K to the mother reduces the risk of postpartum haemorrhage

C. Meconium in the liquor during labour can be ignored as it is to be expected

D. The condition can run in families

E. The recurrence risk in a subsequent pregnancy is over 50%

Although meconium liquor can occur in pregnancies affected by cholestasis it should not be ignored because it is sometimes an indication of fetal hypoxia.

The recurrence risk is quoted as between 45 and 90% in the next pregnancy.
Source: RCOG Green-top guideline number 43. *Obstetric Cholestasis.*

3.12 Which of the following statements concerning HIV in pregnancy is true:

A. In HIV positive mothers on antiretroviral treatment breastfeeding is safe
B. Interventions can reduce the risk of vertical HIV transmission from 30% to zero
C. All infants born to women who are HIV positive should be treated with antiretroviral therapy from birth
D. Women who do not require treatment for their own health do not need to take antiretroviral therapy during pregnancy
E. The use of short-term steroids to promote fetal lung maturation is inadvisable

In order to reduce the chance of passing on HIV to the baby, the mother should take antiretroviral drugs during pregnancy, be delivered by caesarean section (unless her viral load is very low) and avoid breastfeeding. The incidence of vertical transmission does not reach zero even with these measures.

The baby should get antiretroviral therapy until it is possible to check HIV status at three months of age.

Source: RCOG Green-top guideline number 39. *The Management of HIV in Pregnancy.*

3.13 A refugee woman from Ethiopia books for antenatal care in her first pregnancy and discloses to the midwife that she has undergone female genital mutilation (FGM) in the past. Which of these statements about FGM is true?

A. UK law states that the suturing can legally be restored after delivery
B. She must be delivered by elective caesarean section
C. The FGM can be surgically 'undone' before delivery
D. A female baby may be at risk of FGM as a teenager in the future
E. It usually involves complete closure of the vaginal introitus except for a tiny hole

If you suspect that a woman has undergone FGM, she should be referred to a clinic with experience of dealing with this as it is entirely possible to 'undo' the introitus so that she can have a vaginal delivery without too much trauma. In the UK it is illegal to resuture the vaginal introitus so that it is closed again. There may be child protection issues; there is often intense cultural pressure to inflict the same procedure on young girls but the surgery is normally carried out well before puberty. There are several different types of FGM resulting in varying degrees of closure of the introitus.

3.14 You see a pregnant woman in your surgery who has just been to the hospital for a dating scan at 11 weeks gestation which reveals that she has monochorionic twins in separate sacs. Which of the following statements is true about this type of twin pregnancy?

A. Monochorionic twins are at lower risk of twin–twin transfusion syndrome (TTTS) than dichorionic twins
B. She will be having regular growth scans from 32 weeks gestation
C. She should be delivered by caesarean section as there is a risk of cord entanglement

D. Delivery should be planned for 37 weeks if she has not laboured

E. She will not be able to have any sort of screening for Down syndrome

Monochorionic twins are at risk of TTTS rather than dichorionic twins and because of this her growth scans will start earlier at 24 weeks. There is a risk of cord entanglement but this is not a reason for caesarean delivery; however, there is a risk of stillbirth if the pregnancy goes to term so we would normally deliver by 37 weeks. She could have nuchal translucency scans to screen for Down syndrome but there is an ethical dilemma regarding the results – what if one of the twins has a thickened nuchal fold and the other one doesn't? The subsequent diagnostic test is also problematic if required.

Source: RCOG Green-top guideline 51. *Management of Monochorionic Twin Pregnancy.*

3.15 You are consulted by a primigravid woman at 24 weeks gestation who has an unbearable headache. She has a history of severe migraine which she has consulted you about before several times. You do a thorough examination and find epigastric tenderness. Testing her urine reveals proteinuria +++. Which one of the following statements about her situation is correct?

A. The diagnosis cannot be pre-eclampsia because of the early gestation

B. If her blood pressure is 125/80 mmHg the diagnosis cannot be pre-eclampsia

C. Fundal height is irrelevant as IUGR will not be apparent at this early gestation

D. She needs assessment by an obstetrician urgently

E. Prescribing antibiotics without awaiting the results of an MSU is not advisable

In general practice you might be consulted about symptoms by patients who actually have pre-eclampsia so it is important to recognize the symptom cluster of unremitting frontal headache, visual disturbance and epigastric pain, sometimes with nausea and vomiting. The measured BP should be compared with the booking blood pressure to quantify the rise although very occasionally patients can develop eclampsia with normal blood pressure so the presence of proteinuria with the above symptoms should prompt referral to the obstetric unit for assessment. Occasionally pre-eclampsia happens at a very early gestation.

3.16 Consultant referral is necessary so that antenatal serial growth scans can be arranged to check on fetal growth if the pregnancy is affected by which one of the following conditions in the mother:

A. 'Slapped cheek' syndrome

B. Recurrent unexplained antepartum haemorrhage

C. Previous delivery by caesarean section

D. History of polycystic ovarian syndrome

E. Maternal vitamin B12 deficiency

Polycystic ovarian syndrome increases the risk of miscarriage and diabetes but not IUGR. The other conditions are good reasons for referring for consultant care but for reasons other than the potential for poor fetal growth.

'Slapped cheek' syndrome is due to parvovirus infection, which can cause severe fetal anaemia and stillbirth but not usually growth restriction. There is no known association between any maternal vitamin deficiency and growth problems.

Source: RCOG Green-top guideline number 31. *The Investigation and Management of the Small-for-Gestational-Age Fetus.*

3.17 A 14-year-old schoolgirl is brought to your surgery by her angry mother, having been sent home with a note from the school nurse suggesting that she might be pregnant. On examination it is obvious that her abdominal swelling is due to a pregnancy of about 36 weeks gestation; fetal movements can be clearly seen and the fetal heart auscultated. Which one of the following statements is true with regard to this teenage pregnancy?

A. She is no more likely to deliver a small-for-dates infant than mothers ten years older

B. You should involve the police because her pregnancy must be the result of rape

C. There is no point in discussing contraception

D. There is a higher incidence of sexually transmitted infections in teenage mothers

E. Her due date can be accurately predicted when she has her first scan at the hospital

Teenagers who get pregnant are far more likely than older mothers to have infections such as chlamydia, and some antenatal clinics routinely screen teenagers for STIs. Although it may seem like 'shutting the stable door after the horse has bolted' a discussion about future contraception is advisable during antenatal clinic appointments so that a method can be prescribed as soon as she delivers; otherwise a proportion of these teenagers will be back in antenatal clinic sooner than everyone would like. Having sexual intercourse with anyone under the age of 16 years is illegal but in practice it does not seem appropriate to refer pregnant teenagers to the police; we want them to engage with services, not conceal their pregnancies until delivery. There is a caveat here – if her partner is much older than her or there is any suspicion of incest, there may be child protection issues and you should take advice from your local Child Protection Lead and Social Services in that case.

Teenage mothers are more at risk of IUGR and should have growth scans. As she is booking late, the dating of the pregnancy from ultrasound will be hopelessly inaccurate so she will need a growth scan two weeks later anyway to check that the baby is growing along the same centile as her first scan.

3.18 A 34-year-old woman who has had two uncomplicated pregnancies before expresses a wish to have a home birth this time. At her 28-week check-up with the midwife she mentions that she has had a couple of minor episodes of vaginal bleeding following intercourse during the previous few weeks. Her blood group is A Rhesus negative. Which one of the following statements about her situation is correct?

A. If she had a normal anomaly scan the diagnosis cannot be placenta praevia

B. The bleeding will not be due to cervical cancer if her prepregnancy smear was normal

C. Kleihauer testing will help diagnose placental abruption

D. This woman could still have a home birth as requested if the placenta is not low

E. She should be referred to consultant-led antenatal care for growth scans

She needs an ultrasound scan to rule out placenta praevia, which is sometimes missed on the anomaly scan. Undiagnosed recurrent antepartum haemorrhage is associated with growth restriction and cerebral palsy so her antenatal care should be transferred to an obstetric consultant for growth scans. We would not advise home birth because of the increased risk of fetal distress in labour. The Kleihauer test is performed to discover how much anti-D a Rhesus-negative mother needs after a potential sensitizing event, not to diagnose abruption.

3.19 You see a primigravid woman in clinic who has just had a 20-week detailed (anomaly) scan which reveals a low-lying placenta. Which of these is the most appropriate advice for her?

A. Take folic acid 5 mg daily
B. Avoid sexual intercourse
C. Take an increased dose of oral iron three times daily
D. Admission to hospital will be necessary later in the pregnancy
E. Delivery will be by caesarean section at 37 weeks

Although the placenta is low lying at this gestation it may not be on a subsequent ultrasound scan so she could still have a vaginal delivery if the placenta is no longer low at term. There is no point in arranging the repeat scan before 32 weeks gestation because the lower segment of the uterus does not start to form until then.

It is worth avoiding anaemia but she does not necessarily need either iron or folic acid. Even if the placenta does turn out to be low lying later on, it is no longer considered mandatory to admit women with a low lying placenta in the third trimester. If there has been no bleeding and the placenta doesn't cover the os she can remain at home until near term, particularly if she lives close to the hospital.

Not having intercourse is sensible advice to avoid causing vaginal bleeding (and the release of prostaglandin in the vagina will make the uterus contract).

3.20 You are looking after a 'grand multip', pregnant with her fifth baby, who has had four normal births before. She is particularly at risk of which pregnancy complication?

A. Anaemia
B. Hypertension
C. Low-lying placenta
D. Postpartum haemorrhage (PPH)
E. Placenta accreta

It is the poor contractility of the myometrium that makes a 'grand multip' more at risk of PPH. This was the cause of death of Mumtaz Mahal who died of haemorrhage giving birth to her 13th child (resulting in the construction of the incredible Taj Mahal).

Hypertension is more common in older mothers but a 'grand multip' is not necessarily older. Placenta accreta is more common after several caesarean sections but not after vaginal births.

EXTENDED MATCHING QUESTIONS

A.	Alpha fetoprotein level
B.	Amniocentesis
C.	Chorionic villus sampling
D.	Combined nuchal translucency scan and serum screening
E.	Cordocentesis

F.	Detailed ultrasound scan
G.	Karyotype both parents for balanced (Robertsonian) translocation
H.	Nuchal translucency scan
I.	Serum screening with hCG/alpha fetoprotein/estriol levels
J.	Third trimester growth scan
K.	3-D ultrasound scan

The clinical scenarios below relate to prenatal screening and diagnostic tests. For each woman select the most appropriate investigation.

Each option may be used once, more than once or not at all.

3.21 The wife of a prominent politician is referred to a private obstetric clinic at ten weeks gestation because she has conceived unexpectedly many years after the birth of her last child and is now aged 42. She wishes to be absolutely reassured that the baby does not have Down syndrome as soon as possible because she feels that it would hamper her contribution to her husband's career.

C. Chorionic villus sampling

If she wishes to have a quick definitive answer from a diagnostic test rather than a screening test, then CVS is the best option in spite of the increased miscarriage risk. The current NHS screening programme would not provide a diagnostic CVS or amniocentesis on the NHS on grounds of maternal age.

3.22 A patient with a history of a previous pregnancy affected by neural tube defect wishes to have the most sensitive test in this current pregnancy.

F. Detailed ultrasound scan

Although the alpha fetoprotein level would give some idea of the likelihood of neural tube defect (NTD) it is not diagnostic and misses some cases, especially closed NTDs, therefore detailed ultrasound is the best option. Very few cases of NTD are missed on ultrasound these days because the scan machines have much improved resolution.

3.23 A 36-year-old woman has conceived after many years of infertility. She wishes to have a screening test for Down syndrome with the least false-positive rate

D. Combined nuchal translucency scan and serum screening

This patient is seeking a screening test rather than a diagnostic test with a risk of miscarriage attached and this combination gives the most accurate option. If the result is in the high-risk category she will have to decide whether to risk miscarriage by opting for a diagnostic test.

3.24 A couple who know that they are both carriers of cystic fibrosis present at nine weeks gestation requesting prenatal diagnosis.

C. Chorionic villus sampling

It is possible to exclude this condition now at an early gestation by offering CVS.

3.25 A 40-year-old woman who has reached 15 weeks gestation having had three previous first-trimester miscarriages wishes to have a diagnostic test for Down syndrome because her partner has a balanced Robertsonian translocation.

B. Amniocentesis

If this patient wishes to have a diagnostic test she will have to accept the risk of miscarriage and have an amniocentesis. Serum screening and detailed scan might suggest a problem but are not diagnostic. The balanced translocation increases the risk of trisomy and we probably know about it because of investigation of recurrent miscarriage in this couple.

A.	Abruptio placentae
B.	Appendicitis
C.	Constipation
D.	Pancreatitis
E.	Pre-eclampsia
F.	Red degeneration of a uterine fibroid
G.	Torsion of an ovarian cyst
H.	Ureteric calculus
I.	Urinary tract infection
J.	Uterine rupture

The clinical scenarios below relate to the emergency presentation of a pregnant woman with abdominal pain. For each woman select the most likely diagnosis for her pain.

Each option may be used once, more than once or not at all.

3.26 Two years after a myomectomy operation, a 42-year-old woman has conceived following IVF treatment. At 32 weeks gestation she is admitted to the obstetric unit with increasing pain in her abdomen for three days, which only responds to opiate analgesia. Apart from nausea she has no systemic symptoms. On examination she is apyrexial and normotensive but has a tachycardia. There is localized tenderness only at the fundus of the uterus.

F. Red degeneration of a uterine fibroid

Apart from a tachycardia her observations are normal and the tenderness is over the uterus. This makes appendicitis, urinary tract infection and pancreatitis less likely. If the cause of the pain was uterine rupture or abruptio placentae it would not have been going on for several days and she would be much more unwell. As she has had a myomectomy previously she may well have another fibroid. Red degeneration happens when a fibroid grows so rapidly that it outgrows its vascular supply and the middle of the fibroid becomes necrotic. This is not uncommon during pregnancy and the pain can be severe.

3.27 An 18-year-old primigravid woman presents in A&E at 16 weeks gestation with lower abdominal pain and vomiting. She has fetor oris and a temperature of 37.8 °C.

B. Appendicitis

The gastrointestinal upset and fetor oris suggests appendicitis rather than urinary tract infection. Appendicitis can be a difficult diagnosis to make in pregnancy.

3.28 At 32 weeks gestation a woman pregnant with her second baby is admitted in an ambulance having collapsed in a supermarket due to sudden onset of severe abdominal pain. Her observations are stable apart from a maternal tachycardia. The uterus is tender and unfortunately no fetal heart beat is detectable.

A. Abruptio placentae

The uterus is described as 'woody hard' if abruption occurs. If there is no vaginal bleeding the diagnosis is concealed abruption.

3.29 At 17 weeks gestation a 38-year-old primigravid woman is rushed in to A&E with severe unilateral colicky loin pain. She was writhing about on the bed but the pain has now subsided following a dose of morphine. Urinalysis reveals haematuria and her temperature is normal.

H. Ureteric calculus

The history of the pain and lack of pyrexia suggest that this is more likely to be ureteric calculus than urinary tract infection (although colic is uncommon in pregnancy because high progesterone levels relax the smooth muscle of the ureters). Torsion of an ovarian cyst would not produce haematuria.

3.30 A primigravid woman on holiday in London attends an NHS 'walk-in' centre with severe epigastric pain and headache. Her pregnancy has been uncomplicated so far and she is now 30 weeks gestation. On admission, urinalysis reveals that there is a lot of protein in her urine.

E. Pre-eclampsia

This could be a urinary tract infection but the symptoms are more suggestive of pre-eclampsia, even at this early gestation. Taking her blood pressure should be the next move.

A.	Aim for vaginal delivery but with a shortened second stage
B.	Await spontaneous labour and aim for vaginal delivery
C.	Classical caesarean section
D.	Elective caesarean section at 39 weeks gestation
E.	Elective caesarean section at 39 weeks gestation and sterilization
F.	Elective caesarean section at 40 weeks gestation
G.	Emergency caesarean section
H.	Induction of labour at 38 weeks gestation and aim for vaginal delivery

I.	Offer external cephalic version and await spontaneous labour
J.	Offer external cephalic version and if successful induce labour

The following scenarios relate to a woman with a complicated pregnancy or underlying medical condition. How would you counsel her with regard to delivery?

Each option may be used once, more than once or not at all.

3.31 Having been delivered by caesarean section in both previous pregnancies a 30-year-old woman books for antenatal care at 17 weeks gestation in her third pregnancy.

D. Elective caesarean section at 39 weeks gestation

It is usual to offer caesarean delivery if the patient has had two previous sections because of the increased risk of scar rupture. In terms of timing, we normally choose 39 weeks gestation because babies rarely develop transient tachypnoea of the newborn if delivery is deferred to then.

3.32 Having had a myomectomy operation a few years ago, a 39-year-old woman is followed up carefully in antenatal clinic because she has several more fibroids in the uterus. Serial growth scans show that the baby is OK but at 37 weeks the ultrasonographer notes that the fibroid in the lower segment has grown to 8 cm diameter and the baby is lying transversely above it.

C. Classical caesarean section

Myomectomy does not necessarily mean that she has to have a caesarean section and vaginal delivery is feasible. However a fibroid occupying the lower segment of the uterus – especially one that is nearly as large as the baby's head – is likely to obstruct labour. It would also make a lower segment caesarean tricky so that the best option would be to open the uterus longitudinally above the fibroid with a classical incision. We very rarely perform classical caesarean sections and there are implications for her next pregnancy, so if you know that your patient has had one before, you should take pains to point that out in your next referral letter.

3.33 A woman with HIV attends antenatal clinic at 36 weeks gestation. She is on antiretroviral medication and her viral load is extremely low < 50 copies per ml.

B. Await spontaneous labour and aim for vaginal delivery

HIV positive patients are normally delivered by caesarean to reduce the chance of vertical transmission. However if her viral load is extremely low, as in this case, we know that the mode of delivery makes no difference to the baby. There are rules to follow which include avoiding prolonged labour and leaving the membranes intact as long as possible; therefore avoiding induction of labour is a good idea.

3.34 A primigravid woman is referred to hospital antenatal clinic at 37 weeks gestation because the presentation is found to be breech. Scan confirms that the baby is of average size and the presentation is flexed breech.

I. Offer external cephalic version (ECV) and await spontaneous labour

There are several 'distractors' in this question. If the presentation remains breech, this woman is likely to be offered elective caesarean; therefore the best option is to try and turn the baby. It is unnecessary to induce labour if ECV is successful as spontaneous labour is more efficient than induced.

3.35 Just prior to conceiving, a 34-year-old woman was treated for a cerebral aneurysm, which was successfully clipped leaving no neurological deficit. Her craniotomy wound has healed well and she is now 36 weeks gestation in her first pregnancy.

A. Aim for vaginal delivery but with a shortened second stage

A history of previous intracranial problems such as bleeding, detached retina, treated aneurysm make it inadvisable for a woman to be performing the Valsalva manoeuvre every couple of minutes for an hour in labour so we would plan to have an elective assisted delivery in order to shorten the second stage. We don't need to consider caesarean delivery because she has had her aneurysm successfully treated.

A.	Admit immediately to a psychiatric 'mother and baby' unit
B.	Advise that depression is common and resolves after delivery
C.	Advise that she should stop medication as it can harm the baby
D.	Arrange specialist counselling
E.	Ask a psychiatric liaison worker to visit at home
F.	Continue medication and seek psychiatric advice
G.	Recommence psychiatric medication immediately
H.	Refer back to her previous psychiatrist
I.	Refer for a routine opinion from a specialist obstetric psychiatric clinic
J.	Refer for an urgent opinion from a specialist obstetric psychiatric clinic
K.	Suggest that she considers short-term use of sleeping tablets
L.	Suggest that she takes an antidepressant

The following scenarios relate to psychiatric problems in pregnant women. In each case decide the most appropriate course of action.

Each option may be used once, more than once or not at all.

3.36 Having been diagnosed with schizophrenia at university many years ago, a 34-year-old woman books for antenatal care very late at 36 weeks gestation as she had not realized that she was pregnant until the third trimester. She has been off medication for many years and has been psychiatrically well since.

J. Refer for an urgent opinion from a specialist obstetric psychiatric clinic

The chance of this woman developing a puerperal psychosis after delivery is very high (around 30%) and she needs surveillance postpartum with easy recourse to urgent specialist obstetric psychiatric advice if she becomes ill. Ordinary psychiatrists sometimes do not appreciate the urgency of the problem and something drastic can happen before psychiatric admission can be organized. As she is very near term, this needs urgent action. This message came over very clearly from the 2000–2002 maternal mortality reports (when maternal suicide was the leading cause of maternal death in the UK).

3.37 A primigravid woman at 28 weeks gestation consults you in surgery about feeling very low in mood and having trouble sleeping following the death of her mother. She denies thoughts of self harm.

D. Arrange specialist counselling

Although this woman does sound depressed, it is a reactive depression and likely to respond to simple measures. The use of antidepressants in pregnancy is OK if the benefits outweigh the risks but there is limited information about the safety of many drugs with regard to the fetus, so it is better if she can cope with non-drug therapy.

3.38 A young woman with bipolar disorder has been well controlled on lithium for a few years and seeks preconceptual counselling. She is planning pregnancy in the near future and has no other medical problems.

F. Continue medication and seek psychiatric advice

Patients on lithium to stabilize their mood can become quite unwell if they stop it abruptly and in this situation the risks of stopping the lithium outweigh the benefits. She needs advice from her psychiatrist to decide if it is advisable to come off her medication in order to reduce the chances of damaging the fetus, especially in the first trimester. It is good that she has come for preconceptual counselling as it gives an opportunity to organize withdrawal before pregnancy if she is well enough.

3.39 The midwife caring for one of your patients contacts you with concerns about a 42-year-old first time mother who has refused to allow her access to the house for the previous three days. The husband reveals on the telephone that his wife has not slept since the baby was born and is making bizarre comments about the health of the baby. Her psychiatric liaison worker has left a written care plan in her obstetric notes.

A. Admit immediately to a psychiatric 'mother and baby' unit

This woman appears to have developed postpartum psychosis and needs inpatient assessment done by an experienced team. If she goes into a specialized unit she can take the baby with her, which is better for bonding as she improves in the long run. If there is a written care plan it is likely that she has previous history and the plan should be accessible to everyone looking after her.

3.40 A woman books for antenatal care at ten weeks in her second pregnancy. She gives a history of postnatal depression, which involved several months of inpatient care following her previous delivery. She is currently well and not on any medication.

I. Refer for a routine opinion from a specialist obstetric psychiatric clinic

This woman has booked early, which provides the obstetric and psychiatric medical team lots of time to look into her past history and assess the risk for this pregnancy. The fact that she was looked after as an inpatient previously increases the likelihood of it having been a psychosis rather than an ordinary depression, but this can be investigated to confirm the previous diagnosis in order to work out her recurrence risk. 'Postnatal depression' is an acceptable diagnosis to many patients so any sort of mental illness may be referred to as depression (when it was actually a psychosis).

A.	Abdominal ultrasound scan
B.	Computed tomogram scan
C.	Doppler measurement
D.	Electronic cardiotocograph fetal monitoring
E.	Fetal growth scan in two weeks
F.	Speculum examination of the cervix with fibronectin swab
G.	Speculum examination of the cervix with microbiology swabs
H.	Transvaginal scan
I.	Ultrasound scan with umbilical artery doppler
J.	Vaginal examination in theatre with the operating team standing by

These clinical scenarios relate to women in the third trimester of pregnancy, presenting with vaginal bleeding. In each case, choose the most appropriate initial investigation.

Each option may be used once, more than once or not at all.

3.41 A woman attends the labour ward at 35 weeks gestation on account of a small amount of vaginal bleeding, which has now stopped. Initially there was some minor abdominal pain but this has settled and there is no uterine activity. There have been reduced fetal movements since the episode of bleeding. On examination the size of the uterus is compatible with dates.

D. Electronic cardiotocograph fetal monitoring

Although the diagnosis here could be placenta praevia, therefore an ultrasound is a good idea, it is important to check that the baby is OK before she goes to scan because another potential diagnosis is placental abruption. At some stage she will also need a speculum examination to exclude a cervical cause of the bleeding – such as chlamydial infection – but this should not be done until after the scan excludes placenta praevia.

3.42 A primigravid 37-year-old woman presents with a heavy vaginal bleed at 39 weeks gestation. The uterus is non-tender and the baby is well grown but appears to be lying transversely. There are no contractions and the condition of both the mother and the baby is stable.

A. Abdominal ultrasound scan

Transverse lie is extremely unusual in a primigravid patient and this makes the diagnosis of placenta praevia very likely – so she needs an abdominal scan. If she were contracting (so you haven't much time to make the diagnosis) you could consider examining her in theatre in case you make her bleed torrentially from a low-lying placenta.

3.43 A primigravid patient is seen in the antenatal assessment unit because of recurrent episodes of antepartum haemorrhage (APH) over the previous few weeks. The uterine fundus measures 'small for dates' at 37 weeks gestation. An ultrasound scan confirms that the baby's abdominal circumference is on the tenth centile of the growth chart and the liquor volume is less than expected.

D. Electronic cardiotocograph fetal monitoring

Recurrent APH is sometimes associated with intrauterine growth restriction. Although a Doppler is indicated here and another growth scan in two weeks' time, it is important to check that the baby is OK now before planning future management.

3.44 Having booked late for antenatal care because she tried to conceal her pregnancy, a 15-year-old primigravid woman comes in to labour ward late one evening with a small amount of postcoital bleeding at term. The baby is moving normally and the uterus is non-tender.

G. Speculum examination of the cervix with microbiology swabs

The lack of uterine tenderness rules out abruption as a diagnosis and it is likely that she has had a scan (which would have picked up placenta praevia) even though she booked late. The rate of chlamydial carriage in teenagers is very high and this infection is the most likely cause of her postcoital bleeding.

3.45 The emergency ambulance brings a 23-year-old woman to hospital at 34 weeks in her second pregnancy because she experienced sudden onset of abdominal pain and vaginal bleeding an hour ago. On examination the uterus is very tender and feels hard.

D. Electronic cardiotocograph fetal monitoring

The diagnosis here is likely to be placental abruption so the first priority is to check that the baby is OK.

A.	Candida albicans
B.	Chlamydia trachomatis
C.	Escherichia coli
D.	Gardnerella vaginalis
E.	Gonococcus
F.	Group B streptococcus
G.	Listeria monocytogenes
H.	Parvovirus B19
I.	Rubella
J.	Streptococcus faecalis
K.	Toxoplasma gondii

The clinical scenarios below relate to women with infectious diseases in pregnancy. For each case select the single most likely infecting organism.

Each option may be used once, more than once or not at all.

3.46 A woman presents in the surgery at 22 weeks gestation complaining of increasing abdominal discomfort and on examination the uterus is tense and large for dates. She gives a history of a mild flu-like illness two weeks previously. The community midwife refers her to hospital for an ultrasound scan, which shows polyhydramnios and fetal hydrops.

H. Parvovirus B19

Rubella, toxoplasma, parvovirus B19 and listeria all cause a mild flu-like illness in pregnancy and all three organisms can cross the placenta and infect the fetus. Parvovirus B19 causes suppression of fetal bone marrow and leads to severe fetal anaemia, which causes the classical picture of hydrops fetalis. The knowledge of how to diagnose and treat hydrops fetalis is clearly not part of the DRCOG syllabus. However the core knowledge being tested is the risk that infectious diseases pose in pregnancy and the dietary advice given to all pregnant women to avoid unpasteurized foods.

3.47 A primigravid woman presents at 34 weeks gestation with a history of feeling increasingly unwell, rigors and right upper quadrant pain. On examination she is flushed, has a tachycardia of 100 bpm and has a temperature of 38 °C. She is tender in the right renal angle.

C. Escherichia coli

This should be a familiar clinical example: the woman clearly has a urinary tract infection and the high pyrexia suggests pyelonephritis. You know that E. coli is the commonest cause of UTI in women. It is tempting to think that the answer is too obvious and look for complexity where there is none, so-called 'over-thinking' the question. Not all questions will have complex answers; pyelonephritis is a risk for premature labour and therefore this is important core knowledge to be tested.

3.48 A 17-year-old woman presents at 30 weeks gestation in her first pregnancy with a history of recurrent postcoital bleeding. Her booking scan at 20 weeks showed a normally sited placenta. Speculum examination reveals a florid ectropion with contact bleeding on taking swabs.

B. Chlamydia trachomatis

There are two possible answers to this question: Chlamydia trachomatis and gonococcus. Both may cause postcoital bleeding (PCB) but chlamydia is significantly more common, especially in younger women. Candida albicans causes vaginal irritation and discharge but rarely causes PCB. The fact that the scenario makes no mention of any symptoms other than PCB should allow you to discount candida as the correct answer.

3.49 In antenatal clinic at 17 weeks gestation a primigravid woman complains of vaginal discharge and soreness. On speculum examination there is a thick white discharge adherent to the vaginal walls.

A. Candida albicans

The nature of the discharge and the symptoms suggest thrush infection, which is exceedingly common in pregnancy.

3.50 A 28-year-old primary school teacher is pregnant for the first time. Several children in her class have 'slapped cheek syndrome' at the start of term and when she comes to hospital for her routine anomaly scan her baby is found to be hydropic.

H. Parvovirus B19

Children with slapped cheek syndrome due to parvovirus do not feel ill and are therefore sent to school where the parvovirus poses a risk to the pregnancy. It causes fetal anaemia, which is why the baby looks hydropic on the scan due to high-output cardiac failure. This also shows that in the real exam the same answer may well be used more than once.

Curriculum module 4: Answers

MULTIPLE CHOICE QUESTIONS

4.1 Considering vaginal birth in women who have previously been delivered by caesarean section (VBAC):

A. The chance of a successful vaginal birth occurring next time is about 70% T

The chances of a successful VBAC vary according to the reasons for the caesarean last time and also depending on how many centimetres dilatation the cervix reached during the previous labour, but a figure of 70% overall is generally quoted to patients. The RCOG Green-top guideline states that 'Women considering their options for birth after a single previous caesarean should be informed that, overall, the chances of successful planned VBAC are 72–76%'.

B. They should never consider vaginal delivery if they have had two previous caesarean sections   F

It is possible to achieve a successful vaginal delivery after two previous sections especially if they have managed a vaginal delivery before, but the risk of scar dehiscence is higher after two sections than after one, so most obstetricians would recommend a repeat section the third time. The Green-top guideline states that 'Women with a prior history of two uncomplicated low transverse caesarean sections, in an otherwise uncomplicated pregnancy at term, with no contraindication for vaginal birth, who have been fully informed by a consultant obstetrician, may be considered suitable for planned VBAC'.

C. If the mother is obese the chance of a successful VBAC is reduced   T

Obesity compromises obstetric performance on many levels. Evidence suggests that patients with a body mass index greater than 30 have a greatly reduced chance of a successful VBAC.

D. The risk of uterine rupture is increased if the previous section was complicated by infection   T

Uterine infection compromises the healing of the uterine scar. There is limited evidence from a case–control study that women who experienced both intrapartum and postpartum fever in their prior caesarean birth were at increased risk of uterine rupture in their subsequent planned VBAC labour (OR 4.02, 95% CI 1.04–15.5).

E. Can have a 'water birth' as long as it is in hospital   F

One of the signs of scar rupture is fetal distress and it is recommended that patients undergoing VBAC should have continuous fetal monitoring as well as IV access. It is also difficult to assess maternal condition in terms of scar tenderness if she is in a birthing pool.

Source: RCOG Green-top guideline number 45. *Birth after Previous Caesarean Birth.*

4.2 A woman who has developed severe pre-eclampsia in pregnancy is at risk of the following problems:

A. Fetal distress in labour   T
B. Reduced uterine response to synthetic oxytocin   F
C. Cerebrovascular accident (stroke)   T
D. Excess bleeding due to disseminated intravascular coagulation   T
E. Renal failure   T

These patients need careful management in labour, which involves blood pressure control to avoid intracerebral bleeding, fluid balance and fetal monitoring as there is often placental insufficiency. The PET causes low-grade DIC and the obstetric anaesthetist will want to know her platelet count before inserting an epidural.

4.3 The following obstetric conditions predispose to cord prolapse during labour:

A. Unstable lie   T
B. Breech presentation   T
C. Maternal diabetes   F
D. Placenta praevia   F
E. Polyhydramnios   T

Cord prolapse is an obstetric emergency necessitating immediate delivery and is more likely where the presenting part is either not in the pelvis (for example with a transverse lie) or does not fit it well (for example with a high head which is 5/5 palpable or a breech presentation as the breech may be smaller than the head, especially before 37 weeks).

4.4 Induction of labour is indicated in the following conditions:

A. Maternal urinary tract infection   F
This is not an indication for induction and active infection in the pelvis during labour may increase the chances of septic complications.

B. Symphysis pubis dysfunction   F
There is no evidence that inducing labour is beneficial to these patients although they usually request induction (or even caesarean!).

C. Pregnancy-induced hypertension   T
D. Pathological CTG tracing   F
A pathological CTG tracing usually indicates the need for immediate delivery (or fetal blood sampling – which is not likely to be possible if labour has not yet started).

E. Undiagnosed antepartum haemorrhage   F
Although antepartum haemorrhage is an indication for induction of labour it is important to exclude placenta praevia before planning induction.

4.5 The following are contraindications to a home delivery:

A. Twin pregnancy   T
B. A woman with a BMI of 37 who has had two normal births before   F
C. Grand multiparity   T
D. Second labour after previous forceps delivery   F
E. Poor rapport with community midwife   F

Women with a significantly raised BMI, i.e. over 35, should be advised against home birth due to increased risk of complications such as shoulder dystocia.

Although this woman's BMI is raised she could opt for home birth if she wishes, in accordance with NMC guidance. Although it is not ideal for a woman who did not manage a normal delivery last time or does not get on well with her midwife to plan a home birth she is still likely to be able to deliver without medical intervention. Twins may need intervention for the delivery of the second twin and a grand multip is more likely to have a postpartum haemorrhage and therefore should be advised to plan delivery in a consultant-led unit.

4.6 Planning to labour in a birthing pool of water in hospital is safe for the following pregnant women:

A. A primigravid woman whose baby is in the occipito-posterior (OP) position at the start of labour   T

Most babies in the OP position will rotate during labour although the labour is often prolonged (which will result in the use of oxytocin out of the pool).

B. A pregnant woman with a BMI of 45   F

This woman should not plan to deliver in the pool because if there is a problem such as maternal collapse or shoulder dystocia the midwife may not be able to get her out of the pool quickly enough.

C. A multiparous woman whose pregnancy is complicated by mild Rhesus disease   T

The main issue for this pregnancy is going to be the baby's haemoglobin and bilirubin levels and as long as the midwife can obtain blood samples from the cord after delivery, labouring in the birthing pool should be OK.

D. A woman with an uncomplicated postmature pregnancy being induced   F

Induction of labour will involve an IVI, usually oxytocin, and continuous electronic monitoring so this excludes the mother from a pool birth.

E. A woman with an otherwise uncomplicated pregnancy who has had a successful external cephalic version (ECV)   T

The ECV was successful so this pregnant woman can be treated the same as any other mother with a cephalic presentation.

4.7 Concerning certification of stillbirth:

A. If a child is born dead, the doctor or midwife will issue a medical certificate of stillbirth   T

B. Any child born in the 20th week of pregnancy that did not breathe or show any other signs of life should be registered as a stillbirth   F

C. The Stillbirth Register is separate from the standard Register of Births   T

D. A fetus papyraceus (one of a twin pregnancy which died in utero many weeks previously) should not be registered as a stillbirth   T

E. Hospitals may provide certification for a fetus lost too early in pregnancy to be classified as a stillbirth if the parents request it   T

The law in England and Wales (Section 41 of the Births and Deaths Registration Act 1953) requires that any child expelled or issued forth from its mother after the 24th week of pregnancy that did not breathe or show any other signs of life be registered as a stillbirth. If a child is born showing signs of life at any gestation and then subsequently dies, the child must be registered as a birth and death regardless of gestation.

In the case of a fetus papyraceus, it is known that the fetus must have died before the 24th week of pregnancy and thus it would be incorrect under the Act to register it as a stillbirth.

Certification of babies who die earlier in pregnancy and would be classified as a late miscarriage is not legally necessary, but is recommended as it provides women or couples with a certificate recording their pregnancy loss before 24 weeks of gestation. Not all couples would want this.

Source: RCOG Good practice guideline number 4. *Registration of Stillbirths and Certification for Pregnancy Loss before 24 Weeks of Gestation.*

4.8 The indications for assisted vaginal delivery (shortening the second stage of labour with forceps or ventouse) include:

A. Maternal cardiac disease   T
B. Fetal prematurity   F
C. Suspected fetal compromise   T
D. Maternal hypertensive disease   T
E. Previous third-degree tear   F

Mothers who are pushing actively are performing the Valsalva manoeuvre frequently which is probably not a good idea if she has raised blood pressure or cardiac problems. If there are concerns about the fetal condition on the cardiotocograph, the options are to perform a fetal blood sample or to expedite delivery. Instrumental delivery is associated with an increased risk of third-degree tear so should only be used if there is failure to progress or fetal compromise in women with a previous third-degree tear.

4.9 Placental abruption:

A. Is associated with pre-eclampsia   T
B. Can cause fetal death   T
C. May occur in the absence of vaginal bleeding   T
D. Makes it difficult to feel fetal parts on examination of the woman's abdomen   T
E. Can cause disseminated intravascular coagulation in the mother   T

This serious condition usually presents with severe continuous pain and vaginal bleeding and will compromise the fetus depending on how much of the placenta has separated. If there is no bleeding, it is called a concealed abruption. The uterus is described as 'woody' hard and the mother is at risk of DIC as a result of thromboplastin release from the placenta so a clotting screen is useful. Abruption is more common in women who have pre-eclampsia.

4.10 An obstetric anaesthetist will be unwilling to site an epidural until they have seen a recent normal platelet count and clotting screen for a woman whose pregnancy is complicated by:

A. Pre-eclampsia   T
B. Maternal diabetes   F
C. Twin pregnancy   F
D. Placental abruption   T
E. Intrauterine fetal death   T

Pre-eclampsia, abruption and IUFD (stillbirth) all put the patient at risk of disseminated intravascular coagulation. If an epidural is inserted in the presence of this condition there is an increased risk of a haematoma in the restricted space within the spinal canal, which could lead to paralysis.

SINGLE BEST ANSWER QUESTIONS

4.11 An ambulance is summoned by a community midwife who is conducting a home delivery for a multiparous woman who has had two normal deliveries before. Half way through the first stage of labour the patient has become increasingly distressed and is complaining of severe abdominal pain. The pain continues between contractions, which are occurring every three minutes, and the midwife has noticed that the uterus is tender and hard on palpation. Which of the following is the most likely complication?

A. Obstructed labour
B. Concealed placental abruption
C. Hyperstimulated labour
D. Chorioamnionitis
E. Uterine rupture

Fresh vaginal bleeding is suggestive of abruption or uterine rupture. Rupture is uncommon – unless oxytocin (or prostaglandins) are being used to stimulate contractions – but if the uterus ruptures the contractions usually cease.

4.12 You are in a labour room trying to cope with a severe postpartum haemorrhage while waiting for the registrar to arrive. The inexperienced student midwife hands you a selection of drugs to choose from to try and stop the uterine bleeding. Which of these drugs has she picked up in error?

A. Atosiban
B. Carboprost
C. Ergometrine
D. Misoprostol
E. Oxytocin

Atosiban is used to stop contractions in the management of preterm labour.

4.13 A woman books for antenatal care in her fourth pregnancy. Her obstetric history includes three previous deliveries by caesarean section. She is predisposed to which obstetric complication?

A. Cord prolapse
B. Haemorrhage
C. Placenta accreta
D. Pre-eclampsia
E. Unstable lie

The risk of placenta praevia increases with increasing number of sections and the chance of that low-lying placenta invading the myometrium and becoming accreta increases markedly with each subsequent caesarean. This is one of the main reasons for trying to keep the caesarean section rate down.

4.14 The most important reason that administration of ergometrine to control postpartum haemorrhage is contraindicated in a woman with pre-eclampsia is:

A. It is likely to make her vomit profusely
B. It does not work as well as oxytocin
C. It gives a sustained effect rather than a quick onset of action
D. It is likely to increase her blood pressure
E. It could decrease her intracranial pressure

Ergometrine does make patients vomit and has a sustained effect but the main reason for not giving it to pre-eclamptic patients is the potential effect on blood pressure. Several patients – whose stories are described in the triennial maternal mortality reports – died because their blood pressure was significantly raised by third-stage administration of syntometrine and they subsequently died from massive intracranial bleeding.

4.15 As a junior doctor on the labour ward, it often feels as though you are being asked to insert an intravenous line on every woman in labour. Which of the following pregnant women does not need a cannula when she is admitted?

A.   A woman with an uncomplicated pregnancy delivering her sixth baby

B.   A primigravid woman whose haemoglobin was 95 g/l two weeks ago

C.   A woman who had a postpartum haemorrhage (PPH) in her last delivery

D.   A woman who had a forceps delivery for fetal distress in her previous pregnancy

E.   A woman who had an emergency caesarean for fetal distress in her last pregnancy

The issue here is which of these women is likely to have a PPH, need a blood transfusion or end up in theatre for an emergency section. For any of these reasons, she could need a cannula and a 'group and save' doing while she is labouring. The only woman on the list above who is not in this situation is the woman who needed a forceps delivery last time.

4.16 Having had a massive postpartum haemorrhage following the delivery of her first baby a 34-year-old woman has received eight units of blood, two units of cryoprecipitate and fresh frozen plasma during the previous couple of hours. She has developed pulmonary oedema with an oxygen saturation of 55%. Currently her temperature is 37.5 °C, her pulse is 110 beats per minute, her blood pressure 90/40 mmHg and her urine output is reduced to only 5 ml per hour. The clotting screen is normal and her haemoglobin is currently 95 g/l. What is likely to be the cause of this clinical situation?

A.   Bacterial contamination of the blood transfused

B.   Adult respiratory distress syndrome

C.   Blood-borne viral infection

D.   Delayed transfusion reaction

E.   Inadequate transfusion

The pulmonary oedema with a low oxygen saturation is the key to this diagnosis, although some of the clinical information given would also fit sepsis.

4.17 You are looking after a woman in labour who has had two fetal blood samples done already because of an abnormal cardiotocograph trace, the results of which are normal so far. The obstetric anaesthetist is keen for her to have an epidural inserted, thereby avoiding a general anaesthetic if emergency delivery becomes necessary later. The most important reason for avoiding general anaesthetic in labour is:

A.   The mother does not have to be kept 'nil by mouth' in labour

B.   General anaesthetic in an emergency takes longer than topping up an epidural

C.   Ventouse delivery is more difficult under GA because the mother cannot push

D. **The mother is at risk of Mendelssohn's syndrome (aspiration pneumonitis)**

E. Epidural can lower her blood pressure and improve placental perfusion

The effect of progesterone is to relax smooth muscle, therefore the lower oesophageal sphincter is relaxed in pregnancy and there is reduced gastric emptying. This leads to a high chance of a pregnant woman aspirating during induction of anaesthesia and developing pneumonitis. Before the widespread use of regional anaesthesia by trained obstetric anaesthetists, this was a common cause of maternal death.

It is true that ventouse delivery is more difficult under GA but this is not as important as avoiding maternal death. Epidural may lower her blood pressure but this will reduce rather than improve placental perfusion, so it is important to make sure that the baby is not hypoxic before she has her epidural.

4.18 When performing a fetal blood sample in the first stage of labour it is preferable to place the mother in the left lateral position for the following reason:

A. The midwife is more easily able to support the mother's legs

B. **Placental perfusion is improved by relieving pressure on maternal vena cava**

C. The cervical os is easier to access with the amnioscope

D. Necessary equipment for the procedure can be placed on the bed within reach

E. The baby may be lying on the placenta, thereby compressing the umbilical cord

The main reason is to improve placental perfusion by preventing the weight of the gravid uterus compressing the inferior vena cava, thereby reducing venous return. It has nothing to do with the comfort of the midwife or obstetrician.

4.19 While on labour ward you notice a commotion in one of the delivery rooms and hear someone shouting for help with shoulder dystocia. Which of the following procedures may help the birth attendants deliver the baby in this life-threatening situation?

A. **McRobert's manoeuvre to hyperflex the maternal hips**

B. Løvset manoeuvre to rotate the baby

C. Delivering the anterior arm of the baby

D. Mauriceau–Smellie–Veit (MSV) manoeuvre to flex the baby's neck

E. Fundal pressure on the uterus

Hyperflexion of the maternal hips changes the incline of her pelvis and makes more room for the impacted shoulder stuck behind the symphysis pubis to enter the pelvis.

If you want to relieve the situation by delivering an arm, it is the posterior arm that is used as it is not possible to reach the anterior one. Løvset manoeuvre is used during a vaginal breech delivery and MSV manoeuvre is for the after-coming head of a breech baby. We do not do fundal pressure because of the risk of rupturing the uterus (although this is done in some countries).

4.20 A primigravid woman has been in labour for nearly 20 hours and actively pushing for 90 minutes so a decision is made to perform an assisted vaginal delivery on account of delay in the second stage. The woman is at increased risk of which complication?

A. Fetal distress

B. Inverted uterus

C.   **Postpartum haemorrhage (PPH)**
D.   Cervical dystocia
E.   Paravaginal haematoma

The uterus does not contract so well after delivery when labour is prolonged and she is at increased risk of PPH due to uterine atony. This risk is increased if there is an element of infection, which may be the case after prolonged labour.

EXTENDED MATCHING QUESTIONS

A.	Amniotomy
B.	Elective caesarean section
C.	Electronic fetal monitoring
D.	Emergency caesarean section
E.	Intermittent auscultation
F.	Request a clotting screen
G.	Routine elective episiotomy
H.	Titrated synthetic oxytocin infusion
I.	Vaginal examination in theatre with the operating team standing by
J.	Ventouse delivery

The following clinical scenarios apply to women delivering in a hospital obstetric unit. In each case, select the most appropriate management plan.

Each option may be used once, more than once or not at all.

4.21 A primigravid 32-year-old woman presents early in the first stage of spontaneous labour at 38 weeks gestation, contracting once every ten minutes. Her membranes have just ruptured spontaneously and fresh meconium is seen in the liquor.

C. Electronic fetal monitoring

Meconium in the liquor becomes more likely as gestation advances, especially in postmature babies. It is, however, sometimes a sign of hypoxia especially if the pregnancy has not reached term, so in any labour where meconium is noted it is imperative to commence electronic fetal monitoring to look for other signs of hypoxia.

4.22 During vaginal examination in a woman's third labour, the midwife finds the cervix to be 8 cm dilated and feels a pulsatile cord alongside the fetal head. The head is below the ischial spines and in the occipito-anterior position.

D. Emergency caesarean section

This is a cord prolapse so delivery of the baby must be expedited. As the cervix is not fully dilated the delivery has to be emergency caesarean section, with a birth attendant lifting the presenting part off the cord until the operator can get the baby out.

4.23 A primigravid woman had had an uncomplicated pregnancy so far under midwifery care and presents with a heavy vaginal bleed at 39 weeks gestation. The uterus is non-tender and the baby is well grown with a cephalic presentation, four-fifths palpable. The condition of both mother and baby is stable but she is contracting strongly every three minutes and the blood continues to trickle from the vagina.

I. Vaginal examination in theatre with the operating team standing by

The baby's head should be engaged after 37 weeks in a primiparous woman, so that the fact that it is 4/5 palpable makes you wonder why and in this situation where there is vaginal bleeding a low-lying placenta is likely. An alternative would be to arrange an ultrasound scan but it is not on the option list and since it sounds as if she is in labour, vaginal examination is more appropriate as an initial plan.

4.24 Having been admitted to labour ward four hours previously experiencing three contractions every ten minutes, a low-risk primigravid patient is examined and her cervix is found to be 6 cm dilated with intact membranes. She mobilizes in her labour room using nitrous oxide for analgesia and four hours later the cervix is 7 cm dilated.

A. Amniotomy

This is primary dysfunctional labour and is common in primigravid women. Although you might choose the oxytocin infusion from the list, this works better if the membranes have been ruptured, so amniotomy is the first thing to do here. There is also a theoretical risk of amniotic fluid embolism if oxytocin is used to augment labour with intact membranes.

4.25 A midwife calls you in to a delivery room because of a small vaginal bleed in a low-risk primigravid woman whose labour has been progressing normally. The midwife is auscultating the baby's heartbeat which has been 70 beats per minute for five minutes. The mother's pulse is 90, her blood pressure is stable and the cervix is 8 cm dilated.

D. Emergency caesarean section

*This is likely to be a placental abruption, so cross matching blood and getting a clotting screen done are both reasonable options. However the baby is bradycardic so the overwhelming urgency is to deliver the baby quickly to avoid brain damage and therefore emergency caesarean section is the **most appropriate** option.*

A.	Arrange emergency caesarean section
B.	Check airway and administer oxygen by facial mask
C.	Check plasma glucose level
D.	Commence electronic fetal monitoring
E.	Contact the consultant haematologist on-call
F.	Cross-match blood
G.	Counsel about postpartum sterilization
H.	Perform a vaginal examination to exclude cord prolapse

I.	Rapid IV administration of 1 litre crystalloid
J.	Request urgent ultrasound scan
K.	Site IV cannula and check haemoglobin

These clinical scenarios relate to an emergency situation involving a woman on the labour ward in the third trimester of pregnancy. In each case, choose the most appropriate initial management plan.

Each option may be used once, more than once or not at all.

4.26 A 28-year-old woman with type 1 diabetes at 30 weeks gestation attends triage on labour ward early one morning because of an antepartum haemorrhage. She collapses in the waiting room and when you attend to sort out the situation she appears confused and is asking where she is.

C. Check plasma glucose level

When someone collapses our immediate response is 'AIRWAY, BREATHING, CIRCULATION'. However, this patient is talking, therefore ABC is unnecessary. In a diabetic the most likely problem is hypoglycaemia, so her blood sugar would be the first thing to do.

4.27 A 34-year-old woman is admitted to delivery suite at term in her eighth pregnancy. She has delivered six live children previously. On examination the cervix is 7 cm dilated and she is involuntarily pushing.

K. Site IV cannula and check haemoglobin

The main risk for this 'grand multip' is postpartum haemorrhage (PPH) so you need to be prepared for that. It is unlikely that you will need to cross-match blood unless she has become anaemic – but the PPH risk will have been identified as a risk factor antenatally so this should not have happened. Discussion of sterilization does not seem appropriate when delivery is imminent!

4.28 The labour ward is very busy when a young primigravid woman is admitted at 38 weeks gestation in labour. Yesterday in the midwifery antenatal clinic she was found to have a breech presentation and is awaiting a consultant outpatient appointment arranged for tomorrow. On admission she experiences spontaneous rupture of membranes and the student midwife in triage tells you that 'the fetal heart is dropping intermittently to 80 beats per minute'

H. Perform a vaginal examination to exclude cord prolapse

Breech presentation increases the risk of cord prolapse so although there are several things you need to do for this woman who needs an emergency caesarean delivery – such as putting up a drip – you need to exclude cord prolapse because if present someone will have to lift the presenting part off the cord on the way to theatre for an urgent (category 1) caesarean section.

4.29 A woman who has just delivered twins collapses in the delivery room at the end of the second stage. The placenta is still *in situ* and the midwife tells you that she has just noticed a large amount of blood in the bed. The patient is unresponsive and has a tachycardia of 120 beats per minute.

B. Check airway and administer oxygen by facial mask

Although you are clearly dealing with a massive postpartum haemorrhage and there are several relevant things on the list which must be done urgently, an obstructed airway will kill her before you have had chance to do any of them. The airway always takes priority. There are other disastrous conditions that could result in the same clinical picture, such as an amniotic fluid embolism.

4.30 Having been admitted with a fresh antepartum haemorrhage, a primiparous patient is diagnosed with a placental abruption at 34 weeks gestation. Both mother and baby are stable at the moment, but the haematology technician has just bleeped you to say that the clotting screen you sent to the lab an hour ago is not normal.

E. Contact the consultant haematologist on-call

Placental abruption can cause disseminated intravascular coagulation and if she is developing this severe complication, you will need the urgent help of the consultant haematologist to decide on the appropriate clotting factors to deal with the clotting abnormality.

A.	Cryoprecipitate
B.	Iron infusion
C.	Iron injections weekly
D.	Oral iron
E.	Platelet transfusion
F.	Recombinant Factor VIIa
G.	Transfuse 'O negative' blood
H.	Transfuse type-specific blood
I.	Transfuse cross-matched blood
J.	Transfuse blood from cell saver

Each of these clinical scenarios describes a pregnant woman whose clinical condition is or could be compromised by haemorrhage; for each patient pick the best management option given the information that you are presented with.

Each option may be used once, more than once or not at all.

4.31 During a routine caesarean section under spinal anaesthetic the consultant you are assisting unexpectedly comes across a low-lying placenta and the woman loses 2500 ml blood before the baby is delivered and the placenta is removed from the uterus. Her haemoglobin done the previous day is 105 g/l. Her blood pressure has dropped to 70/40 mmHg and she has become unresponsive to questions.

G. Transfuse 'O negative' blood

This woman is in hypovolaemic shock and needs the 'O negative' blood stored on every labour ward. Unless you were expecting placenta praevia, there will only be a 'group and save' in the lab for this woman. The maternal mortality reports often criticize management of severe haemorrhage as 'too little, too late'.

4.32 A primigravid woman has a blood test at 36 weeks gestation and is found to have a haemoglobin level of 69 gm/l. She has not been taking the iron tablets prescribed by her GP because of severe nausea, and has tried three different preparations.

B. Iron infusion

There is still enough time for her to increase her haemoglobin to reasonable levels before labour if she can get her iron stores replenished. If she can't tolerate oral iron, it will have to be parenteral and oral iron will only increase her haemoglobin at about 1 g per month anyway. There is an increased risk of skin discolouration and pain at the injection site with intramuscular iron. This needs to be balanced with the risk of anaphylaxis and a possible increased risk of venous thrombosis with intravenous iron dextran. The use of IM iron requires a test dose and a Z-track technique of injection so for the majority of women IV iron is preferred, according to the British Committee for Standards in Haematology.

4.33 A 31-year-old primigravid woman is known to have beta-thalassaemia and has a haemoglobin level of 80 g/l by the time she reaches 38 weeks gestation. She is symptomatic, feeling very tired and slightly breathless.

I. Transfuse cross-matched blood

It will not be long before this woman is in labour so transfusion should be considered even if she is not symptomatic. Anaemia related to haemoglobinopathy should be managed by blood transfusion with advice from a haematologist. Women with haemoglobinopathy may have a problem with iron overload.

Source: RCOG Green-top guideline 47. *Blood Transfusion in Obstetrics.*

4.34 You are the junior doctor on labour ward assisting the registrar dealing with a manual removal of placenta under general anaesthetic. During the last 15 minutes the woman started having a major haemorrhage and so far has lost 3 litres of blood. The consultant obstetrician has been called and the two units of blood stored on the labour ward have already been transfused. Her heart rate is 120 bpm and her blood pressure is 90/50 mmHg.

H. Transfuse type-specific blood

The haematology laboratory will be able to supply type-specific blood in about 20 minutes but a full cross-match takes longer. She is becoming haemodynamically unstable and therefore type-specific blood should be transfused pending the fully cross-matched units.

4.35 A 35-year-old woman pregnant with twins attends antenatal clinic at 28 weeks gestation for a growth scan. She has a routine blood test done and her haemoglobin is 90 g/l.

D. Oral iron

There is plenty of time for this woman to increase her haemoglobin with oral iron and you don't need to worry about parenteral iron (even though twins often arrive early and there is a chance she might go into labour anytime).

A.	Attempt to turn the baby (version) for vaginal delivery
B.	Arrange an emergency caesarean section
C.	Arrange an elective caesarean section

D.	Ask the anaesthetist to site an epidural
E.	Conduct an assisted vaginal delivery with ventouse or forceps
F.	Conduct a breech extraction
G.	Obtain a fetal blood sample from the scalp
H.	Obtain a fetal blood sample from the cord
I.	Obtain maternal serum for cross-matching blood
J.	Obtain maternal serum for a clotting screen
K.	Perform a vaginal examination to exclude cord prolapse
L.	Put up a syntocinon drip to increase the contractions
M.	Rupture the membranes with an amnihook

As the junior doctor on the labour ward you have been called to assist the midwives with the management of labouring women experiencing a complication.

In each scenario, choose the most appropriate immediate action that you think the obstetric team (not necessarily you personally) should take.

Each option may be used once, more than once or not at all.

4.36 One hour after administration of a prostaglandin pessary to induce labour for postmaturity, a primigravid woman is found to be having more than six contractions in ten minutes. You are asked to site an intravenous cannula while the midwife removes the pessary. Although the contractions lessen in frequency to three in ten the baby becomes bradycardic and you can hear that the fetal heart rate has been running at 90 beats per minute for four minutes so far.

B. Arrange an emergency caesarean section

The prostaglandin pessary has caused hyperstimulation of the uterus. If it does not resolve on removing the pessary, you could give her a drug such as terbutaline to relax the uterus; however, this option isn't on the list.

As there is a persistent bradycardia, this baby must be delivered with all haste to avoid possible cerebral palsy. The confounding option is to check for cord prolapse as a possible cause of the bradycardia, but since the membranes are intact this would be termed a cord presentation and therefore the most likely cause of the bradycardia is uterine hyperstimulation. The practicalities are that you only have a few minutes to save the baby, hence the correct option is caesarean section.

4.37 A 21-year-old primigravid woman was admitted in spontaneous labour six hours previously when the cervix was 7 cm dilated and has been relaxing in the birthing pool, coping without formal analgesia. The liquor is clear and intermittent auscultation of the fetal heart is reassuring. The cervix is now 8 cm dilated and the baby appears to be lying in the occipito-posterior position.

L. Put up a syntocinon drip to increase the contractions

This woman has primary dysfunctional labour with delay in the first stage due to malposition of the fetal head, with ruptured membranes. There are no concerns about the condition of the baby and the problem should respond to oxytocin.

4.38 A multiparous woman has delivered her first twin vaginally 15 minutes ago and there is no sign of the second twin appearing, although the contractions are continuing every two minutes. On examination it is apparent that the second twin is lying transversely in the uterus.

A. Attempt to turn the baby (version) for vaginal delivery

We often use a syntocinon drip in between the delivery of the first and second twin to ensure that contractions continue. However, the second twin is lying transversely and the options are caesarean section or that a version must be performed to convert to a longitudinal lie. As she is multiparous, the second option is quicker and safer than a second-stage caesarean section and therefore external version is the correct answer even though some obstetric trainees do not have the practical skill or experience to perform version.

4.39 A rather frightened 17-year-old primigravid woman is in spontaneous labour and the cervix is 6 cm dilated. The midwife has noted meconium in the liquor and there are late decelerations on the cardiotocograph. The woman has asked for more analgesia and the midwife says that she is becoming more and more uncooperative.

G. Obtain a fetal blood sample from the scalp

You might be thinking that this woman needs an epidural but before that is offered, there is a need to address the suspected fetal distress by performing a fetal blood sample. An epidural may drop her blood pressure resulting in reduced placental perfusion and worsening the situation for the fetus. Likewise, if the baby is already acidotic an emergency caesarean may be indicated so the prime imperative is to establish fetal wellbeing with an FBS.

4.40 A multiparous woman who has had three previous uncomplicated vaginal births is admitted in advanced labour at term and to everyone's surprise the presentation of the baby is found to be breech, station at the ischial spines and the cervix 9 cm dilated. The membranes rupture just after the vaginal examination and the liquor is clear. The midwife commences a cardiotocograph trace, which shows occasional early decelerations.

K. Perform a vaginal examination to exclude cord prolapse

The first stage of labour is progressing well and she is nearly ready for second stage, so a vaginal breech delivery is likely. However the cause of the early decelerations should be considered – it cannot be head compression because the presentation is breech. Cord prolapse is more common with breech presentation so this obstetric emergency must be excluded before anything else is done. If there is a clinical suspicion of fetal distress then caesarean section may well be the next course of action as fetal blood samples cannot be taken from the breech.

A.	Abruption of the placenta
B.	Cervical laceration
C.	Disseminated intravascular coagulation
D.	Placenta accreta
E.	Placenta praevia
F.	Retained succenturiate lobe of placenta

G.	Rupture of the uterus
H.	Uterine atony
I.	Vasa praevia
J.	Velamentous insertion of the cord

Given the clinical information provided, select the most likely diagnosis for each of these obstetric patients experiencing vaginal bleeding.

Each option may be used once, more than once or not at all.

4.41 A woman has just delivered her first baby and while the midwife is inspecting the placenta the patient has a brisk vaginal bleed of about 600 ml. Maternal observations are stable and the uterus feels well contracted. The midwife points out to you that there are blood vessels running through the membranes.

F. Retained succenturiate lobe of placenta

This situation sounds like a velamentous insertion of the cord, where the vessels are attached to the membranes instead of being inserted directly into the placenta. However, if the vessels are running off the edge of the membranes, they must be carrying blood to something, which suggests an extra lobe of placenta. If it is left in the uterus, it will cause haemorrhage and/or infection and must be retrieved.

Uterine atony is the confounding option but those blood vessels are the key to this answer.

4.42 A primigravid woman aged 21 presents to labour ward at 39 weeks gestation because of a brisk painless vaginal bleed of about 100 ml following intercourse. The uterus is non-tender with a transverse fetal lie. The fetal heart is steady at 140 beats per minute.

E. Placenta praevia

The fact that the baby is lying transversely at 39 weeks in a primigravid woman is a clue to the possibility that the placenta is in the way. Also the bleeding is painless, which suggests praevia as placental abruption is usually associated with pain.

4.43 You are called to see a primigravid woman who has started bleeding half way through the first stage of labour, losing 200 ml in a couple of minutes. In spite of her epidural she seems to be in a lot of pain and there are unmistakeable signs of severe fetal distress on the cardiotocograph.

A. Abruption of the placenta

It is very rare for a primigravid patient to have a ruptured uterus and the only other cause of pain on this list is abruption. Both would cause an abnormal CTG. Ruptured uterus is usually associated with a uterine scar such as previous caesarean section or myomectomy. The unscarred uterus can rupture in multiparous women with obstructed labour, particularly with syntocinon use, but again this is very rare in the UK.

4.44 During her second labour a 35-year-old woman starts to lose fresh blood per vaginam. Her first baby was delivered by caesarean section because of fetal distress related to chorioamnionitis at 6 cm dilatation in the first stage.

This time the cervix has reached 7 cm dilatation but the contractions have stopped.

G. Rupture of the uterus

Cessation of contractions is an ominous sign which suggests rupture of the uterus, especially in a woman who is labouring with a previous section scar. Other features of scar rupture are bleeding as in this case, pain continuing between contractions, CTG abnormalities, a sudden change in the presentation as the baby is expelled from the uterus into the abdominal cavity or even fetal death.

4.45 The midwife looking after a primigravid woman in labour at term ruptured the membranes five minutes ago with an amnihook to speed up the progress of the first stage of labour, as cervical dilatation has been stuck at 5 cm for the last four hours. You are called because the midwife is concerned that the liquor is very heavily bloodstained. The uterus is non-tender, contracting four in ten minutes and the fetal heart rate has risen from a baseline of 120 before amniotomy to 180 beats per minute with late decelerations.

I. Vasa praevia

Your first thought might be that the midwife has lacerated the cervix with the amnihook and that is where the bleeding is coming from. However, there are ominous signs of the CTG which suggest that the baby is in trouble and the tachycardia may be occurring because of acute fetal blood loss. This is a very rare situation but there are only minutes to save the baby's life before it exsanguinates and suspected vasa praevia should be mentioned to the resuscitating paediatrician as they should give blood to the baby early on or resuscitation may be unsuccessful.

A.	Administer oral benzylpenicillin
B.	High vaginal swab on admission
C.	Induction of labour and intrapartum IV benzylpenicillin
D.	Prescribe intrapartum IV benzylpenicillin
E.	Prescribe intrapartum IV erythromycin
F.	Prescribe intrapartum IV clindamycin
G.	Prescribe intrapartum IV metronidazole
H.	Reassure the patient that no action is necessary
I.	Vaginal cleansing with chlorhexidine on admission in labour

Each of these pregnant women has been found to be carrying group B streptococcus on vaginal swabs at some stage in this or a previous pregnancy. For each patient select the most appropriate management plan to prevent early-onset neonatal group B streptococcal disease.

Each option may be used once, more than once or not at all.

4.46 A primigravid woman has been admitted to labour ward for elective caesarean delivery for persistent breech presentation. She had a swab taken last week by her GP which has grown group B streptococcus (GBS).

H. Reassure the patient that no action is necessary

This is an elective caesarean and you should assume that there are intact membranes therefore the guidance given in the Green-top guideline is that antibiotic treatment is unnecessary for the prevention of early onset neonatal GBS disease.

4.47 A woman is admitted in established labour at term. A swab done at 12 weeks gestation when she had a threatened miscarriage grew group B streptococcus.

D. Prescribe intrapartum IV benzylpenicillin

The background risk of neonatal early onset GBS disease is 0.5/1000 births. The risk rises to 2.3/1000 births if GBS is detected in the current pregnancy even if she received antibiotic treatment earlier in the pregnancy. The significantly increased risk justifies antibiotic treatment in labour and benzylpenicillin is the first-line drug of choice. The intravenous route is preferred due to variable absorption of oral antibiotics during labour.

4.48 At 37 weeks gestation a multiparous woman is admitted with prelabour rupture of the membranes (PROM). She was found to have group B streptococcus on a high vaginal swab done a few weeks previously when she was seen in another maternity unit in Skegness on holiday.

C. Induction of labour and intrapartum IV benzylpenicillin

Routine care would be to offer induction of labour 24 hours after PROM, however the risk of ascending GBS infection in colonized women with PROM justifies immediate induction with IV antibiotic cover. The aim is to ensure that the first dose of IV antibiotics are given at least two hours prior to delivery. The IV antibiotics should be continued four-hourly throughout labour until delivery. If the delivery takes place within two hours of the first dose of antibiotics, then the baby needs IV treatment instead.

4.49 A woman presents in spontaneous labour at term with her second baby. In her previous pregnancy she had a swab done in the first trimester which grew group B streptococcus; then she delivered at term and the baby was fine. She has not had any swabs done in this pregnancy.

H. Reassure the patient that no action is necessary

If GBS was detected in a previous pregnancy the chance of the woman being colonized in this pregnancy rises from the background incidence of 21% to around 38%. However, the risk of early onset neonatal GBS only rises from 0.5/1000 to 0.9/1000 births and therefore the guidance is to only offer antibiotics to women with a previously affected child.

4.50 A woman is admitted in established labour at 38 weeks with ruptured membranes. Her previous baby developed meningitis after delivery, which was subsequently found to be due to group B streptococcus. Following that delivery she developed a rash when she was given penicillin in the puerperium to prevent her developing endometritis.

F. Prescribe intrapartum IV clindamycin

We frequently meet patients claiming to have a penicillin allergy when in fact they had GI upset or a candida infection following treatment. However, a clear

description of a rash should be taken seriously and the guideline recommends clindamycin as an alternative to benzylpenicillin for women colonized by GBS.
Source: RCOG Green-top guideline number 36. *The Prevention of Early Onset Neonatal Group B Streptococcal Disease.*

This guideline was introduced following a Cochrane review and discussion by the UK National Screening Committee, as it is routine practice to screen for group B streptococcal colonization in the USA. The review concluded that it was not necessary to copy the USA in this regard, but that women who are at higher risk of colonization should be offered IV penicillin in labour (clindamycin if they are allergic to penicillin).

Curriculum module 5: Answers

MULTIPLE CHOICE QUESTIONS

5.1 Concerning maternal mental health in the puerperium:

A. The incidence of puerperal psychosis is 0.02 per 1000 births   F

The incidence is actually much higher than this at two per thousand births.

B. Women who suffer from depression in pregnancy are less likely to breastfeed   T

Babies of mothers who are depressed do less well than their peers, with fewer of them being breastfed and a higher chance of 'failure to thrive'.

C. Psychosis typically presents within the first 90 days postnatally   T

50% present within the first week after birth, 75% within the first six weeks and 90% within 90 days.

D. Suicide is an important preventable cause of maternal death in the UK   T

The mode of suicide in puerperal psychosis is often violent, unlike the way in which women 'normally' kill themselves, i.e. overdose. Unfortunately these mothers commit suicide in such a way that they cannot be rescued. In the 2006–2008 CEMACE Report, 31% of suicide deaths were due to hanging, another 31% due to jumping from a height, whereas only 10% were associated with taking an overdose. However, the overall numbers are small – 29 in that triennium.

E. Less than 1% of recently delivered women will develop a depressive illness   F

The figure is very much higher at 10%.

Source: CEMACE report on maternal deaths in the UK.
Review of postnatal affective disorders. *The Obstetrician and Gynaecologist,* 10(3), 2008.

5.2 A primigravid woman sustains a fourth-degree tear during a normal delivery, which is repaired by the registrar on duty. With regard to her perineal trauma:

A. The tear should be repaired as soon as possible in the delivery room   F
B. There is likely to be damage to the anorectal mucosa   T
C. Laxatives will be needed postpartum   T
D. She should be followed up in secondary care   T
E. She may experience deep dyspareunia as a result   F

A third-degree tear involves damage to the anal sphincter – if the mucosa is involved it is a fourth-degree tear. Although it seems sensible to repair it as soon as possible to avoid unnecessary blood loss, it is important that the repair takes place in theatre with good assistance and adequate lighting. Postnatal laxatives and antibiotic cover are important. At follow-up, if she has symptoms then physiotherapy and possibly imaging of the sphincter is organized. If she does get dyspareunia it will be superficial and not deep (which is due to pathology within the pelvis).

5.3 Potentially fatal causes of maternal pyrexia in the puerperium include:

A.	Endometritis	T
B.	Mastitis	T
C.	Deep vein thrombosis	T
D.	Streptococcal sore throat	T
E.	Breast abscess	T

Maternal mortality reports have underlined the importance of taking puerperal infections seriously and having a low threshold for prescribing antibiotics and referring ill patients back to tertiary care. There has been an increase in the number of deaths from severe infections, especially Group A streptococcal infections originating in the pharynx, which can cause systemic sepsis and death within a few hours of onset. It is recommended that all new mothers are warned about the signs and symptoms of sepsis.

5.4 A woman who delivered her first baby two days ago is having problems breastfeeding because of sore nipples. She is considering bottle feeding instead and the midwife asks you to discuss breastfeeding with the woman. Which of the following statements are true or relevant to her situation?

A.	She should stop breastfeeding until the soreness has resolved	F
B.	Sore nipples mean that she is already developing mastitis	F
C.	She will need antibiotics in order to continue breastfeeding	F
D.	She is not likely to resume menstruation while she is breastfeeding	T
E.	She does not need to use contraception while she is breastfeeding	F

The organism that causes mastitis can enter via cracks or fissures in the nipples but it is important to continue to empty the breast as mastitis is due to milk stasis with superimposed infection. Cracked nipples should be treated with lanolin ointment and breastfeeding continued in order to prevent mastitis.

Full breastfeeding may prevent ovulation but this cannot be relied on for contraception.

5.5 Babies born to mothers who have used cocaine in pregnancy are at increased risk of the following:

A.	Low birthweight	T
B.	Placental abruption	T
C.	Neonatal abstinence (withdrawal) syndrome	F
D.	Nasal septum defect	F
E.	Abnormal brain development	T

Cocaine use in pregnancy is a serious issue for the fetus, causing placental insufficiency and abruption. Recreational drug use is common amongst women of child bearing age and it is possible that they may consult their GP for advice when they find out they are pregnant.

Neonatal abstinence syndrome does not occur in babies exposed to cocaine alone in utero, although they may suffer withdrawal if the cocaine is taken in the context of other drugs of dependence, e.g. heroin.

There is ongoing research into the brain development of babies exposed in utero to cocaine. Several mechanisms are postulated for the abnormal brain development that is seen in those babies.

5.6 You are asked to review a woman who had a forceps delivery of her first baby 12 hours ago after a long labour, because she is keen to go home. The midwives are unhappy to let her leave the hospital because she has not yet passed urine.

With regard to the management of her bladder and urine output:

A. Dehydration is the most likely cause   F
B. She should be catheterized   T
C. A referral to urology is indicated   F
D. The problem is likely to be related to damage to her bladder from the forceps   F
E. She is at risk of long-term voiding problems   T

Retention of urine postpartum may go unrecognized unless midwifery staff are vigilant. Overdistension of the bladder can result in detrusor failure and long-term voiding problems, which could result in the woman having to self-catheterize. Midwives will normally catheterize a woman who has not passed urine by six hours postpartum to prevent this happening. There is no need to involve urology at this stage.

5.7 A woman who had just been delivered by caesarean section weighs 130 kg. She runs an excess risk of the following complications compared with mothers who have a normal BMI:

A. Pulmonary embolus   T
B. Wound infection   T
C. Pressure sore   T
D. Urinary tract infection   F
E. Postpartum haemorrhage   T

Morbid obesity is increasingly challenging maternity services and we have had to modify our protocols and practices to cope with this as these mothers are at increased risk of complications.

Women who have a significant layer of fat are prone to wound infection and also pressure sores because they are less mobile than their slimmer counterparts. Primary postpartum haemorrhage is increased in obese women. Their myometrium seems to behave differently.

In the 2003–2005 maternal mortality reports, more than half the mothers who died were obese and this finding prompted further study of the issue, resulting in the production of a CMACE / RCOG Joint Guideline in 2010 'Management of Women with Obesity in Pregnancy'.

5.8 A woman who is HIV positive has just been delivered of her first baby by caesarean section. With regard to the postnatal care of the neonate:

A. She should be advised against breastfeeding the baby   T
B. The baby should not have any invasive tests such as blood tests   F
C. Cord blood should be sent for viral load   F
D. The baby should receive antiretroviral therapy   T
E. The baby should be isolated from the mother until she has stopped bleeding   F

All neonates should receive antiretroviral therapy within four hours of birth and HIV tests on the baby are performed at day one, six weeks and 12 weeks of age. A confirmatory HIV antibody test is performed at 18 months of age. If these tests are negative (and the baby is not being breastfed) the parents can be informed that the baby is HIV-negative. Breastfeeding doubles the risk of mother-to-child transmission.

Source: RCOG Green-top guideline number 39. *Management of HIV in Pregnancy.*

5.9 You are asked to review a woman on the postnatal ward because the midwives suspect that she has had a pulmonary embolus 48 hours after an emergency caesarean section for slow progress in labour.

Regarding her clinical situation:

A. A renal and liver function test should be requested before commencing anticoagulation treatment   T
B. She should be fully anticoagulated while awaiting the results of tests   T
C. Breathlessness may be the only symptom   T
D. She cannot breastfeed while on heparin   F
E. Anticoagulation should be delayed as it may cause her section wound to bleed   F

If you suspect that a woman has a pulmonary embolus from her history and examination, you should not delay anticoagulation – it can always be stopped if investigations are negative. She is not likely to bleed excessively from anywhere more than six hours after her surgery. The maternal mortality reports highlight how easy it is to misdiagnose thromboembolism and we should be wary if a woman is breathless as this is sometimes the only symptom.

The use of anticoagulant therapy can be influenced by renal and hepatic function so the guideline recommends LFT, U&E and clotting screen before commencing treatment.

Neither heparin nor warfarin is contraindicated during breastfeeding.

Source: RCOG Green-top guideline number 37b. *The Acute Management of Thrombosis and Embolism during Pregnancy and the Puerperium.*

5.10 You are reviewing a woman on the postnatal ward whose first pregnancy was complicated by intrahepatic cholestasis of pregnancy (obstetric cholestasis). Her labour was induced because of it and her baby was born without complications eight hours ago. With regard to her condition:

A. She is likely to have a persistent skin rash as well as severe itching   F
B. The pruritus will have mainly affected her hands and feet   T
C. She should have another liver function test done ten days postpartum   T
D. There is a high recurrence rate of over 50% in subsequent pregnancies   T
E. She should not use a contraceptive method containing estrogen   T

The diagnosis of cholestasis is suspected if the woman has severe itching without a skin rash and is confirmed by finding abnormal liver function and raised bile acid levels. If the levels do not return to normal after delivery then the diagnosis is not cholestasis but repeat measurements should be deferred until at least ten days after delivery because there is often an initial transient rise in liver enzymes postpartum. The recurrence risk is very high (up to 90% in some studies) and a postnatal follow-up appointment should be offered to discuss this as well as checking that her liver function has returned to normal and sorting out contraception.

Source: RCOG Green-top guideline number 43. *Obstetric Cholestasis.*

SINGLE BEST ANSWER QUESTIONS

5.11 A woman has just delivered her second baby yesterday and requests sterilization before she goes home. Her partner is not keen for her to have this done as he is having trouble coping with their toddler and wants her to go home immediately. While you are counselling her about puerperal sterilization, which of the following statements is correct about this situation?

A. **Clip sterilization is more likely to fail as the fallopian tubes are thicker**
B. If she is sterilized now it will take longer for the uterus to involute
C. Laparoscopic sterilization is feasible immediately postpartum
D. Puerperal sterilization requires the written consent of both partners
E. She should defer the decision 24 hours for further discussion to avoid regret

Puerperal sterilization is feasible but not via the laparoscope as the fundus of the uterus is still high – a 'mini-laparotomy' will be needed with the incision just below the umbilicus to reach both the tubes. The failure rate is higher as it is more difficult to get the whole fallopian tube securely included in the clip. The chance of her changing her mind is also higher and it is worth pointing out that if the decision is delayed until after the baby's first birthday, the chance of cot death will have declined and regret is less likely.

5.12 A woman is recovering on the postnatal ward following an emergency caesarean section. On the third day she complains of discomfort and swelling in her right leg, which is clearly larger than the left leg, with a tender calf. The most appropriate medication while awaiting the results of further investigation is:

A. Enoxaparin 20 mg daily
B. Enoxaparin 40 mg daily
C. **Enoxaparin 1 mg per kg twice daily**
D. TED stockings
E. Loading dose of warfarin

You need to protect her against VTE while you are awaiting the results of investigations. The first two doses in the list above are prophylactic rather than treatment so this is not enough heparin. In pregnancy the advice is still to give twice daily treatment doses despite the change in management for non-pregnant patients on medical wards to use once-daily treatment doses. It is better to use heparin rather than warfarin as it is easier to manage and TED stockings alone are not enough.

5.13 You are called to the obstetric postnatal ward to see a recently delivered patient with a swelling on her vulva. The delivery was normal and she had an episiotomy sutured by the midwife four hours ago. She seems to be in severe discomfort and cannot pass urine. The most likely diagnosis is:

A. Acute herpes infection of the vulva
B. **Paravaginal haematoma**
C. Bartholin's abscess
D. Thrombosed haemorrhoid
E. An infection in the episiotomy wound

Paravaginal haematomas usually develop slowly during the first couple of hours after delivery and are extremely painful. There may be a large amount of blood in the haematoma by the time it presents with vulval swelling as most of the haematoma is in the paravaginal space and will not be noticed unless you digitally examine the vagina.

Although acute herpes infection can cause retention of urine it would be unusual for it to present in the immediate postpartum period; it would have been noticed in labour, as would a Bartholin's abscess. A thrombosed pile is unlikely to cause retention of urine, although retention sometimes happens just due to pain, e.g. after a posterior repair operation.

5.14 A community midwife asks you to attend a home delivery because she cannot determine the sex of the baby. On examination the newborn infant is well but the genitalia are ambiguous with a small phallus and some scrotal-like development of the skin. Bilateral swellings palpable in the inguinal canals might be gonads. Which is the most appropriate course of action?

A. Advise the parents to choose a name that could be either male or female

B. Reassure the parents that the child is male with undescended testes

C. Send a referral letter to paediatric clinic so karyotyping can be arranged

D. Send the baby into hospital for urgent paediatric review

E. Take the baby's blood for 17-hydroxyprogesterone levels

This baby is likely to be a girl with congenital adrenal hyperplasia due to 21-hydroxylase deficiency. The ambiguous genitalia are due to exposure to high levels of androgen in utero.

Although there will be high levels of 17-hydroxyprogesterone in the baby's blood, it is important to check that the baby does not have the salt-losing form of this condition, which can lead to severe dehydration and death so hospital admission is advisable.

5.15 A woman consults you in surgery about feeling very low in mood for the last four weeks. She is experiencing bouts of crying, is off her food and having trouble sleeping. She delivered her first baby six weeks ago and is very upset that she has had to give up breastfeeding as she felt unable to cope.

What is the most appropriate course of action to deal with her symptoms?

A. Suggest that she takes an antidepressant and monitor her progress

B. Inform her that her symptoms are very common and will resolve shortly

C. Inform her that she has a mental illness and should see a psychiatrist

D. Admit her urgently to a 'mother and baby unit'

E. Refer to a breastfeeding counsellor

This woman clearly has a mild depressive illness and it is not just about the breastfeeding. However she does not need formal psychiatric input at this stage.

5.16 You have just finished assisting at a difficult caesarean section during which the woman sustained a massive haemorrhage. She is at present on the High Dependency Unit having a blood transfusion but her condition seems to have stabilized and her husband is at her bedside looking after the newborn baby. His mother came into hospital with them but only one person was allowed into the operating theatre with her. In the hospital coffee bar you meet the mother-in-law, who is anxiously waiting for news and asks you why the delivery is taking so long.

You have to deal with her enquiry but what should you tell her?

A. That the mother and baby are both fine

B. That she is not on labour ward but you are not allowed to tell her why

C. That you will send the husband to give her information

D. The delivery has been complicated but everything is all right now

E. To go to the High Dependency Unit to see the new mother and baby

This is an ethical challenge. It is a breach of confidentiality even to acknowledge that the patient is in the hospital but the mother-in-law came in with her, so it is slightly ridiculous to pretend otherwise. However you are absolutely not allowed to give her any information – family dynamics can sometimes be surprisingly awkward – and the safest thing to do is to send the husband to tell his mother what is going on.

5.17 The highest risk factor for the occurrence of puerperal psychosis is:

A. A history of postnatal depression in a previous pregnancy

B. A previous history of bipolar disorder

C. Eating disorder as a teenager

D. Family history of puerperal psychosis

E. Personality disorder

A family history of puerperal psychosis is a risk factor but the highest risk is for those patients with a personal history of severe mental illness (which gives about a 50% chance of developing puerperal psychosis).

Source: SIGN guideline number 127. *Management of Perinatal Mood Disorders, 2012.*

5.18 On the evening shift you go to the postnatal ward and find that the midwives have been waiting for you to complete a list of prescribing tasks they have been saving up. Which one takes priority?

A. A woman who delivered a stillborn baby this morning is waiting for a prescription for cabergoline to suppress lactation

B. A woman who had a caesarean section three days ago is ready to be discharged and is awaiting a prescription for analgesic drugs to take home

C. A woman who has just been readmitted with puerperal sepsis is waiting for antibiotics. Her temperature is 35.8 °C, BP 90/60 mmHg and pulse 120 bpm

D. A woman who suffered a major postpartum haemorrhage yesterday is waiting for you to prescribe a blood transfusion. Her haemoglobin is 60 g/l

E. A woman who had an emergency caesarean section two hours ago is waiting for a prescription of low molecular weight heparin prophylaxis

The woman with sepsis is urgent because her clinical condition is serious, as evidenced by her low temperature and blood pressure. She shouldn't even be on the postnatal ward and transferring her to a high-dependency ward would be a priority too. She should get her antibiotics immediately as she may deteriorate rapidly.

Source: RCOG Green-top guideline number 64b. *Bacterial Sepsis following Pregnancy.*

5.19 A 34-year-old primigravid Jehovah's Witness signed an advance directive refusing blood transfusion when she first booked for antenatal care. She has just been readmitted a week postpartum with a massive haemorrhage and is on the operating table where the consultant is having difficulty stopping the bleeding. Her haemoglobin is currently 30 g/l and her life hangs in the balance. Which of the following statements is correct with regard to the management of this situation?

A. Her husband can give consent for her to have a blood transfusion

B. Transfuse her without consent because it is in her best interests

C. Get an emergency court order to transfuse

D. Respect advance directive and withhold transfusion

E. Transfuse her own blood from the cell saver

Unfortunately there is nothing you can do if she has signed an advanced directive unless you can prove that she was not of sound mind when she did that. This must be one of the most distressing situations medical staff can find themselves in but she cannot be rescued by a blood transfusion.

5.20 This morning a woman was delivered of her first baby using forceps because of fetal distress in the second stage of labour. The baby is doing fine but the mother sustained a third-degree tear which has been repaired by your consultant. When debriefing her about the third-degree tear, which of the following statements is true?

A. The tear will have involved the anal mucosa as well as the sphincter muscle

B. She will be given antibiotics and laxatives postpartum

C. She is very likely to be incontinent of flatus in the future

D. If she has another baby she will need a caesarean section

E. Third-degree tears do not occur with normal deliveries

Third-degree tears usually heal very well and it is uncommon for women to have problems with anal incontinence afterwards. Studies show that 60 to 80% of women are asymptomatic at 12 months postpartum. These tears can happen during a normal birth but are more common with assisted delivery (forceps more so than ventouse). We are uncertain how to advise women to deliver in the next pregnancy and some obstetricians only advise caesarean if she has residual symptoms after the previous repair. There is a paucity of research evidence in this area.

Source: RCOG Green-top guidelines number 26, *Operative Vaginal Delivery*, and number 29, *The Management of Third- and Fourth-degree Perineal Tears*.

EXTENDED MATCHING QUESTIONS

A.	Combined oral contraceptive pill
B.	Condoms
C.	Copper intrauterine device
D.	Depot medroxy progesterone acetate
E.	Diaphragm
F.	Female sterilization
G.	Levonorgestrel intrauterine system
H.	Progesterone-only pill
I.	Spermicide gel
J.	Vasectomy

The clinical scenarios below describe mothers requesting contraceptive advice in the postpartum period. Select the most appropriate method of contraception for each woman.

Each option may be used once, more than once or not at all.

5.21 Having just delivered her first baby a 15-year-old schoolgirl is very keen to avoid getting pregnant again.

D. Depot medroxy progesterone acetate

LARCs (long-acting reversible contraception) are recommended for teenagers as they need secure contraception. The best option from the list is to give her depot medroxy progesterone acetate, which you would review after two years. In the long term she would do well to consider an implant.

5.22 A 40-year-old woman who was delivered by caesarean section yesterday has now had two children. She wishes to start secure contraception immediately before she leaves hospital but does not want to rule out having another child in the future.

H. Progesterone-only pill

If she wants to start contraception immediately this rules out the various IUCDs because they cannot be inserted until the uterus has healed. As she is over 35 years, the POP is a safer option than the combined pill although she may opt for that if the side effects of the POP become a problem. The COC would also add to the risk of DVT, which is high because of her age and recent pregnancy as well as the caesarean section.

5.23 An overweight 35-year-old woman with a BMI of 45 attends for her postnatal check-up with her first baby. She conceived after IVF treatment because of infertility due to polycystic ovarian syndrome. She still has some frozen embryos in storage but does not want to conceive again just yet as she has been advised to lose a lot of weight first.

G. Levonorgestrel intrauterine system

This patient is at risk of endometrial hyperplasia due to her PCO and if she wishes to use contraception a levonorgestrel IUS is a good idea because it will protect her against that problem until she is ready to conceive again.

5.24 Having used the pill with no problems in the past, a 25-year-old wishes to restart contraception after delivering her first baby a week ago. She had a normal delivery, her lochia is normal and she is successfully breastfeeding.

H. Progesterone-only pill

She is likely to be keen to use the pill again but will need the POP instead of the combined pill while she is breastfeeding. Exogenous estrogen interferes with milk production.

5.25 A woman who used to suffer from premenstrual syndrome wishes to have a secure form of contraception after delivering her first baby. She has decided that she is very sensitive to hormones and requests a method that does not involve using hormones.

C. Copper intrauterine device

The only secure method of contraception without hormones on the list is the copper coil. Barrier methods have too high a Pearl index to be described as secure.

A.	Arrange a district nurse to supervise dressings
B.	Arrange a visit from a breastfeeding peer support group
C.	Arrange readmission to the obstetric unit for review

D.	Arrange urgent admission to the emergency medical ward
E.	Ask the community midwife to visit at home
F.	Prescribe broad-spectrum antibiotics
G.	Send her in to A&E
H.	Take the sutures out and allow the wound to drain

These clinical scenarios describe recently delivered women who have developed complications. In each case, select the most appropriate management plan.

Each option may be used once, more than once or not at all.

5.26 A woman who had a caesarean section two days ago was discharged home yesterday. She has asked for a home visit this morning because there is copious sero-sanguinous fluid discharging from the wound.

C. Arrange readmission to the obstetric unit for review

The nature of the discharge suggests the possibility of wound dehiscence although it could be a wound infection or haematoma about to discharge: this patient needs reviewing at the hospital.

5.27 Two days after a normal delivery, a primiparous women telephones the surgery to report heavy vaginal bleeding with clots.

C. Arrange readmission to the obstetric unit for review

This patient either has retained products of conception or endometritis or both. She needs readmission and possibly an evacuation of uterus.

5.28 You are asked to do a home visit to look at the caesarean wound of a patient who has been out of hospital for four days. She has an absorbable subcuticular suture *in situ* in the skin and there is a spreading cellulitis around the scar.

F. Prescribe broad-spectrum antibiotics

This is a superficial spreading wound infection rather than an abscess. Antibiotics should resolve the problem providing they will cover staph aureus. The distractor is H., 'take the sutures out'.

5.29 A primiparous patient who delivered four days ago is having problems with breastfeeding due to pain. On examination her nipples are cracked and sore but there is no unusual swelling of the breasts.

E. Ask the community midwife to visit at home

Cracked nipples are very painful and this woman is going to need extra help to continue breastfeeding. Peer support can be very helpful but she is likely to need clinical help until the situation improves. It is not an abscess so she does not need admission. It is not mastitis so she does not need antibiotics.

5.30 The community midwife is doing a home visit for a woman who has been discharged from hospital two days after a forceps delivery. She is struggling with breastfeeding and has asked for help. The midwife telephones you because she has noticed that the woman's left leg is swollen.

C. Arrange readmission to the obstetric unit for review

She probably has a DVT so she needs to go back into hospital for investigation and anticoagulation. As she is trying to establish breastfeeding, she will want to take the baby in with her and the obstetric unit is more likely to admit her baby too.

A.	Blood transfusion
B.	Evacuation of retained products of conception
C.	Examination under anaesthetic
D.	Full blood count
E.	Intravenous antibiotics
F.	Norethisterone 5 mg tds
G.	Oral antibiotics
H.	Pelvic ultrasound scan
I.	Reassure the patient
J.	Resuture the perineum

The clinical scenarios below relate to women in the puerperium with problems following a vaginal delivery. For each scenario select the most appropriate course of action from the list above.

Each option may be used once, more than once or not at all.

5.31 You are seeing a 24-year-old woman in your GP surgery for her postnatal check. She had a normal vaginal delivery six weeks ago with a small second-degree perineal tear. She is breastfeeding and is feeling well. She tells you that she still has a pink loss vaginally but there have been no clots and the loss is not offensive.

I. Reassure the patient

Lochia is a red loss initially, then becomes red/brown followed by pink and finally becomes a white discharge. The mean duration of lochia is 24 days but 13% of women will still have pink or red lochia at eight weeks postpartum. Unless the lochia is increasing in amount, is associated with clots or is offensive then this is unlikely to indicate infection or retained products of conception so the patient can be reassured that it will settle spontaneously.

5.32 You are the junior obstetric doctor on-call overnight and at midnight are asked to see a woman who has been readmitted three days after the delivery of her third child. Over the last few hours her lochia has become heavier and she is passing clots vaginally. Her observations are: pulse 90 bpm, blood pressure 125/85, temperature 37.5 °C, respiratory rate 14. The midwife has already taken a high vaginal swab.

E. Intravenous antibiotics

The change in her lochia associated with a pyrexia and tachycardia suggests that she has either sepsis or retained placental tissue. The initial management is to treat aggressively with intravenous antibiotics. She does also need an ultrasound scan but this should be done by an experienced practitioner. It is unlikely that this would be available out of hours so this isn't the correct answer. A full blood count could be helpful but the scenario above is one of sepsis rather than postpartum haemorrhage which is why IV antibiotics is the correct answer here.

5.33 The midwives ask you to review a woman on the postnatal ward one day after delivery. She had a right mediolateral episiotomy which was repaired by the registrar and now she is complaining of severe perineal pain so she can't sit comfortably. On examination her temperature is 36.5 °C, pulse 75 bpm, blood pressure 110/65. The episiotomy sutures are intact and the perineum is bruised with a 3 cm swelling underlying the sutures. The vaginal sutures are also intact and there is no swelling in the vagina.

G. Oral antibiotics

Perineal haematomas usually present within 24 hours of delivery. This is a small haematoma as it is less than 5 cm and therefore, unless it is rapidly enlarging, it is likely to resolve spontaneously. The blood is an obvious focus for infection, hence the need to treat with oral antibiotics. The indications for taking the woman to theatre are if the haematoma is large, if she is haemodynamically unstable or if the haematoma is infected.

5.34 Eight hours after delivery a woman who has just arrived on the postnatal ward suddenly starts to bleed heavily per vaginam, losing another 200 ml on top of the 300 ml estimated blood loss at delivery. Her predelivery haemoglobin done on admission in labour was 115 g/l. The notes indicate that the placenta was removed in pieces after the cord came off during controlled cord traction.

B. Evacuation of retained products of conception

It is likely that there is still some placental tissue in this woman's uterus and if nothing is done to remove it, she is likely to bleed again. Having experienced a blood loss of 500 ml in total, she is unlikely to need blood transfusion unless she continues to bleed and the point of evacuating the uterus is to stop her bleeding. Ultrasound scan will not help here.

5.35 A woman is readmitted by her community midwife because she is worried about the appearance of the perineal wound a week after delivery. On examination you find that the wound has broken down and the tissues are covered in a sloughy yellow-green exudate, which smells offensive.

G. Oral antibiotics

If the wound is resutured while it is infected like this, it will not heal and will break down again. It is best to let it heal by secondary intention and the oral antibiotics will speed this process.

A.	Bimanual pressure to compress the uterus
B.	Controlled cord traction (Brandt–Andrews method)
C.	Ergometrine 500 milligrams IM
D.	Evacuation of uterus
E.	Inject carboprost (Hemabate®) into the uterus
F.	IV infusion of 40 units of oxytocin over four hours

G.	IV dose of 40 units of oxytocin stat
H.	Manual removal of placenta
I.	Place a Bakri balloon into the uterine cavity

Each of these obstetric patients has either bled heavily after delivery or is at risk of doing so and this question refers to the prevention or treatment of postpartum haemorrhage. Choose the most appropriate management plan for each woman.

Each option may be used once, more than once or not at all.

5.36 A 35-year-old woman has just had an emergency caesarean section for failure to progress in labour and the baby weighed 4.8 kg. During the delivery the blood loss was estimated at nearly a litre but she is no longer bleeding actively. As they are suturing the skin at the end of the operation, the registrar asks you to prescribe something in order to keep the uterus contracted.

F. IV infusion of 40 units of oxytocin over four hours

Ergometrine does have a sustained effect compared with oxytocin but in this case we want the effect to last much longer so the four-hour option is best.

5.37 A woman has delivered her third baby at home two hours ago but the community midwife has transferred her in to hospital because she has not been able to deliver the placenta in spite of active management of the third stage. There is quite a big blood clot in the bed, which amounts to about 600 ml.

H. Manual removal of placenta

The distractor answer here is controlled cord traction but the midwife will already have been doing this and failed. As it is two hours since delivery and she has already lost quite a bit of blood she needs to go to theatre urgently for manual removal of placenta.

5.38 A woman is urgently brought back to labour ward six hours after a normal delivery because she suddenly bleeds heavily vaginally, losing 500 ml in a couple of minutes. Looking through her previous notes you see that a succenturiate lobe was mentioned on her anomaly scan at 21 weeks gestation.

D. Evacuation of uterus

Unless the succenturiate lobe was found at delivery it is probably still in the uterus so this woman needs an evacuation.

5.39 You are the only doctor on labour ward when a woman who was being induced for pre-eclampsia unexpectedly starts pushing and rapidly delivers the baby and placenta. She has a brisk postpartum haemorrhage of 500 ml. She has already had ten units of oxytocin given as the baby was delivering and you have put up an oxytocin infusion with another 40 units so she is now nearing the maximum dose. The registrar is in the gynaecology emergency theatre dealing with a woman in extremis due to a ruptured ectopic pregnancy and you are waiting for the obstetric consultant to arrive from home. She continues to bleed heavily, so you must select the best course of action to save her life.

A. Bimanual pressure to compress the uterus

This is an emergency situation where squashing the uterus between your hands can slow the bleeding down for long enough for the consultant to arrive and take over. Compressing the uterus against the sacrum abdominally may also have the same effect. You cannot give her ergometrine because it can cause an uncontrolled rise in her blood pressure (although if you don't stop this woman bleeding, her blood pressure is going to drop dramatically shortly).

5.40 The midwives ask you to put up an intravenous infusion on a woman who is bleeding heavily after delivery of her placenta. You are sure the bleeding is coming from the uterus but every time the senior midwife stops massaging the uterus the bleeding starts again. You are having trouble getting a cannula into a vein so you send for the anaesthetist and ask the midwife to continue rubbing the fundus. The registrar is on the way but you need to give something quickly to make the uterus contract.

C. Ergometrine 500 milligrams IM

As you have not yet got IV access, intramuscular ergometrine is the obvious answer. We do also use carboprost but IM, not directly into the uterus.

A.	Arterial blood gas
B.	Blood cultures
C.	CT pulmonary angiogram
D.	CT brain
E.	Chest x-ray
F.	D-dimer
G.	Electrophoresis
H.	Haemoglobin
I.	Liver function test daily until results are normal
J.	Liver function test ten days after delivery
K.	Liver ultrasound
L.	Lumbar puncture
M.	Pelvic x-ray
N.	Pulmonary V/Q scan

These clinical scenarios relate to postpartum women with complicated pregnancies experiencing problems or seeking advice after delivery. For each woman, select the most appropriate initial investigation that will help you make a diagnosis.

Each option may be used once, more than once or not at all.

5.41 You are asked to see an unwell 27-year-old woman on the postnatal ward who delivered yesterday. She is complaining of a fronto-occipital headache which is so severe that she can hardly move and is associated with nausea. She had an epidural in labour which was initially ineffective and while it was being resited the dura was inadvertently punctured. Her temperature is 38 °C.

L. Lumbar puncture

Although the most likely cause of this woman's headache is a so-called 'spinal headache' she might also have meningitis. If there are no indicators of infection, she could have a 'blood patch' done to stop the CSF leak, which will cure her headache. The distractor is CT brain.

5.42 A woman whose labour was induced for obstetric cholestasis has returned home from hospital and you are asked to review her by the community midwife. She asks you what tests she needs now that the baby is safely delivered.

J. Liver function test ten days after delivery

The diagnosis of cholestasis is made if the liver function tests return to normal after delivery and other causes such as hepatitis have been ruled out. The distractor is daily liver function tests and ultrasound of liver (which will already have been done antenatally to rule out gallstones etc.).

Source: RCOG Green-top guideline number 43. *Obstetric Cholestasis.*

5.43 A woman with sickle cell disease is on the postnatal ward after a caesarean section for the delivery of her first baby. She complains of pain at the top of her right leg near the hip joint and cannot stand up comfortably. There is no swelling of either leg on examination.

M. Pelvic x-ray

Women with sickle cell disease are at risk of avascular necrosis of the femoral head, although you would be initially concerned about the possibility of deep vein thrombosis or sickle crisis. Having had a caesarean section, she is likely to be fully anticoagulated for six weeks prophylactically.

Source: RCOG Green-top guideline number 61. *Management of Sickle Cell Disease in Pregnancy.*

5.44 Following an unsuccessful attempt at induction of labour over three days, a primigravid woman has an emergency caesarean section at 42 weeks gestation. The baby has been admitted to the Special Care Baby Unit (SCBU) with meconium aspiration and you are asked by the SCBU staff to review the mother there the following day because she has become increasingly short of breath.

A. Arterial blood gas

Postoperative pulmonary embolism (PE) is still a major cause of death in pregnant women. A woman with risk factors should be commenced on treatment dosage of low molecular weight heparin if there is a suspicion of a PE while awaiting further investigation. The symptoms and signs can be subtle such as shortness of breath or an unexplained tachycardia and a drop in oxygen saturation may be an important clue.

5.45 A primigravid woman has a rather prolonged second stage but achieves a normal delivery of a 4 kg baby after pushing really hard for two hours. Shortly after delivery she becomes progressively short of breath and complains of mild left-sided chest pain on inspiration. On examination there is decreased air entry on the left side of her chest. Her midwife brings the saturation probe from theatre and tells you that her oxygen levels are normal.

E. Chest x-ray

This sounds like a pneumothorax and a chest x-ray is appropriate especially as you already know that her oxygen saturation is normal. The other distractors are the

more expensive chest imaging such as CTPA and V/Q scan used to diagnose pulmonary embolism.

A.	Elective caesarean section at 37 weeks
B.	Elective caesarean section at 39 weeks
C.	External cephalic version
D.	Induce labour before term
E.	Vaginal birth and consider episiotomy
F.	Vaginal birth with CTG monitoring
G.	Vaginal birth with oxytocin drip
H.	Take low-dose aspirin 75 mg in pregnancy
I.	Terminate the pregnancy

These clinical scenarios relate to women who have recently delivered and have returned to the hospital postnatal clinic for debriefing. In each case, select the most appropriate advice with regard to her next pregnancy.

Each option may be used once, more than once or not at all.

5.46 After being induced for severe pre-eclampsia at 34 weeks gestation, a primigravid woman is delivered by emergency caesarean section for fetal distress at 8 cm dilatation. She is thinking of embarking on another pregnancy in about a year's time as her husband is keen to have another baby soon.

H. Take low-dose aspirin 75 mg in pregnancy

Although you need to have the discussion about VBAC with this woman, it would be beneficial to try and prevent her getting early onset pre-eclampsia again as she is more likely to have a vaginal birth if the pregnancy is uncomplicated and the baby well grown. The distractor is vaginal birth with monitoring.

5.47 After a very prolonged first stage of labour, the registrar unsuccessfully attempts a forceps delivery in theatre for a primigravid woman who has been pushing for two hours. The position of the baby's head was occipito-anterior at the ischial spines with moulding ++. A caesarean section was performed after three strong pulls, during which there was no descent of the fetal head. The baby weighed 3.8 kg and was two weeks overdue.

B. Elective caesarean section at 39 weeks

The clinical details here are suggestive of cephalopelvic disproportion, which may well recur in a subsequent pregnancy unless she spontaneously labours early for some reason. The distractor is induction of labour before term but we prefer not to induce women with section scars as the drugs used increase the risk of scar rupture.

If she did present in spontaneous labour before term in her next pregnancy, she could attempt a vaginal birth with continuous monitoring.

5.48 Half way through her labour, when the membranes ruptured at 5 cm dilatation, a primigravid woman was found to have a breech presentation and therefore had her first baby delivered by caesarean section. You note from the operation notes that there was a bicornuate uterus, which might lead to another breech presentation next pregnancy. Choose the best course of action if the next baby is breech too.

B. Elective caesarean section at 39 weeks

The distractor is external cephalic version which is contraindicated when there is a major uterine malformation and relatively contraindicated if there is a scar on the uterus.

Source: RCOG Green-top guideline number 20a. *External Cephalic Version (ECV) and Reducing the Incidence of Breech Presentation;* 2006, reviewed 2010.

5.49 During a forceps delivery performed for fetal distress, a primigravid woman sustains a third-degree tear. At her follow-up appointment it has healed well and she has made a full recovery with no symptoms related to the anal sphincter. She wishes to discuss plans for her next birth.

E. Vaginal birth and consider episiotomy

We are actually unsure as to how to advise women who have sustained a third-degree tear previously. If she has residual symptoms such as faecal incontinence, most obstetricians would suggest elective section but there is no hard evidence to back up that opinion – it is merely a worry that next time a repeat third-degree tear might make things worse. A compromise (also not evidence-based) is to offer an elective episiotomy next time.

Source: RCOG Green-top guideline number 29. *The Management of Third- and Fourth-degree Perineal Tears.*

5.50 Having reached 8 cm cervical dilation in her first labour, a primigravid woman was delivered by emergency caesarean section because of a fetal bradycardia associated with fresh vaginal bleeding. The labour was progressing well up to that point but unfortunately the bradycardia turned out to be due to placental abruption and the baby did not survive. She does not feel strong enough to contemplate another pregnancy just yet, but is wondering about the mode of delivery next time.

F. Vaginal birth with CTG monitoring

This is slightly difficult because we might be considering induction before term (as soon as the baby's head is safely engaged in the pelvis, reducing the risk of cord prolapse) in a woman who had suffered a placental abruption before. However, induction will increase the risk of scar rupture so the correct answer here is vaginal birth with monitoring, which is safer if labour is spontaneous rather than induced.

Curriculum module 6: Answers

MULTIPLE CHOICE QUESTIONS

6.1 The following gynaecological problems can present with intermenstrual bleeding:

A.	Genital chlamydia infection	T
B.	Nabothian follicle on the cervix	F
C.	Subserous fibroids	F
D.	Granulosa cell tumour of the ovary	T
E.	Endometrial polyp	T

Chlamydia causes cervicitis, which can make the cervix bleed. The ovarian granulosa cell tumour secretes estrogen, which can cause the endometrium to become unstable or even hyperplastic so that the woman bleeds erratically. Endometrial polyps are affected by the hormonal changes of the menstrual cycle but tend to be a bit more fragile than normal endometrium and can bleed at any time.

6.2 An asymptomatic nulliparous 39-year-old woman attends for a routine cervical smear and the practice nurse discovers a large pelvic mass making the cervix difficult to access. The following are possible differential diagnoses for this mass:

A.	Uterine fibroid	T
B.	Diverticular abscess	F
C.	Ovarian cyst	T
D.	Urethral diverticulum	F
E.	Haematocolpos	F

An asymptomatic mass in the pelvis (and it is likely to be asymptomatic as this is a routine smear) is either a fibroid or an ovarian cyst. It is not uncommon for a practice nurse to find such a mass, especially if it makes the cervix difficult to get at, although they do not routinely do bimanual examinations. A diverticular abscess would be tender on examination and diverticular disease is uncommon in women in their 30s anyway. A urethral diverticulum can be found on the anterior wall of the vagina rather than in the pelvis. Haematocolpos refers to a vagina full of blood due to an intact hymen and presents at menarche.

6.3 Bacterial vaginosis:

A.	Causes vaginal discharge with a characteristic fishy smell	T
B.	Is associated with pruritus and vulvovaginitis	F
C.	Is associated with a lowered vaginal pH	F
D.	May be treated with metronidazole	T
E.	Should be treated if detected during pregnancy	T

The main reason for treating bacterial vaginosis in pregnancy is that it can cause miscarriage or premature labour. One of the ways of preventing or treating it is to lower the pH of the vagina using acid jelly. Clindamycin cream and metronidazole are effective treatments. It does not usually cause irritation.

6.4   Women with polycystic ovarian syndrome:

A.   Are always overweight   F

B.   May develop gestational diabetes   T

C.   Cannot conceive without ovulation induction   F

D.   Are more likely to miscarry than women without the syndrome   T

E.   During an IVF cycle are more likely to develop hyperstimulation
       syndrome   T

A history of PCO is a good reason for organizing a GTT in pregnancy. Unfortunately there is no PCO treatment that reduces the increased risk of miscarriage. Many women with PCO conceive spontaneously but some need help, e.g. clomifene, gonadotrophins, metformin or ovarian drilling.

6.5   Regarding hormone replacement therapy (HRT):

A.   It should be offered to patients with premature ovarian failure   T

B.   Protects against unwanted pregnancy in perimenopausal women   F

C.   The incidence of cardiovascular disease is reduced in the first year of use F

D.   Is first-line management in a patient at risk of osteoporosis   F

E.   The risk of breast cancer returns to baseline five years after stopping HRT T

Women with premature ovarian failure should be offered HRT until the natural age of the menopause. The dose of hormones is not contraceptive and perimenopausal women on HRT should also use a non-hormonal method of contraception such as barrier or coil. It used to be advised in patients at risk of osteoporosis but this is no longer the case because of the cardiovascular and breast cancer risks of long-term use and the advice is to use the lowest possible dose for the shortest possible time.

6.6   A 29-year-old woman attends surgery complaining of urinary leakage on coughing since the birth of her first son 14 months ago. On examination there is demonstrable stress incontinence but no vaginal wall prolapse and urodynamic study shows a stable bladder. The following are appropriate treatments to consider in her case:

A.   Duloxetine tablets   T

B.   Oxybutynin tablets   F

C.   Bladder drill (retraining)   F

D.   Pelvic floor muscle training   T

E.   Pelvic floor repair operation   F

This patient has genuine stress incontinence and oxybutynin and bladder drill are all treatments designed for unstable bladder. She does not have a prolapse so pelvic floor surgery is not indicated.

6.7   Features of premenstrual syndrome include:

A.   Occurrence in anovulatory cycles   F

B.   Relief of symptoms at menstruation   T

C.   An association with dysmenorrhoea   F

D.   Abnormally high progesterone levels   F

E. Cyclical pelvic pain F

Most gynaecologists believe that PMS represents an abnormal sensitivity to normal levels of progesterone in the second half of the menstrual cycle and by definition it should not occur in cycles where there is no ovulation.

Source: RCOG Green-top guideline number 48. *Management of Premenstrual Syndrome.*

6.8 A woman from Somalia brings her four-year-old daughter to paediatric A&E as she has become acutely unwell on return from a holiday to visit family back home. The child seems to be unable to talk and is sweaty, shivering and incontinent of urine. You can see that there is blood on her pyjamas.

The following conditions should be considered in the differential diagnosis:

A. Genital mutilation T
B. Malaria T
C. Sexual abuse T
D. Tetanus T
E. Urinary tract infection T

It is quite common for families from countries where female genital mutilation is practised to take their small daughters back to have this procedure done as it is illegal in this country. We should have a low threshold for suspecting it, and tetanus is one of the possible sequelae as it is usually performed in primitive conditions.

6.9 The following are features of human papilloma virus infection:

A. Koilocytes on a cervical biopsy T
B. Genital warts T
C. Intermenstrual bleeding F
D. Painful ulcers on the vulva F
E. Cervical stenosis F

Human papilloma virus causes cervical cancer, CIN or genital warts – depending on the subtype. Painful ulcers on the vulva will be herpes, not HPV. Both wart virus and CIN on the cervix are asymptomatic.

6.10 In your GP surgery you see a woman aged 32 with severe premenstrual syndrome (premenstrual dysphoric syndrome). She has regular periods which are not heavy and does not need contraception because her husband has had a vasectomy. She is hoping for a solution for her mood changes.

The following treatments have been shown to be effective in PMS:

A. Transdermal estradiol F
B. Progesterone given in the luteal phase of the menstrual cycle F
C. Psychological treatment in the form of cognitive behavioural therapy (CBT) T
D. Combined oral contraceptive pill T
E. Selective serotonin reuptake inhibitors (SSRIs) given in the luteal phase T

If considering any hormonal treatment, the idea is to wipe out cyclical changes as PMS is thought to be a result of hypersensitivity to normal cyclical progesterone levels. Transdermal estradiol cannot be given on its own to a woman with an intact uterus in case she develops endometrial hyperplasia.

Source: RCOG Green-top guideline number 48. *Management of Premenstrual Syndrome.*

SINGLE BEST ANSWER QUESTIONS

6.11 A 68-year-old woman with a BMI of 30 presents to her GP with a history of urinary urgency and frequency almost every hour with occasional urge incontinence. She has to wear a pad all the time and rarely leaves the house as a result. Vaginal examination reveals no prolapse and urinalysis is negative. Which one of the following management options is most likely to ameliorate her symptoms?

A. Colposuspension operation

B. Electrical stimulation of pelvic floor muscle

C. Weight loss

D. Prescription of duloxetine

E. Bladder drill (retraining)

This patient probably has detrusor instability from the symptoms, although you are not told the results of a bladder pressure study (which would be the next step if you were looking after this woman because the bladder is an unreliable witness).

Colposuspension and duloxetine are treatments for genuine stress incontinence. Pelvic floor physiotherapy (including electrical stimulation) and weight loss may help but the best treatment here for instability is bladder drill.

6.12 A 38-year-old woman attended for a routine cervical smear during which an asymptomatic polyp is noted on the surface of the cervix. The result of the smear was normal. In counselling her about the polyp, which one of the following statements is true?

A. It could be caused by chlamydia

B. It is unlikely to be associated with endometrial pathology

C. It is most likely to be a nabothian follicle

D. It is associated with human papilloma virus infection

E. It should be removed because it is likely to be malignant

If the polyp is obviously an endometrial polyp – bright red and coming through the cervix instead of being on the surface – then there might be further polyps within the uterus. Cervical polyps are usually benign and not associated with endometrial problems. Nabothian follicles sit within the substance of the cervix; they are mucus retention cysts.

6.13 When you are on-call for gynaecological emergencies in your hospital, you are frequently asked to organize management for women attending the Early Pregnancy Clinic. Which one of these statements is correct with regard to the management of miscarriage?

A. Medical management is associated with an increased incidence of pelvic infection

B. Women having a surgical evacuation should be screened for chlamydia

C. Expectant management is the treatment of choice if the uterus is septic

D. Histological proof that the uterus contained trophoblastic tissue will always exclude ectopic pregnancy

E. Perforation of the uterus during surgical evacuation is more likely in incomplete rather than missed miscarriage

There is a reduction in clinical pelvic infection after medical evacuation compared with surgical (7.1% vs. 13.2% $p < 0.001$). The chance of a patient developing an infection after surgical evacuation with subsequent fertility problems can be

reduced if screening for chlamydia is undertaken routinely. If the uterus is already septic, she is at risk of systemic sepsis and the uterus should be evacuated with antibiotic cover. Ectopic cannot be completely excluded by finding trophoblastic tissue in the uterus, although the chance of a coexistent ectopic and intrauterine pregnancy – heterotopic pregnancy – is rare (somewhere between 1 in 10 000 to 1 in 30 000 pregnancies).

In missed miscarriage the cervix is often tightly closed and difficult to dilate, making perforation of the uterus much more likely during surgical evacuation. Having said that, surgical evacuation is more effective than medical management in this group of patients.

Source: RCOG Green-top guideline number 25. *The Management of Early Pregnancy Loss.*

6.14 You see a woman in clinic with urinary frequency and urgency who you suspect might have overactive bladder (detrusor instability) and counsel her about it. Which of these statements is not correct in this context with regard to detrusor instability?

A. **It can be confidently diagnosed from the history without further investigation**

B. Bladder drill (retraining) is recommended treatment

C. It may be a symptom of multiple sclerosis

D. It will respond to oral anticholinergics

E. It can be improved by pelvic floor exercises

It can be difficult to tell from her symptoms whether the diagnosis is unstable bladder or genuine stress incontinence. The bladder is an unreliable witness. For example, in patients with instability, a cough will provoke a detrusor contraction, which results in urinary leakage. If the woman has mixed symptoms, a bladder pressure study is usually indicated to sort out the diagnosis.

Pelvic floor physiotherapy helps both genuine stress incontinence and instability.

6.15 A routine 'dating' scan arranged by the midwife shows that a primigravid woman has suffered a missed miscarriage. The sac contains a fetus about 9 weeks size but there is no fetal heart pulsation seen. She was not expecting this as she has not had any bleeding at all during the pregnancy, so is extremely upset and would like to deal with the problem as quickly as possible. Which would be the best management plan in her case?

A. Admit to hospital for medical management with methotrexate

B. **Evacuate the uterus with cervical preparation**

C. Expectant management with another scan in two weeks to see if she has miscarried

D. Give 800 micrograms of misoprostol

E. Prescribe mifepristone orally and follow up after two weeks

The quickest way to complete this episode for her is surgical management. Missed miscarriages are different from other miscarriages because there has been no bleeding and often the cervix is tightly closed, being difficult to dilate at evacuation. Expectant management is not as successful compared with incomplete miscarriage and if medical management is chosen the doses of misoprostol prescribed is usually higher (800 micrograms instead of 600). The guidance from NICE recommends that mifepristone should not be offered as treatment. Methotrexate is used for ectopic pregnancy.

Sources: RCOG green top guideline number 25. *The Management of Early Pregnancy Loss.* NICE guideline CG154. *Ectopic Pregnancy and Miscarriage, 2012.*

6.16 A 24-year-old woman whose scan reveals polycystic ovarian syndrome (PCO) consults you about management of her facial hirsutism. Her serum testosterone is within normal limits and she does not wish to conceive. Which of these treatments for PCO is the most appropriate management option?

A. Clomifene citrate
B. Co-cyprindiol combined oral contraceptive pill
C. Cyproterone acetate
D. Metformin
E. Ovarian drilling

Clomifene, metformin and ovarian drilling are all treatments designed to produce ovulation so are used to treat fertility problems. Cyproterone is an antiandrogen which can be used in large doses (when it might cause menstrual irregularity and liver tumours, although it is effective against hirsutism) or small doses in the form of the co-cyprindiol pill – the latter will be more suitable because she needs contraception.

6.17 In your GP surgery you see a diabetic woman aged 49 years who seeks treatment for irregular heavy menstrual bleeding. Her pelvis feels normal on examination and speculum reveals a healthy cervix. Which of the following statements about her management is correct?

A. LH/FSH levels are a useful investigation
B. Serum ferritin should be measured as well as haemoglobin at the first visit
C. She should be referred to gynaecology clinic
D. Testing for coagulation disorders should be done prior to commencing treatment
E. Tranexamic acid can be prescribed as first-line therapy without referral

This woman should be referred because the bleeding is irregular, which makes the chances of serious endometrial pathology higher. Diabetes is a risk factor for endometrial cancer.

It is unlikely that a coagulation disorder will present in this age group – the problem will have been noticed at menarche. The LH and FSH levels do not reliably go up until she has finished menstruating; therefore they are a good test to diagnose premature menopause in a woman with secondary amenorrhoea but do not predict the menopause.

6.18 You are seeing a 48-year-old woman for a preoperative check-up. She is due to have a hysterectomy for fibroids next week and is thinking of having her normal ovaries removed at the same time as the uterus. She wishes to discuss the possible benefits and problems associated with a surgical menopause. Which one of her ideas about the bilateral oophorectomy operation is actually correct?

A. Oophorectomy will not affect her libido
B. She will need sequential HRT to get rid of her menopausal symptoms
C. It will completely prevent her from getting any gynaecological cancer in later life
D. She should consider oophorectomy if her mother had ovarian cancer
E. Oophorectomy will increase the operating time substantially

The loss of the testosterone-producing ovaries could decrease her libido and some women ask for testosterone replacement therapy because of this. She will be able to take estrogen-only HRT instead of sequential HRT (with all its progestogen side effects) as she has no uterus. It will not completely protect her against ovarian cancer as there are patients who develop a condition called primary peritoneal cancer which looks and behaves like ovarian cancer even though their ovaries have been removed. Removing the ovaries does not add anything to the operating time and family history is a strong predisposing factor for ovarian cancer.

6.19 A 23-year-old woman with a BMI of 50 attends your GP surgery to discuss her fertility problems because she and her husband have been trying to conceive for 18 months. She has irregular periods with a cycle varying from 35 to 42 days and the ovulation predictor kits she has purchased from the chemist indicate that she is not ovulating. Her husband has two children from his previous marriage. Which of the following is the most appropriate piece of advice?

A. Continue trying for six more months then you will refer her to infertility clinic
B. Commence taking folic acid 10 mcg daily
C. Make an appointment for her husband to arrange a semen analysis
D. Prescribe clomifene citrate to be taken on days two to six of the cycle
E. To avoid pregnancy until she has lost weight

She is likely to be anovulatory because of her weight, and fertility treatments do not work well in women with such a high BMI. In addition pregnancy poses a great risk to her health when she is at risk of developing problems such as diabetes, hypertension, pre-eclampsia etc. In the recent CMACE maternal mortality report over half the patients who died were morbidly obese.

6.20 A young woman attends her GP's surgery with a positive pregnancy test after seven weeks of amenorrhoea. She is anxious because has suffered two previous early pregnancy losses; a miscarriage at ten weeks followed by an ectopic pregnancy, which was managed surgically. Which course of action is most appropriate?

A. Admit to gynaecology ward
B. Arrange midwifery booking
C. Refer for early scan
D. Refer to antenatal clinic
E. Take blood for serum hCG in the surgery

The main worry here is the ectopic pregnancy history which carries a recurrence risk of 10%, so she needs an early scan to confirm intrauterine pregnancy.

EXTENDED MATCHING QUESTIONS

A.	Ascorbic acid
B.	Clomifene citrate
C.	Danazol
D.	Depot medroxy progesterone acetate
E.	Dianette®

F.	LHRH analogues
G.	Medroxyprogesterone acetate
H.	Mefenamic acid
I.	Tamoxifen
J.	Tibolone
K.	Tranexamic acid

Each of these clinical scenarios describes a woman presenting to her GP requesting help with menstrual problems; for each patient pick the most appropriate treatment option given the information that you are presented with.

Each option may be used once, more than once or not at all.

6.21 A 22-year-old nulliparous lady who is not currently sexually active seeking treatment for menorrhagia and primary dysmenorrhoea.

H. Mefenamic acid

This woman does not need contraception, therefore your choices are between mefenamic and tranexamic acid. Mefenamic acid is better for this patient as it would also treat her dysmenorrhoea.

6.22 An obese teenager with acne and frequent heavy periods seeking secure contraception.

E. Dianette®

This girl may have PCO but in any case she has androgenic problems in terms of her acne. She needs secure contraception and a cyproterone-containing combined pill will give her that as well as helping with her skin.

6.23 A 34-year-old overweight woman with irregular heavy bleeding whose endometrial biopsy reveals cystic hyperplasia with no atypia.

G. Medroxyprogesterone acetate

Endometrial hyperplasia should be treated with progestogen. The usual management plan is for her to take it for six months and then have a repeat endometrial biopsy to check that it has been adequately treated. A Mirena® would also be suitable although it is not licensed for this.

If there had been atypia on the histology report, she should have a hysterectomy as this is a premalignant condition and some of these women already have endometrial cancer.

6.24 A 30-year-old woman with three children has just undergone a third termination of pregnancy without complications. She has attended the surgery twice in the past for help with her menorrhagia and dysmenorrhoea.

D. Depot medroxy progesterone acetate

This woman clearly needs a secure method of contraception as well as help with her periods. Depot medroxy progesterone acetate would be an appropriate option to deliver both, although the effect on her periods may be unpredictable.

6.25 A sterilized 32-year-old woman whose menorrhagia has not responded to treatment with non-steroidal anti-inflammatory drugs.

K. Tranexamic acid

This woman does not need contraception and if her period problems do not respond to mefenamic acid, tranexamic acid is the next option.

A.	Anterior colporrhaphy operation
B.	Antibiotics
C.	Biofeedback
D.	Bladder drill (retraining)
E.	Helmstein bladder distension
F.	Injection of phenol into the bladder trigone
G.	Sacrocolpopexy operation
H.	Supervised pelvic floor physiotherapy
I.	Tension-free vaginal tape (TVT) operation

Each of these scenarios describes a woman presenting to gynaecology clinic with urinary incontinence; for each patient pick the most appropriate treatment option given the clinical information that you are presented with.

Each option may be used once, more than once or not at all.

6.26 Eighteen months after a colposuspension operation for stress incontinence, a 60-year-old woman presents with a recurrence of her incontinence. She brings with her the results of a private urodynamic study that she had done after surfing the internet. This shows that she has a compliant bladder on filling in a sitting position, but when she stands up there is demonstrable leakage of urine associated with spikes of high detrusor pressure measurements > 30 cm water.

D. Bladder drill (retraining)

This woman has an unstable bladder – likely to be a de novo problem following her stress incontinence surgery. The first-line management would be bladder drill; anticholinergics could also help but we haven't given you this option.

6.27 Less than a week after her bladder pressure study where she was diagnosed as having detrusor instability, a 51-year-old postmenopausal woman comes to the surgery seeking treatment on account of a marked deterioration in her symptoms of dysuria, urinary frequency and urgency with urge incontinence.

B. Antibiotics

Urinary tract infection is a complication of a bladder pressure study because of the catheterization involved.

6.28 Six months after the normal vaginal birth of her first child, a 37-year-old teacher complains of urinary incontinence when doing her aerobic classes. On examination she does have a moderate cystocoele and minor rectocoele but no uterine descent.

H. Supervised pelvic floor physiotherapy

A young woman with a minor prolapse like this is likely to respond to intensive physiotherapy.

6.29 A bladder pressure study excludes detrusor instability in a 55-year-old woman with a mixed picture of stress and urge urinary incontinence. Her symptoms are getting worse with frequent leakage in spite of intensive supervised pelvic floor physiotherapy.

I. Tension-free vaginal tape (TVT) operation

If her symptoms have not responded to physiotherapy, she should consider surgery and the TVT is the only operation on the list that fits the bill.

6.30 A fit 62-year-old woman has had a vaginal hysterectomy done years ago for menorrhagia. She presents with 'something coming down' and on examination of the external genitalia you can see the vaginal vault protruding.

G. Sacrocolpopexy operation

The only treatment option on this list that would deal adequately with vault prolapse is this operation where the vaginal vault is fixed to the sacral promontory.

A.	Appendicitis
B.	Ectopic pregnancy
C.	Haemorrhage into an ovarian cyst
D.	Incomplete miscarriage
E.	Missed miscarriage
F.	Normal intrauterine pregnancy
G.	Partial hydatidiform mole
H.	Threatened miscarriage
I.	Urinary tract infection

The clinical scenarios below describe women presenting with pain in early pregnancy. For each case select the most likely diagnosis.

Each option may be used once, more than once or not at all.

6.31 A 23-year-old woman comes in to the Gynaecological Admission Unit complaining of left iliac fossa pain. She is very tender on the left side of her abdomen and on pelvic examination you find cervical excitation. She has had seven weeks of amenorrhoea and her serum βhCG is 5000 IU/ml. The transvaginal ultrasound scan shows a small empty rounded structure (thought to be a gestational sac) in the uterus.

B. Ectopic pregnancy

The history and examination findings would make you suspect ectopic pregnancy. The rounded structure in the uterus on the scan could just as easily be a decidual ring as a gestational sac and does not rule out ectopic.

6.32 A week after her 12-week dating scan, a 24-year-old woman presents to A&E with an acute onset of central abdominal pain and nausea. On examination you find severe lower abdominal tenderness with generalized guarding and rebound. Her white cell count is 14×10^6/l, and urinalysis is negative.

A. Appendicitis

Just because someone is pregnant does not mean that their symptoms have to be related to the pregnancy. Appendicitis can be difficult to diagnose in more advanced pregnancy because the position of the appendix can alter.

6.33 An obese 35-year-old who had her Mirena® intrauterine system removed five months ago on account of breast tenderness attends her GP to complain of lower abdominal discomfort and that her breast tenderness persists. She remains amenorrhoeic. On examination you can feel a mass in her lower abdomen above the symphysis pubis.

F. Normal intrauterine pregnancy

The mass could be an ovarian cyst but in the absence of contraception it is more likely to be a pregnant uterus.

6.34 A 21-year-old woman is admitted to A&E by ambulance having collapsed while out shopping. On arrival at hospital she is complaining of shoulder tip pain, and examination shows a tender abdomen with guarding. She had a coil fitted a month after the delivery of her two-year-old son, and thinks her last menstrual period was two weeks ago although it was lighter than usual.

B. Ectopic pregnancy

The fact that she has collapsed and has shoulder tip pain suggests ectopic.

6.35 A primigravid woman presents to the Early Pregnancy Unit with a history of 11 weeks amenorrhoea, minor lower abdominal discomfort and a small amount of vaginal bleeding. A urine pregnancy test is positive. Pelvic examination reveals no tenderness and the uterus is the correct size with a closed cervical os.

H. Threatened miscarriage

You won't know whether it is a viable pregnancy or not until you get the scan result. The absence of pelvic tenderness makes ectopic less likely and the fact that the uterus is the right size for dates means that the diagnosis is not likely to be missed miscarriage either.

A.	Adenomyosis
B.	Appendicitis
C.	Chronic pelvic inflammatory disease
D.	Endometriosis
E.	Interstitial cystitis
F.	Irritable bowel syndrome
G.	Ovarian cyst
H.	Polycystic ovarian syndrome
I.	Urinary tract infection
J.	Uterine fibroids

The clinical scenarios below describe non-pregnant women presenting in the gynaecology clinic with lower abdominal or pelvic pain. For each case select the most likely diagnosis.

Each option may be used once, more than once or not at all.

6.36 A 22-year-old student with an 18-month history of non-cyclical intermittent lower abdominal pain and deep dyspareunia. She is tender in both adnexae and the uterus is retroverted.

C. Chronic pelvic inflammatory disease

As her pain is non-cyclical, this suggests PID rather than endometriosis.

6.37 As well as experiencing deep dyspareunia for six months, a 48-year-old woman has pain when her bladder is full, which is associated with urinary frequency and nocturia.

E. Interstitial cystitis

Interstitial cystitis produces pain which is always worse when the bladder is full and is often mistaken for endometriosis and chronic PID. The bladder will be very tender on bimanual examination and it is sometimes refractory to treatment. It is diagnosed at cystoscopy.

6.38 After years of being on the pill, a 35-year-old woman has developed gradually increasing severe dysmenorrhoea, intermittent pelvic pain and dyspareunia in her first pill-free year. On examination her uterus is normal size but both adnexae are tender.

D. Endometriosis

The pill often protects women from the manifestations of endometriosis until they stop taking it in later life.

6.39 A woman who has had five normal deliveries complains of increasingly severe secondary dysmenorrhoea. Her periods are regular but becoming heavier. The uterus is bulky and very tender on pelvic examination.

A. Adenomyosis

If the uterus is very tender on examination this suggests adenomyosis, which is more common in multiparous women. It produces severe secondary dysmenorrhoea. If the uterus is irregularly enlarged, this suggests fibroids instead.

6.40 A 24-year-old woman has been using the pill since her teenage years to control her heavy periods as well as for contraception. She seeks help on account of intermittent pain in both iliac fossae associated with abdominal bloating and deep dyspareunia.

F. Irritable bowel syndrome

The bloating is the clue to this diagnosis. There is a useful description of the management of women with pelvic pain in the Green-top guideline number 41, 'The Initial Management of Chronic Pelvic Pain' 2012.

A.	Reassurance only
B.	Repeat pelvic ultrasound at beginning of next cycle
C.	Repeat pelvic ultrasound in three months

D.	Repeat serum CA125
E.	Routine referral to a gynaecological oncologist
F.	Routine referral to a gynaecologist
G.	Serum CA125 and repeat pelvic ultrasound scan
H.	Serum CA125 and urgent (two-week wait) referral to gynaecologist
I.	Urgent (two-week wait) referral to gynaecological oncologist
J.	Urgent (two-week wait) referral to gynaecologist

Each of these clinical scenarios relates to a woman presenting in a general practice surgery with an ovarian cyst. In each case select the most appropriate management plan for that patient.

Each option may be used once, more than once or not at all.

6.41 A 54-year-old postmenopausal woman presents to your surgery with irregular vaginal bleeding over the last six months. An ultrasound scan shows an endometrial thickness of 8 mm and large bilateral multiloculated ovarian cysts. There are no other abnormal features on the scan.

H. Serum CA125 and urgent (two-week wait (2ww)) referral to gynaecologist

The cysts and the thickened endometrium might be related (granulosa cell tumours secreting estrogen and causing endometrial stimulation) but in any case she requires a 2ww referral because she may have endometrial cancer. The CA125 will help work out the Risk of Malignancy Index which guides the treatment plan for the ovarian cysts. It might not be malignant, so referral to a gynaecologist initially rather than oncology is indicated.

6.42 A 27-year-old woman gives a history of longstanding dysmenorrhoea and deep dyspareunia. A pelvic ultrasound shows a unilocular 4 cm diameter cyst on the left ovary consistent with a 'chocolate cyst'.

F. Routine referral to a gynaecologist

This woman probably has endometriosis and should be referred for further investigation and management of her symptoms. The CA125 level doesn't usually help that much with the diagnosis as it is often mildly raised in cases of endometriosis.

6.43 A 19-year-old woman attends surgery with right iliac fossa pain, nausea and vomiting. Her last menstrual period was three weeks before and an ultrasound scan shows a 3 cm diameter right ovarian cyst with internal echoes consistent with haemorrhage. Her pain settles with simple analgesia.

C. Repeat pelvic ultrasound in three months

This cyst is likely to disappear over the next few months as the most likely diagnosis is an ovulatory cyst. The beginning of the next cycle is a little too early to rescan to check it has disappeared. Persistence of the cyst would require referral.

6.44 A 39-year-old woman complains of left iliac fossa pain radiating down her left leg. The ultrasound shows a 9 cm diameter complex cyst on her left ovary and her CA125 level is 470.

I. Urgent (two-week wait) referral to gynaecological oncologist

The high CA125 level increases the chance of this cyst being malignant, therefore she requires urgent referral to a gynaecological oncology service.

6.45 A 65-year-old woman presents to the surgery with loss of appetite and abdominal distension, 12 years after her menopause. It started with a bout of 'gastroenteritis', which has just settled. You organize a CA125 level, which is slightly raised at 55, and an ultrasound scan of the pelvis, which is normal.

D. Repeat serum CA125

This scenario has become increasingly common since the recommendation that GPs 'think ovarian cancer' and request CA125 levels on women presenting with nebulous distension symptoms. The problem is that other conditions such as bowel problems (diverticulitis, gastroenteritis, inflammatory bowel disease) can also raise the levels. In this case a repeat CA125 level is indicated as it will have decreased if the bowel problem has resolved. If the level is increasing a repeat ultrasound is indicated to see if anything is developing on the ovaries.

A.	Ergometrine infusion over four hours
B.	Evacuation of uterus on routine consultant list tomorrow
C.	Evacuation of uterus immediately on emergency list
D.	Evacuation of uterus after cervical priming
E.	Gemeprost pessaries
F.	Intravenous antibiotics
G.	Methotrexate injection
H.	Mifepristone and misoprostol
I.	Oxytocin infusion over four hours
J.	Repeat βhCG level in 48 hours

These clinical scenarios describe women experiencing complications in the first trimester of pregnancy. For each case, select the most appropriate management plan for that patient.

Each option may be used once, more than once or not at all.

6.46 Having developed hyperemesis, a 39-year-old primigravid patient has an ultrasound scan during her hospital admission which shows a 'snowstorm appearance'. You are asked to review the scan and plan management when you take over the night shift at 8 pm.

B. Evacuation of uterus on routine consultant list tomorrow

The scan shows the typical appearance of a hydatidiform molar pregnancy. She requires a careful evacuation of the uterus to remove all the abnormal tissue and histological classification of the type of molar pregnancy. These are difficult evacuation operations to perform and a senior surgeon is required.

Follow-up with βhCG measurements is arranged in conjunction with the appropriate National Gestational Trophoblast Disease Surveillance Centre.

The distractors are immediate evacuation or cervical preparation, but not medical evacuation.

6.47 A 20-year-old shop assistant presents to Early Pregnancy Unit at seven weeks gestation in her second pregnancy complaining of left-sided abdominal pain. She had an ectopic pregnancy a year ago which was treated by laparoscopic right salpingectomy. Her BP and pulse are normal and scan shows an empty uterus with a mixed echo mass in the left adnexa which is 2 cm in diameter. The βhCG level is 2150 IU/ml and haemoglobin is 117 g/l.

G. Methotrexate injection

This woman only has one fallopian tube left and the clinical information suggests that she has another ectopic pregnancy in that remaining tube. Her only chance of achieving a pregnancy in the future without assisted conception is to retain that tube so medical management of ectopic is more appropriate than surgical here. Awaiting a repeat βhCG level before organizing treatment is not sensible because the diagnosis is clear.

6.48 A routine 'dating' ultrasound scan shows that a 21-year-old woman who had a ventouse delivery for her previous child nine months ago, has suffered a missed miscarriage.

D. Evacuation of uterus after cervical priming

The history indicates that there was no warning symptom that might have prompted earlier investigation. With missed miscarriage, the cervix is more resistant to dilatation so cervical priming is needed and surgical evacuation is preferred to medical management.

6.49 On admission to the gynaecology ward, you note that a young woman admitted with bleeding at ten weeks gestation has a temperature of 38.5 °C and a tender uterus. There is a small amount of bleeding on speculum examination but the cervical os is open and you can see what looks like a gestation sac protruding through.

F. Intravenous antibiotics

The pyrexia and tenderness suggest a diagnosis of sepsis and although the uterus needs to be evacuated at some point, administering antibiotics is the first priority.

6.50 At 2 am you are summoned to A&E urgently to see a 23-year-old woman who is having a miscarriage. There is a lot of blood all over the bed and someone has initiated an intravenous infusion as she is hypotensive. On speculum examination you have to remove clots from the vagina to visualize the cervix and find that the cervical os is wide open.

C. Evacuation of uterus immediately on emergency list

You have to do something to stop her bleeding and the best way to do this is to evacuate the uterus, which needs doing as an emergency because of the severity of her bleeding.

Curriculum module 7: Answers

7.1 If a 15-year-old schoolgirl consults you for contraception provision:

A. You must inform her parents or legal guardians before prescribing   F

B. There are unlikely to be child protection issues if she is deemed competent to give consent for treatment   F

C. She should be advised to have a cervical smear as she has become sexually active   F

D. She cannot attend a family planning clinic until she reaches the age of 16 years   F

E. You must enquire about her sexual history regarding partners   T

If you think she is mentally competent to understand the implications of the course of action she is embarking on and the complications and side effects of the proposed contraceptive method, then she can give consent. Obviously it is better if her parents are aware of the situation but you cannot insist on that. You should enquire about the age of her partner(s) because you may need to consider child protection issues and you also have a duty of care to consider the possibility of sexually transmitted diseases. Even though she has become sexually active at a very young age, she does not have a smear until the age of 25 years under the current screening programme rules.

7.2 In women who are thinking of using the combined pill for contraception:

A. The risk of venous thromboembolism (VTE) is about the same as in pregnancy   F

B. The risk of mortality from large bowel cancer is reduced   T

C. A family history of breast cancer is an absolute contraindication   F

D. An alternative method should be sought if they are planning a long high-altitude trek   T

E. The failure rate in typical use rather than in ideal use is 9%   T

The risk of VTE in COC users is about ten times less than pregnancy (29 per 10 000 women years against 300–400 per 10 000 women years). A large cohort study found a significantly lower mortality from bowel cancer in COC users. Women with a family history of breast cancer already have an increased risk compared to the background risk but there is no evidence that taking the COC increases this risk.

High-altitude trekking (above 4500 metres) is associated with an increased risk of VTE and if planning to do this for more than a week, women should plan to change their contraceptive method.

Typical use represents actual use involving inconsistent or incorrect pill taking as opposed to perfect or ideal use. The failure rate with ideal use is 0.3% but in real life it is more like 9%.

Source: Bateson, McNamee and Briggs (2013). Combined hormonal contraception: Clinical Guidance, Faculty of Sexual and Reproductive Healthcare Clinical Effectiveness Unit. *BMJ*; 346: p.341.

7.3 A woman comes to see you in your GP surgery requesting female sterilization as she has had trouble with various other forms of contraception. She is not in a stable relationship currently but has had six pregnancies; five children and one ectopic pregnancy. You agree to write a referral letter to the hospital but should counsel her regarding:

A. A lifetime failure rate of 1 in 2000   F
B. Future risk of ectopic pregnancy   T
C. Mirena® IUS has a much lower Pearl index   F
D. A history of previous ectopic pregnancy is a contraindication   F
E. If she regrets her decision, reversal involves laparoscopic clip removal   F

The chance of a sterilization operation failing in a woman's lifetime is reckoned to be about 1 in 200 and if it does fail, there is a substantial chance of the pregnancy being tubal. In terms of contraceptive reliability (Pearl index) it is about the same as Mirena®. If she regrets having it done, a laparotomy will be needed to reconstruct the fallopian tubes and restore patency as the portion of the tube under the clip is irretrievably crushed. Reversal operations are rarely available on the NHS.

7.4 Regarding non-oral hormonal contraception:

A. The combined transdermal patch (Evra®) works primarily by inhibiting ovulation   T
B. With the progesterone implant the release of hormone is highest just after insertion   T
C. The levonorgestrel intrauterine system (Mirena®) should normally be changed every five years to maintain contraceptive efficiency   T
D. The effectiveness of Mirena® is reduced by liver enzyme-inducing drugs   F
E. The vaginal contraceptive ring (NuvaRing®) is inserted at the beginning of the cycle and removed on day 22   T

The combined patch works mainly by ovulation inhibition but there is a secondary effect on cervical mucus and on the endometrium too. The implant releases 25–70 µg daily via a rate-limiting membrane but the release of hormone is maximal immediately after insertion. The efficacy of the Mirena® is not affected by liver excretion because its main effect is local rather than systemic.

Source: British National Formulary.

7.5 Possible complications of vasectomy include:

A. Scrotal haematoma   T
B. Recanalization of the vasa   T
C. Loss of libido   F
D. Formation of antisperm antibodies   T
E. High testosterone levels   F

The presence of antisperm antibodies can reduce the chances of a successful vasectomy reversal.

7.6 In combined oral contraception formulations, the following may be found as the estrogen component:

A.	Mestranol	T
B.	Estriol	F
C.	Estradiol valerate	T
D.	Conjugated equine estrogen	F
E.	Ethinylestradiol	T

Conjugated equine estrogen is used in HRT preparations. Estriol is the estrogen produced by the placenta in pregnancy and used to be measured as a placental function test many years ago. The others are all used in COCs.

7.7 A woman who has had two children has a copper IUCD fitted in the Family Planning Clinic. She turns up in the surgery for a check-up six weeks later but on speculum examination you cannot find the coil strings. Which of the following statements are true with regard to her situation?

A.	She could be pregnant with the coil in the uterus	T
B.	The coil could have been extruded per vaginam without her noticing	T
C.	The next step is to try and retrieve the coil strings with a thread retriever	F
D.	An ultrasound scan is indicated	T
E.	She is not covered for contraception	T

Until you know where the coil is, she cannot assume that she has a secure method of contraception. The coil could be in the uterus and the strings could have disappeared because the uterus is enlarging (she is pregnant) or because the strings are alongside the coil in the cavity. Alternatively it could have fallen out of the uterus or have perforated the uterus at insertion. You need to ascertain her LMP and exclude pregnancy before proceeding further. A scan will show whether the coil is in the uterus.

7.8 When advising women about copper intrauterine devices:

A.	They are considered unsuitable for nulliparous teenage girls	F
B.	Additional contraceptive measures are required when they are first fitted	F
C.	Women should be screened preinsertion for sexually transmitted infections	T
D.	Most IUDs are impregnated with barium so they can be located on x-ray	T
E.	All copper IUDs are licensed for five years use	F

They are considered suitable for women of all ages regardless of parity; however, analgesia may be needed for insertion in the nulliparous woman as the cervix may need dilating. No additional contraceptive measures are required and there are only two that do not have barium (Multiload Cu375® and Gynefix®). As far as infection risk is concerned there is a higher chance of STIs in women under the age of 25 years or older women with a new partner/multiple partners/partner who has multiple partners and preinsertion screening can be applied selectively.

Manufacturers recommend replacing IUDs every five years except T-Safe 380A Quickload® and TT380 Slimline®, which have a ten-year licence.

7.9 In women using progesterone-only pill (POP) oral contraception:

A.	There is no need to stop taking POP prior to major surgery	T
B.	The window for missed pill taking is only three hours for all formulations	F
C.	There is a link between POP use and breast cancer	F

D. Additional measures are not required if the method is initiated on days 1 to 5 of the menstrual cycle   T

E. There is no proven evidence of weight gain associated with POP use   T

All progesterone methods including injectables are suitable for women having major surgery or immobilized, e.g. due to lower limb trauma. The missed pill window is three hours except for Cerazette®, where it is 12 hours. There is no published evidence linking the POP with breast cancer or weight gain.

If the POP is initiated after day 5 of the menstrual cycle or if the woman is amenorrhoeic, additional measures are recommended for 48 hours.

7.10 When advising women about postcoital emergency contraception:

A. The levonorgestrel pill (Levonelle®) can be used more than once in a cycle T

B. The copper device should be fitted within five days of unprotected intercourse   T

C. Ulipristal (EllaOne®) works primarily by altering the endometrium to prevent implantation   F

D. Women experiencing pain having used any method of emergency contraception within the previous few weeks should seek medical advice T

E. Women with poorly controlled asthma should avoid ulipristal (EllaOne®)   T

Repeated doses of levonorgestrel can be used during the same cycle on a named patient basis but are likely to interfere with the bleeding pattern. Ulipristal works by inhibiting ovulation mainly but there is some effect on the endometrium too.

There is a risk of ectopic pregnancy with progesterone methods and the IUD may perforate the uterus on insertion, so pain needs investigating further.

Ulipristal can provoke an asthma attack.

SINGLE BEST ANSWER QUESTIONS

7.11 Which is the single best course of action if a woman presents to your surgery at 12 weeks gestation, having conceived with an IUCD *in situ*?

A. Repeat the pregnancy test to check for miscarriage

B. Remove the coil if the strings can be visualized

C. Request an x-ray to localize the coil

D. Take triple swabs as infection is likely in this situation

E. Do serial βhCG estimations to exclude ectopic pregnancy

An ultrasound scan is better than a repeat pregnancy test to check for viability of the pregnancy.

The reason for removing the coil is that the risk of miscarriage is higher if it stays in the uterus and there is an increased risk of sepsis, risking the health and possibly even the life of the mother.

X-ray is contraindicated especially in the first trimester of pregnancy.

Although screening for infection is reasonable, the best answer is to remove the coil.

If this pregnancy were ectopic it is likely to have caused symptoms by the time the pregnancy has reached 12 weeks and in any case at this gestation ultrasound scan is a better investigation than serial βhCG in excluding ectopic pregnancy. We tend to use serial βhCG much earlier in pregnancy (< six weeks) if the gestation is too early to see an intrauterine sac on scan.

7.12 A woman whose pelvic ultrasound scan indicates that she has polycystic ovarian syndrome consults you because she does not wish to conceive for a

couple of years. She has sought help previously for management of her facial hirsutism and her serum testosterone is within normal limits.

Select the most appropriate management option in her case from the list below:

A. Clomifene citrate
B. Cyproterone acetate
C. Co-cyprindiol (cyproterone acetate and 35 mcg ethinylestradiol)
D. Levonorgestrel-releasing intrauterine system
E. Metformin

As this woman is requesting contraception, your options are co-cyprindiol or the IUS, because the other preparations are not contraceptive. The IUS will not treat her hirsutism.

7.13 Which one of the following statements about laparoscopic female sterilization is correct?

A. The patient should regard it as an irreversible method of contraception
B. The operation is usually done under local anaesthetic
C. The clips are made of nickel so can't be used if a woman is allergic to base metal
D. Diathermy sterilization increases the chances of successful reversal
E. Applying two clips to each tube is advisable to improve efficacy

Some women seem to think that you can just remove the clips from the tubes and they will be fertile again. The reversal operation involves a painstaking reanastomosis of each tube with a variable success rate, depending on many factors including the length of tube remaining after reversal. Diathermy destroys the structure of the tube along most if its length, thereby reducing the chance of successful reversal. Applying two clips to the tube can cause a hydrosalpinx to form between the clips which could be painful – better to ensure correct application of one clip (to the tube, the whole tube and nothing but the tube).

The operation can be done under local but takes much longer and requires a stoical patient!

7.14 A 28-year-old woman who is virgo intacta wishes to start contraception in advance of her marriage which is arranged for a few months' time. She has polycystic ovarian syndrome, which was diagnosed when she saw a gynaecologist with oligomenorrhoea, and she is worried that she will develop hirsutism, which would spoil her wedding photographs.

From the list given below, select the most appropriate form of contraception for her in these unusual circumstances:

A. Cerazette®
B. Dianette®
C. Marvelon®
D. Nexplanon®
E. NuvaRing®

Hirsutism is a secondary issue to contraception for this woman, but combined hormonal contraception increases the level of sex hormone-binding globulin which over time can reduce the level of free testosterone and improve hirsutism. Dianette® should only be used if she has significant hirsutism and other options are not tolerated or effective because of the potential effects of cyproterone on the liver.

Progesterone-only contraception would have no effect on the potential hirsutism. As she is virgo intact, NuvaRing® would not be suitable in her case.

7.15 A woman has unprotected intercourse with a stranger at a party two days before she consults you for emergency contraception. She has since heard that he is HIV positive and she has made herself an appointment with the local GUM clinic this afternoon.

Choose the best option for emergency contraception in her case:

A. Levonelle 1500®
B. Mirena®
C. EllaOne®
D. Marvelon®
E. Multiload Cu375®

The woman is at risk of both unplanned pregnancy and contracting HIV. She will require postexposure HIV prophylaxis and these drugs are inhibitors of liver enzyme inhibitors so oral hormonal emergency contraception methods are not recommended. The Multiload Cu375® can be inserted up to 120 hours after unprotected intercourse.

Neither Mirena® nor Marvelon® are licensed for emergency contraception.

Without the HIV problem, Levonelle® could be used up to 72 hours and EllaOne® up to 120 hours after unprotected intercourse.

Source: UK guideline for the use of postexposure prophylaxis for HIV following sexual exposure: www.bashh.org.documents/4076.pdf; www.fsrh.org/pdfs/CEUguidanceEmergencyContraception11.pdf.

7.16 A 26-year-old woman had her first smear three weeks ago. She is using a copper IUD for contraception and asks you to check on the smear result when she attends your surgery for her family planning check-up. She is asymptomatic and pelvic examination is normal. Her LMP was two weeks ago and she had intercourse yesterday. Her smear result shows no cytological abnormality but mentions the presence of actinomycosis-like organisms. What is the correct course of action?

A. Remove the IUD immediately and admit to gynaecology ward
B. Remove the IUD and prescribe emergency contraception
C. Remove the IUD, prescribe emergency contraception and penicillin
D. Leave the IUD in place and reassure her as she is asymptomatic
E. Leave the IUD in place and arrange ultrasound to exclude pelvic abscess

Actinomycosis is an uncommon cause of infection that cannot be diagnosed on routine swabs. The infection is spotted on cytology or histology because of the presence of hyphae with sulphur granules.

It can colonize the oral, gastrointestinal and genitourinary tracts and is associated with the presence of a foreign body in the female genital tract.

It can cause abscesses which sometimes resemble tumours and pathology books describe the organism as 'the great mimicker' as the lesion can be mistaken for cancer until the histology is revealed.

If the woman is asymptomatic you do not need to do anything and the IUD can be left in place. If she has pelvic pain, tenderness or a mass the device must be removed and referral for urgent gynaecological opinion is indicated.

Source of further reading: www.patient.co.uk/doctor/Actinomycosis.htm.

7.17 A neurology consultant colleague has written to you about an epileptic patient on your surgery list whose compliance with her phenytoin medication is poor so that she is having frequent fits. She attends surgery asking for contraceptive advice, having found a new partner. What is the best method of contraception for her?

A. Cerazette®
B. Evra®
C. Marvelon®
D. Mirena®
E. NuvaRing®

Phenytoin is an enzyme inducer and all forms of contraception on the list are metabolized in the liver except for Mirena®. She is a poor tablet taker as well and you want to avoid pregnancy in someone on phenytoin.

7.18 Which of the following statements is true of abortions performed in the UK?

A. Patients are routinely scanned to check gestational age of the pregnancy
B. Patients are not usually screened for STIs if undergoing medical rather than surgical termination
C. Over 90% of terminations are performed in the first trimester below 13 weeks gestation
D. Subsequent subfertility can be reliably prevented by administering routine antibiotic prophylaxis effective against chlamydia
E. Simultaneous sterilization should be carried out on request if the patient is having a general anaesthetic

Scanning is available in most termination clinics but not routinely recommended unless there is a discrepancy between the gestational age and clinical findings. The risk of infection is the same for medical and surgical termination.

Government statistics collected for 2012 showed that 91% of terminations are carried out below 13 weeks in the UK, presumably due to the increasing use of early medical termination. Antibiotic prophylaxis does not always prevent subsequent pelvic inflammatory disease especially if no contact tracing is undertaken or if the patient is non-compliant with treatment.

Some patients who are sterilized at the same time regret having it done especially if they experience regret about the termination and it may not be advisable to make such an important decision when under pressure. Many women who have a termination replace the unwanted pregnancy with another one within months. The failure rate of sterilization is higher when it is undertaken during pregnancy as the tubes are hypertrophied and there is a risk that a clip will not completely occlude the tubes.

7.19 A 40-year-old woman with mild learning difficulties needs contraception because she is having a sexual relationship with another patient in the same residential accommodation. An ultrasound scan is requested because her periods are known to be heavy and this reveals multiple small submucosal fibroids distorting her uterine cavity.

Select the most appropriate form of contraception in her case:

A. Copper IUD
B. Hysterectomy
C. Mercilon®
D. Mirena®
E. Nexplanon®

Long-acting reversible contraception offers the best option because her learning difficulties might result in non-compliance. An assessment of mental capacity would be needed when taking consent. As her uterine cavity is distorted Nexplanon® would be more suitable than Mirena®.

7.20 Which of the following statements is not true about the use of the combined oral contraceptive pill?

A.   It will reduce primary dysmenorrhoea

B.   It ameliorates the symptoms of premenstrual syndrome

C.   **It is associated with an increased risk of pelvic inflammatory disease**

D.   It reduces the incidence of benign breast disease

E.   It reduces the risk of ovarian cancer in later life

There is known to be a positive effect on the incidence of benign breast disease and pelvic inflammatory disease and the COC is recognized as an effective treatment for women with PMS or dysmenorrhoea. Ovarian cancer is linked to 'incessant ovulation', e.g. early menarche and late menopause.

EXTENDED MATCHING QUESTIONS

A.	Combined oral contraceptive pill
B.	Depot medroxy progesterone acetate
C.	Etonogestrel subdermal implant
D.	Female sterilization
E.	Intrauterine contraceptive device
F.	Levonelle®
G.	Levonorgestrel intrauterine system
H.	Male condom
I.	Progesterone-only pill
J.	Vasectomy

These clinical scenarios relate to women attending your surgery for contraceptive provision. In each case select the most appropriate method for her.

Each option may be used once, more than once or not at all.

7.21 An 18-year-old student is about to go abroad on a 'gap year' and wishes to organize effective contraception while she is away. She has regular periods and no relevant medical or family history

C. Etonogestrel subdermal implant

It may be difficult for this student to access supplies of contraception while she is away so a long-acting method with a low Pearl index seems appropriate.

7.22 The development of a latex-allergy rash on the vulva results in a 38-year-old woman requesting a change in her contraceptive plans. She has four children and has consulted you recently for heavy periods.

G. Levonorgestrel intrauterine system

The IUS is ideal as she would get treatment for her menorrhagia as well as contraceptive cover.

7.23 A 17-year-old hairdresser has just had her second termination of pregnancy. Both pregnancies occurred as a result of running out of supplies of the pill.

C. Etonogestrel subdermal implant

Feckless and erratic use of contraception is common amongst teenagers and this is a situation where long-acting progestogens are more suitable.

7.24 At her postnatal appointment, a 38-year-old mother of three children seeks advice about a reliable method of contraception. She had severe breast tenderness on the Progesterone only pill and is therefore not keen on taking any hormones.

E. Intrauterine contraceptive device

She would have the choice of an IUCD or permanent methods such as sterilization if she doesn't wish to take hormones in any form. The question says reliable rather than permanent and many doctors recommend delaying permanent methods of contraception until the baby is aged one and the risk of cot death is minimal.

7.25 A 32-year-old woman attends gynaecology clinic, having been referred by her GP for sterilization. She reveals that her husband and father of her two children has just found out about her extramarital affair and left the family home. Her lifestyle is rather chaotic and she needs a very secure method of contraception.

G. Levonorgestrel intrauterine system

Choosing an irreversible permanent method does not seem appropriate for a woman whose husband has just left her, as she is likely to find herself in a new relationship at some stage in the future when she may regret having been sterilized. The IUS has a similar Pearl index to sterilization but is obviously reversible.

A.	Three months
B.	Six months
C.	12 months
D.	24 months
E.	Five years
F.	Seven years
G.	Ten years
H.	15 years
I.	20 years

These statements refer to a 47-year-old woman seeking contraceptive advice. Choose the most appropriate time option given the clinical information in each scenario.

Each option may be used once, more than once or not at all.

7.26 If the 47-year-old woman chooses the Mirena® how long will it be effective as a contraceptive in her particular case?

F. Seven years

The licence is only for five years but a woman of 47 will be much less fertile when she reaches 52 and could continue to rely on it for another two years. As this time limit is 'off licence' you would have to discuss this fully with the patient and record that discussion in the notes.

7.27 If the 47-year-old woman chooses a non-hormonal method, how long should she continue to use the method if she has her menopause (last ever period) next year?

D. 24 months

The time recommended depends on the age at which she has her last ever period. If a woman reaches her menopause under the age of 50 years, a time span of two years of amenorrhoea is required before cessation of contraception because there could still be some residual ovarian activity. Over the age of 50 years a time span of one year will be sufficient.

7.28 The 47-year-old woman makes an informed decision to choose the combined pill as she has no cardiovascular risk factors. When she eventually stops taking the pill, for how long after cessation could she expect a protective effect against ovarian cancer?

H. 15 years

No method is contraindicated on age alone. The combined pill may increase the risk of breast cancer but it has a protective effect against both endometrial and ovarian cancer which lasts for up to 15 years from cessation of use.

7.29 If the 47-year-old woman makes an informed decision to choose the combined pill, how soon should you check her blood pressure after initiating the prescription?

B. Six months

7.30 If the 47-year-old woman makes an informed decision to choose the combined pill, how often should she attend for blood pressure checks?

C. 12 months

Source: Faculty of Family Planning guidance on contraception for women aged over 40 years (2010).

A.	Administer a GnRH analogue
B.	Commence antibiotics
C.	Commence the combined oral contraceptive pill (COC)
D.	Commence oral progestogens for 25 days
E.	Continue with the next pack of the COC without a pill-free period
F.	Insert an intrauterine contraceptive device (IUD)
G.	No intervention is required
H.	Remove the IUD
I.	Use condoms as an additional form of contraception

These clinical scenarios relate to women seeking advice in the Family Planning Clinic in your surgery. For each case, select the most appropriate management plan.

Each option may be used once, more than once or not at all.

7.31 A 26-year-old woman using depot medroxy progesterone acetate who has a BMI of 27 kg/m^2 is suffering from breakthrough bleeding. This is now causing relationship difficulties as she does not want to have intercourse when she is bleeding and she is annoyed that she needs to carry pads around with her all the time. She wishes to control the bleeding if possible.

C. Commence the combined oral contraceptive pill (COC)

When there is breakthrough bleeding with depot medroxy progesterone acetate one suggestion is to commence the combined oral contraception pill for two to three months after excluding causes of bleeding such as sexually transmitted infection.
Source: http://www.fsrh.org/pdfs/CEUGuidanceProgestogenOnly Injectables09.pdf.

7.32 A 32-year-old woman attends surgery because she is feeling unwell and on examination she has a large boil in her left armpit after shaving. You prescribe flucloxacillin 500 mg qds for seven days. She is using Microgynon® for contraception and has five pills left in her pack.

G. No intervention is required

The latest advice states that neither continuation of the combined pill pack nor additional contraception is required when antibiotics are commenced, even within a week of the pill-free week. The only situation in which an additional method needs to be considered is when the use of antibiotics results in diarrhoea, except if the antibiotic is an enzyme inducer, e.g. rifampicin.

7.33 A 29-year-old woman attends surgery. She has a BMI of 34 kg/m^2. She has bought the antiobesity drug orlistat over the counter at a chemist and is worried as she has developed severe diarrhoea since taking it. You discover that she is using Mercilon® for contraception but she has not had sexual intercourse since the commencement of orlistat.

I. Use condoms as an additional form of contraception

In the presence of diarrhoea then additional contraception is recommended.
Source: fsrh.org/pdfs/CEUGuidanceCombinedHormonalContraception.pdf.

7.34 A 27-year-old woman attends surgery having discovered that she is eight weeks pregnant via a scan organized by the local Accident and Emergency Department where she went complaining of severe nausea. This has confirmed an intrauterine pregnancy and she has a Multiload Cu375® in place. She is shocked to find herself pregnant but wishes to continue with the pregnancy.

H. Remove the IUD

If an intrauterine pregnancy occurs with an IUD in situ then the advice is that the IUCD is removed if the pregnancy is less than 12 weeks gestation unless the strings cannot be seen.

7.35 A 34-year-old woman attends your surgery. She has a Nova T380® copper intrauterine device *in situ* for contraceptive purposes. She had a casual sexual encounter with a stranger four days ago and now she is suffering from abdominal pain. On examination she is apyrexial, a yellow discharge is noted and the uterus is tender to palpate.

B. Commence antibiotics

If PID is suspected but not confirmed the advice from the Faculty of Family Planning and Sexual Health is to commence appropriate antibiotics and leave the IUD in place.

Source: http://www.fsrh.org/pdfs/CEUGuidanceIntrauterine ContraceptionNov07.pdf.

A.	At any time in the menstrual cycle
B.	After three weeks
C.	After six weeks
D.	After eight weeks
E.	After 12 weeks
F.	After three months
G.	After three years
H.	After five years
I.	After seven years
J.	Day 1–5 of cycle
K.	Day 19 of cycle
L.	Day 21 of cycle

Each of the clinical scenarios below relate to women requesting contraceptive advice. For each patient select the single most appropriate advice to give from the list above.

Each option may be used once, more than once or not at all.

7.36 An 18-year-old woman attends for repeat emergency contraception having had a second episode of unprotected intercourse in this menstrual cycle. You offer her levonorgestrel 1.5 mg orally and counsel her about the need for contraception. She is keen to have the etonogestrel implant (Nexplanon®) inserted and asks you when is the most appropriate time that this can be done.

J. Day 1–5 of cycle

The advice from the Faculty of Sexual and Reproductive Health (FSRH) is that the progestogen implant can be started immediately after emergency contraception (EC) for women who are likely to continue to have unprotected intercourse, but the disadvantage is the difficulty in removing the implant if EC fails and she is pregnant. They therefore recommend bridging contraception with oral contraceptives until pregnancy has been excluded and then proceeding with the Nexplanon® in days 1–5 of her next period.

7.37 A 23-year-old woman has opted to use injection depot medroxy progesterone acetate for contraception. She enquires when she will need her second injection.

E. After 12 weeks

The licence for depot medroxy progesterone acetate clearly states an injection interval of 12 weeks and if longer than 12 weeks and five days, that pregnancy must be ruled out. The answer is not three months because three calendar months can be longer than 12 weeks.

7.38 A 45-year-old woman attends for replacement of her levonorgestrel intrauterine system (Mirena IUS®) which she uses both for contraception and control of her heavy menstrual bleeding. She is currently amenorrhoeic with the IUS in place. She asks you when she will need the next IUS if she hasn't gone through the menopause.

I. After seven years

The FSRH advises that although the licence for the Mirena IUS® specifies replacement every five years, after the age of 45 women can retain the Mirena IUS® for up to seven years and only need replacement if they haven't become menopausal or have an FSH less than 30 IU/l on two occasions.

7.39 A 25-year-old woman is requesting the combined oral contraceptive pill (COC) for contraception postnatally. She had a normal vaginal delivery and is bottle feeding her baby. When should she commence the COC?

B. After three weeks

The COC is licensed for postnatal use from day 21 after delivery in women who are not breastfeeding. Delaying longer than that increases the risk of unplanned pregnancy as ovulation may occur as soon as 21 days after delivery; however, if the COC is commenced before this there is an increased risk of venous thromboembolism.

7.40 A 25-year-old woman attends your surgery requesting to commence the combined oral contraceptive pill for the first time. She has been amenorrhoeic for some time but her pregnancy test is negative. When can she commence her pill?

A. At any time in the menstrual cycle

The FRSH recommend that the COC may be commenced any time within the cycle but with seven days additional contraception or nine days for estradiol valerate/ dienogest pill (Qlaira®).

A.	Copper IUCD delayed until chlamydia swab results available
B.	Copper IUCD with chlamydia antibiotic prophylaxis
C.	Depot medroxy progesterone acetate injection
D.	Levonorgestrel (Levonelle®) 1.5 mg oral dose
E.	Levonorgestrel intrauterine system (Mirena®)
F.	Nexplanon® etonogestrel implant
G.	No prescription needed; reassure
H.	Ulipristal acetate (EllaOne®) 30 mg oral dose
I.	Repeat ulipristal acetate (EllaOne®) 30 mg oral dose

These clinical scenarios relate to women seeking emergency contraception. For each case, select the most appropriate method.

Each option may be used once, more than once or not at all.

7.41 A shy 35-year-old woman presents to her local police station the morning after an alleged rape and is seen at the Sexual Assault Referral Centre (SARC). She has had a full infection screen done and thinks that her last period was about 12 days ago. She does not usually use contraception as she has never been sexually active and is very distressed at the thought of possible pregnancy as a result of the attack.

H. Ulipristal acetate (EllaOne®) 30 mg oral dose

This woman does not need ongoing contraception, otherwise the IUCD would have the lowest failure rate. Ulipristal seems to have a lower failure rate than levonorgestrel, although both could be used within this time frame.

7.42 The same shy 35-year-old woman returns to the SARC three hours later having just vomited in the car on the way home.

I. Repeat ulipristal acetate (EllaOne®) 30 mg oral dose

Women should be advised to seek medical advice if they vomit within three hours of taking ulipristal (two hours if they have taken levonorgestrel).

7.43 Three months after her first delivery, a woman is still fully breastfeeding her baby. She has not had a period yet and thought that she didn't need to use contraception at all so had unprotected intercourse two days ago. It took her a long time to get pregnant and you suspect that her subfertility might have been due to previous episodes of pelvic inflammatory disease related to proven chlamydia infection.

D. Levonorgestrel (Levonelle®) 1.5 mg oral dose

She cannot take ulipristal because of feeding her baby (breastfeeding is not recommended up to 36 hours after taking it) and her gynaecological history precludes the use of a copper IUCD as first choice. She does need ongoing contraceptive advice too.

7.44 A 24-year-old woman normally uses depot medroxy progesterone acetate for contraception but has forgotten to return for her usual injection which is now over a month overdue. She has been amenorrhoeic since she started on depot medroxy progesterone acetate three years ago and she is keen to continue using it because her periods had been heavy previously. She had unprotected intercourse three days ago.

H. Ulipristal acetate (EllaOne®) 30 mg oral dose

It is too late for her to use levonorgestrel as this is only licensed for use within 72 hours. She should have a pregnancy test done now anyway as you would have no idea whether she was already pregnant or not.

7.45 On return from her holidays, a teenage woman seeks help four days after a condom failure abroad. She is now on day 18 of an irregular cycle and uses a Ventolin inhaler several times a day for her asthma (which has been severe enough to necessitate hospital admission in the past).

B. Copper IUCD with chlamydia antibiotic prophylaxis

It is too late for her to use levonorgestrel as this is only licensed for use within 72 hours and she cannot use ulipristal because of her asthma. You should not wait for the results of the chlamydia swab – and you might also counsel her about being screened for other STIs if she has had sex with a stranger on holiday – so it is best to prescribe prophylaxis alongside inserting a copper IUCD straight away.

Source: Faculty of Sexual and Reproductive Healthcare Clinical Guidance on Emergency Contraception (updated January 2012).

A.	24 hours
B.	72 hours
C.	120 hours
D.	Any time in the cycle
E.	Day 1–5 of the menstrual cycle
F.	Day 1–7 of the menstrual cycle
G.	Five days after expected ovulation
H.	Immediately
I.	Next expected menses
J.	Two weeks
K.	Three to four weeks

The following clinical scenarios relate to timing of commencement of contraceptive methods. For each scenario select the most appropriate option.

Each option may be used once, more than once or not at all.

7.46 A 19-year-old drug user had a vaginal delivery yesterday and the baby has been taken into care. She has a chaotic lifestyle and this was her third unplanned pregnancy. She is happy to have an etonogestrel implant but is keen to leave hospital and asks you when is the soonest that the device can be inserted.

H. Immediately

The UKMEC guidance recommends inserting the etonogestrel implant between 21 and 28 days postpartum in non-breastfeeding women but also advises that the implant can be inserted immediately if the woman is unlikely to attend for medical care and is at risk of pregnancy. Given her lifestyle and drug habit it is far better to take the opportunity to insert the implant now and accept that she may have irregular bleeding initially.

7.47 A 19-year-old woman has just completed the second part of a medical abortion. Following counselling she has requested the etonogestrel subdermal implant (Nexplanon®) for ongoing contraception. When should she have this inserted?

H. Immediately

The FRSH recommend that the progesterone-only implant can be inserted on the day of surgical abortion or the second part of a medical abortion or immediately following miscarriage. No additional contraception is required unless the method is started more than seven days after the abortion or miscarriage, at which time additional contraception is required for seven days.

7.48 A woman using medroxyprogesterone acetate (depot medroxy progesterone acetate) for contraception has forgotten to attend her appointment for her next injection. She telephones the surgery to make another appointment and asks how much time she has got before she cannot rely on the injection for effective contraception.

C. 120 hours

If the woman is more than five days late when she attends for her injection (more than 89 days after the previous dose) she should use another method of contraception for 14 days as she is not protected against pregnancy.

7.49 A 32-year-old woman has been using a progesterone-only pill (POP) for a year following the birth of her second child. She has stopped breastfeeding now and is unhappy with the intermenstrual bleeding that she has with the POP. She is keen to switch to the combined oral contraceptive (COC) and asks how long after finishing her POP packet she should start the COC.

H. Immediately

The advice in the British National Formulary is to start the COC without a break after the last progesterone-only pill and to use additional contraception, e.g. condoms, for seven days.

7.50 A 16-year-old woman requests emergency contraception for her first episode of unprotected intercourse due to condom failure. She is in a steady relationship and is keen to start the combined oral contraceptive pill (COC). When would you advise her to start taking the COC?

H. Immediately

The FSRH advises that although starting the COC immediately after EC is unlicensed, it is preferable to start the pill immediately but to recommend avoiding intercourse or to use condoms as well for seven days. The advantages of 'quick starting' COC is to reduce the time in which she is at risk of pregnancy, to ensure she remembers the advice given on starting the COC and to avoid 'waning enthusiasm' for contraception.

Mock exam paper 1: EMQs and SBAs

A.	Anomaly scan at 20 weeks gestation
B.	Laparoscopy
C.	Midstream urine specimen for culture
D.	Repeat ultrasound scan in one week
E.	Repeat ultrasound scan in one month
F.	Routine booking scan
G.	Serum βhCG assay
H.	Serum lactate
I.	Serum progesterone levels
J.	Thyroid function test
K.	Viability scan

These pregnant women have been admitted to hospital with excessive vomiting. For each patient select an appropriate investigation.

Each option may be used once, more than once or not at all.

1. A 39-year-old primigravid woman is admitted to hospital with vomiting at eight weeks gestation. Her ultrasound scan shows a 'snowstorm' appearance.

    Answer [　]

2. A primigravid woman is admitted to hospital with intractable vomiting for the first time at 16 weeks gestation. She has seen her midwife a few times during the pregnancy already and everything seemed to be fine.

    Answer [　]

3. Having been treated for hyperemesis twice before, a primigravid woman is readmitted with further vomiting at 13 weeks gestation. She is very dehydrated and her urine contains a lot of ketones but nothing else. On her first admission at eight weeks she had a scan which showed a twin pregnancy.

    Answer [　]

A.	Chorioamnionitis
B.	Pelvic girdle pain
C.	Placental abruption
D.	Preterm labour
E.	Pyelonephritis
F.	Red degeneration of fibroid
G.	Torsion of ovarian cyst
H.	Urinary tract infection
I.	Uterine rupture

The following clinical scenarios relate to women experiencing pain in pregnancy. For each case suggest the single most likely diagnosis from the list above.

Each option may be used once, more than once or not at all.

4. A 35-year-old African woman presents at 34 weeks gestation with severe continuous abdominal pain. There is no vaginal bleeding or history suggestive of ruptured membranes and fetal movements are normal. On examination the uterus is irregular, large for dates and tender. The cardiotocograph is reassuring.

Answer [　]

5. A woman presents at 28 weeks gestation feeling unwell with generalized abdominal pain for the last 12 hours. She gives a history of losing fluid per vaginam intermittently over the preceding three days. Fetal movements are present but reduced. On examination she is apyrexial and normotensive but has a tachycardia of 120 bpm. On examination the uterus is tender and the symphysis–fundal height is 24 cm.

Answer [　]

6. A 20-year-old woman in her first pregnancy presents to the labour ward complaining of a sudden onset of severe abdominal pain six hours ago. She hasn't felt any fetal movements since the pain started. There is no history of vaginal loss or bleeding. On examination her blood pressure is 170/110 mmHg, pulse 100 bpm and she is apyrexial. Urinalysis shows protein ++++. On abdominal palpation the uterus is hard and tender and the fetal heart cannot be detected.

Answer [　]

A.	Await result of fetal anomaly scan at 20 weeks gestation
B.	Inform the woman that Down syndrome is confirmed
C.	Inform the woman that Down syndrome is excluded
D.	Inform the woman that the risk for this pregnancy is low

E.	Nuchal translucency scan at 11–13 weeks gestation
F.	Offer amniocentesis
G.	Offer chorionic villus sampling
H.	Offer cordocentesis
I.	Serum screening at 15–17 weeks gestation

These clinical scenarios relate to women seeking prenatal testing for Down syndrome. For each woman select the most appropriate option.

Each option may be used once, more than once or not at all.

7. A 38-year-old woman has a nuchal translucency test at 11 weeks of gestation and the risk of Down syndrome is calculated at 1 in 80. She requests a diagnostic test to be done as soon as possible.

Answer [   ]

8. A primigravid 40-year-old woman is ten weeks pregnant after many years of fertility investigations and she consults an obstetrician in private practice for antenatal care. She is concerned about the risk of having a baby affected by Down syndrome and wishes to have a diagnostic test with lowest possible risk of miscarriage.

Answer [   ]

9. A 36-year-old woman presents late for antenatal care at 15 weeks gestation in her first pregnancy because she was unaware that she was pregnant on account of irregular cycles. She has serum screening only done for Down syndrome and the result shows a 1 in 5000 risk of the pregnancy being affected.

Answer [   ]

A.	Delivery by caesarean section at 37 weeks gestation is recommended
B.	Elective caesarean section carries less fetal risks than vaginal birth
C.	Emergency caesarean section in labour is as safe as elective section
D.	Induction of labour is contraindicated
E.	Induction of labour is recommended at 40 weeks of gestation
F.	Pregnancy could continue to await spontaneous labour
G.	The risk of scar rupture/dehiscence in labour is 10%
H.	Vaginal delivery is contraindicated for maternal reasons
I.	Vaginal delivery is only possible if expected fetal weight is < 4000 g

Each of these pregnant women is seeking advice about the management of their delivery. Select the most appropriate advice in each case.

Each option may be used once, more than once or not at all.

10. A 22-year-old woman attends antenatal clinic at 36 weeks gestation in her second pregnancy, worried about her mode of delivery. Her current pregnancy is uncomplicated and she previously had an elective caesarean section for placenta praevia.

Answer [   ]

11. A 25-year-old woman attends your clinic at 37 weeks gestation in her first pregnancy to discuss mode of delivery. She is anxious because the scan confirms a breech presentation and she refuses to consider external cephalic version.

Answer [   ]

12. A 34-year-old primigravid woman with a singleton uncomplicated pregnancy attends your clinic wishing to discuss mode of delivery. She is 38 weeks pregnant, having conceived following her third cycle of IVF. She has no complications and the baby is well grown.

Answer [   ]

A.	Anorexia nervosa
B.	Anovulatory cycles
C.	Asherman syndrome
D.	Haematocolpos
E.	Juvenile-type granulosa cell tumour of the ovary
F.	Kallman syndrome
G.	Munchausen syndrome by proxy
H.	Polycystic ovarian syndrome
I.	Pregnancy
J.	Sheehan syndrome

These teenage patients are referred by their GPs to gynaecology outpatients with amenorrhoea. For each patient select the most likely diagnosis based on the clinical information given.

Each option may be used once, more than once or not at all.

13. Six months of secondary amenorrhoea in a 19-year-old professional model with a BMI of 16. Examination of the abdomen and pelvis is normal.

Answer [   ]

14. Secondary amenorrhoea of four months duration followed by a week of intermittent light vaginal bleeding in a shy 18-year-old shop worker who weighs 68 kg. She has a mass palpable in the suprapubic region arising from the pelvis.

Answer [   ]

15. A 15-year-old girl who has not yet started menstruating complains of lower abdominal pain for three days. You note that she has been admitted to hospital twice already during the previous three months with pain and suspect that she is avoiding school as exams are imminent. Her younger sister also has frequent episodes of pain but attained menarche recently at the age of 14 years.

Answer [ ]

A.	Admission to isolation ward
B.	Admission to maternity ward
C.	Advise termination of pregnancy
D.	Prescribe antibiotics
E.	Prescribe acyclovir
F.	Reassurance that no action necessary
G.	Send blood for varicella zoster IgG levels
H.	Varicella zoster immunoglobulin (VZIG)
I.	Varicella zoster vaccination

These clinical scenarios relate to chickenpox in pregnancy. For each pregnant woman select the most appropriate management option.

Each option may be used once, more than once or not at all.

16. A woman whose first pregnancy is 28 weeks advanced is in the surgery for a routine check with the midwife. She sees a poster about chickenpox in pregnancy on the surgery wall and realizes that she was exposed to a toddler with chickenpox six weeks ago at a birthday party. She had chickenpox herself as a child and is currently well.

Answer [ ]

17. A newly qualified teacher is exposed to chickenpox at 20 weeks gestation when a child in her class is sent home from school unwell with a fever and a rash. She did have some routine screening tests when she started her job six months ago but was not given any results. She visits her GP that afternoon, who contacts occupational health and discovers that the teacher is not immune to varicella zoster.

Answer [ ]

18. A woman whose current pregnancy is 15 weeks advanced takes her three-year-old daughter to the GP because the child is unwell with a maculopapular rash. The GP diagnoses chickenpox and checks in her own medical notes in the surgery to discover that the patient may have had it herself as a child.

Answer [ ]

A.	CT scan of the pelvis
B.	Barium enema
C.	Diagnostic laparoscopy
D.	Erythrocyte sedimentation rate
E.	Faecal occult bloods
F.	Laparoscopy and dye test
G.	MRI scan of the pelvis
H.	Serum estradiol levels
I.	Transvaginal ultrasound scan
J.	Triple swabs

Each of these clinical scenarios describes a woman presenting in primary care with pain which is likely to be gynaecological in origin. For each patient pick the most appropriate investigation given the clinical information provided.

Each option may be used once, more than once or not at all.

19. An 18-year-old woman presents to her GP with cyclical pain for the previous nine months. She is not yet sexually active and her mother had similar problems before starting a family.

Answer [ ]

20. An 18-year-old biology student presents to the University Student Health Centre for contraceptive advice. She mentions that she has experienced severe deep dyspareunia for several weeks and wishes to stop using depot medroxy progesterone acetate as she has read that it can cause low estrogen levels, which she thinks is responsible for her problem.

Answer [ ]

21. When she attends the surgery for a routine smear a 51-year-old woman mentions to the practice nurse that she has had lower abdominal pain for several months associated with bloating and episodes of diarrhoea. Her symptoms have not responded to mebeverine which one of your colleagues has prescribed recently. The nurse arranges for her to have a CA125 blood test and the result is 66 IU/l.

Answer [ ]

A.	Cervical biopsy
B.	Cervical smear at three months postpartum
C.	Colposcopy within four weeks
D.	Counselling regarding increased risk of preterm labour
E.	High vaginal swab
F.	Large loop excision of the transformation zone (LLETZ)

G.	Repeat cervical smear in 12 months
H.	Routine colposcopy
I.	Routine smear for liquid-based cytology
J.	Urgent smear for liquid-based cytology
K.	Urine or endocervical swab for *Chlamydia trachomatis* screen

These scenarios relate to women who have presented for cervical screening. For each woman select the most appropriate management plan based on the clinical information given.

Each option may be used once, more than once or not at all.

22. A 26-year-old nulliparous woman recently had her first cervical smear which is reported as showing severe dyskaryosis. She tells you she is delighted to have discovered that she is about eight weeks pregnant.

Answer [   ]

23. A 26-year-old nulliparous woman complains of postcoital bleeding for the last three weeks. She has been recently assessed at the colposcopy clinic because her second smear showed mild dyskaryosis.

Answer [   ]

24. A 26-year-old nulliparous woman attends for contraceptive advice. She has never had a cervical smear but as the whole family attend your GP practice you are aware that her sister had a hysterectomy for cervical cancer at the age of 28 years.

Answer [   ]

A.	Abdominal x-ray (KUB) to look for calculus
B.	Creatinine clearance
C.	Flexible cystoscopy
D.	FSH and LH levels
E.	Intravenous urogram (IVU)
F.	Micturating cystogram
G.	Renal perfusion study
H.	Serum urea and electrolytes
I.	Three early-morning urine specimens for culture
J.	Urodynamics (bladder pressure study)

Each of these clinical scenarios describes a woman presenting in primary care with urinary symptoms. For each patient pick the most appropriate investigation based on the clinical information given.

Each option may be used once, more than once or not at all.

25. A perimenopausal woman who is seeing you for hormone replacement therapy complains of urge and stress incontinence which is beginning to affect her social life as she cannot leave home without a pad.

Answer [　]

26. Since arriving in the country three months ago, a 47-year-old immigrant agricultural worker has experienced urinary frequency and urgency. She is at risk of losing her job as she cannot continue to work in the fields on account of her symptoms. She is still menstruating regularly but wonders if she is menopausal because she has night sweats. Pelvic examination reveals a minor cystocoele and a tender bladder.

Answer [　]

27. The nurse running your smoking cessation programme sends a 61-year-old woman to see you on account of longstanding urinary incontinence, which is made worse by her chronic cough. On testing her urine you find microscopic haematuria.

Answer [　]

A.	Arrange to see the woman on her own to ask her about domestic abuse
B.	Arrange an independent translator and ask about domestic abuse
C.	Ask the relatives if she is experiencing domestic abuse
D.	Ask the community midwife to visit her at home
E.	Contact the adult safeguarding team
F.	Contact the police
G.	Discuss child protection issues with the on-call social work team
H.	Encourage the woman to confide in a close relative if she is being abused
I.	Give the woman a card with contact numbers of agencies and refuges
J.	Offer immediate admission to hospital

You are concerned about the possibility of domestic violence in each of these women who are attending the hospital for antenatal care. In each case select the best course of action.

Each option may be used once, more than once or not at all.

28. While performing an anomaly scan at 20 weeks gestation, the ultrasonographer notices several bruises of different colours on the abdomen of a timid 17-year-old primigravid woman. Her 25-year-old boyfriend is also present to watch the scan and when she is asked questions (such as her address and date of birth) he supplies the answers.

Answer [　]

29. At 02.30 hours in the morning a 19-year-old primigravid woman presents to labour ward with postcoital bleeding. Her pregnancy is 32 weeks gestation and she is unaccompanied. On examination you notice that she has a 'black eye' and some circular bruises on her arms. Speculum examination reveals a tear in the posterior vaginal fornix which is not actively bleeding and the cervix is healthy. The baby is moving well, the uterus is not tender and the cardiotocograph is normal.

Answer [　]

30. A 26-year-old immigrant woman attends antenatal clinic at 34 weeks with her sister-in-law who translates for her, as she speaks no English at all. This is her first pregnancy and she is having growth scans on account of recurrent antepartum haemorrhage. The growth of the baby is fine, but when you are auscultating the fetal heart you notice some circular lesions on the maternal abdomen which look like cigarette burns.

Answer [　]

SINGLE BEST ANSWER QUESTIONS

31. A woman who has three children has unfortunately conceived while wearing a copper coil for contraception. She comes to see you in surgery having had a positive pregnancy test at the chemists and reports that she is probably seven weeks gestation. Having talked to her husband, she is not too upset and is intending to keep the pregnancy.

Select the most appropriate course of action:

A. Perform a full STI screen as infection is likely to cause miscarriage
B. Prescribe a course of antibiotics prophylactically
C. Remind the midwife that the coil needs removing at her postnatal appointment
D. Send her for a routine booking scan, mentioning the coil on the scan request form
E. Take the coil out as there is a risk of septic miscarriage

Answer [　]

32. As she is completing the hospital discharge paperwork for a recently delivered mother on the maternity ward one of the midwives accidentally puts her copy of the list of current patients on the ward into the hand-held notes, so that the woman takes the list home with her. Which of these options is the most appropriate course of action for the midwife in charge of the ward to take?

A. Ask the woman's community midwife to visit and retrieve the list
B. Complete an incident form and inform the Information Governance Lead
C. Send the police to retrieve the list from the patient's house
D. Telephone the woman and ask her to shred the list
E. Write to the woman and ask her to return the list

Answer [　]

33. A 26-year-old primigravid woman has a routine appointment with her community midwife at 32 weeks gestation. Her ankles and feet are so swollen that she has had to wear sandals instead of shoes to work and can no longer

wear her rings. Her BP at booking was 120/70 and it is now 130/80. Urinalysis is negative. On examination she does have bilateral varicose veins and both ankles are mildly oedematous but there is no redness or tenderness in either leg. Which is the most appropriate management option?

A. Advise the use of compression stockings
B. Arrange lower limb venous Doppler studies
C. Commence low-dose aspirin
D. Refer to an obstetrician
E. Request serum U&E and urate testing

Answer [ ]

34. A 20-year-old woman is admitted to the gynaecology ward over a bank holiday weekend with lower abdominal pain, deep dyspareunia, vaginal discharge and a fever of 38 °C. She has no gastrointestinal symptoms, is using the pill for contraception and is half way through a packet. On examination there is suprapubic tenderness and bimanual pelvic examination elicits cervical motion tenderness. Urinalysis is negative as is her pregnancy test. Which of the following is the most appropriate management plan?

A. Take triple swabs and prescribe appropriate antibiotics according to sensitivities
B. Prescribe doxycycline 100 mg twice daily for 14 days
C. Prescribe metronidazole 400 mg and cefalexin 50 mg tds for 14 days
D. Prescribe metronidazole and ofloxacin 400 mg bd for 14 days
E. Administer azithromycin 1 g intramuscular injection and refer to the GUM clinic

Answer [ ]

35. The reason that obstetric units utilize a 'maternity dashboard' which describes items such as the caesarean section rate and the number of third-degree tears in the month is:

A. To keep track of the costs incurred on labour ward
B. To reduce the risk of litigation in relation to labour
C. To check on the performance of individual obstetricians for revalidation
D. To present the data to the CNST inspectors
E. To compare the outcomes of their maternity services with other units

Answer [ ]

36. Following the realization that suicide is an important cause of maternal death, GPs are expected to be aware of issues concerning the mental health of pregnant women. Which one of the following statements is true?

A. A previous history of puerperal psychosis carries a recurrence risk of 5%
B. A woman with a history of depression should always be referred for a formal psychiatric opinion during pregnancy
C. The risk of suicide increases during pregnancy

D. New mothers who commit suicide are more likely to die by violent means rather than overdose

E. The Edinburgh Depression Scale may be used to screen for the risk of a psychotic depressive illness occurring

Answer [　]

37. Following a ward round with the registrar on labour ward you are left with a list of tasks to do. Which job takes priority over the rest?

A. Inserting an IV line for a patient labouring with a previous caesarean scar

B. Performing a fetal blood sample on account of late decelerations on the CTG at 5 cm dilatation

C. Clerking a new patient admitted with raised blood pressure at 39 weeks gestation

D. Discharging a patient who has been treated for severe postpartum haemorrhage to the postnatal ward

E. Obtaining consent for postmortem from a mother who is waiting to be discharged, having delivered her stillborn baby six hours ago

Answer [　]

38. Six days after a hysterectomy operation, one of your patients presents to the surgery with right loin pain. She reports that she felt 'tired and shivery' when she was discharged from hospital three days before but now looks very unwell with a temperature of 38 °C. There is no vaginal bleeding or discharge. On examination she is tender in the right renal angle and right hypochondrium. You send off a midstream urine specimen and can see that she needs readmission for antibiotic treatment, but what will be the most appropriate investigation to make a diagnosis when she gets to hospital?

A. Intravenous urogram

B. Laparoscopy

C. Serum amylase

D. Three-swab test with methylene blue in the bladder

E. MRI scan of the gallbladder and liver

Answer [　]

39. You are clerking a new patient in gynaecology clinic with pelvic pain and trying to sort out a differential diagnosis. Which one of the following is a recognized symptom of endometriosis?

A. Abdominal bloating

B. Postcoital bleeding

C. Secondary dysmenorrhoea

D. Superficial dyspareunia

E. Weight loss

Answer [　]

40. Two years after her last menstrual period a woman aged 51 is referred to a menopause clinic because of severe dyspareunia which is so bad that she can no longer tolerate intercourse. She was glad to see the end of her periods because they were becoming increasingly troublesome and has not

experienced any vasomotor symptoms. On speculum examination the vulva and vagina look very atrophic and opening the speculum causes a small amount of bleeding by splitting the skin at the introitus. What is the most appropriate treatment in her case?

A. Fenton's operation to enlarge the vaginal introitus
B. Oral combined sequential estradiol and progesterone
C. Psychosexual counselling
D. Transdermal estradiol gel 1 mg daily
E. Vaginal estradiol pessaries

Answer [   ]

41. In a postmenopausal patient presenting to gynaecology clinic with an advanced uterovaginal prolapse, which of the following clinical problems is **not** likely to be attributable to the prolapse?

A. Bleeding
B. Constipation
C. Digitation
D. Recurrent cystitis
E. Ulceration of the vaginal walls

Answer [   ]

42. You are seeing a woman in antenatal clinic who has developed obstetric cholestasis in her second pregnancy at 34 weeks gestation. She wishes to discuss her birth plan as she wanted a home birth with 'everything as natural as possible', having had a lot of medical intervention with a forceps delivery in her first labour. Which of the following plans is **not** correct or appropriate advice for her?

A. Continuous electronic fetal monitoring is advisable in labour
B. Daily fetal monitoring with CTG until delivery will predict the possibility of stillbirth
C. She may be offered induction of labour after 37 weeks to avoid the risk of stillbirth
D. She should deliver in the consultant unit rather than at home
E. She should have repeat liver function tests done a couple of weeks postpartum

Answer [   ]

43. The main purpose of organizing a bladder pressure (urodynamic) study for a woman presenting with a mixed picture of stress and urge incontinence with nocturia is:

A. To check for urinary fistula
B. To differentiate detrusor instability from genuine stress incontinence
C. To find out whether her symptoms are due to uterovaginal prolapse
D. To gauge the results of anticholinergic treatment
E. To prevent subsequent medicolegal problems if she does not respond to treatment

Answer [   ]

44. A primigravid woman presents to labour ward at 32 weeks gestation with vaginal bleeding. She is stable and the baby is well, but she is known to be Rhesus negative. Her clinical notes confirm that she had her prophylactic anti-D injection at 28 weeks gestation administered by her midwife.

Select the most appropriate management option:

A. Administer 250 IU anti-D and perform Kleihauer test
B. Administer 500 IU anti-D
C. Administer 500 IU anti-D and perform Kleihauer test
D. Ask the lab to check for residual anti-D from her prophylactic injection
E. No action necessary

Answer [ ]

45. One of the following is **not** a fetal risk factor for intrauterine growth restriction:

A. Congenital rubella infection
B. Chromosomal abnormalities
C. Cytomegalovirus infection in utero
D. Female sex
E. Multiple gestation

Answer [ ]

46. A 25-year-old woman presents to the Early Pregnancy Unit with brown vaginal discharge. She is unsure of her last menstrual period but thinks the gestational age might be about seven weeks. The ultrasound scan has shown a small sac in the uterus with no contents. On vaginal examination you find no pelvic tenderness. What is the most suitable management plan?

A. Booking scan at 12 weeks gestation
B. Evacuate the uterus and send the contents for histological examination
C. Laparoscopy
D. Repeat ultrasound scan in one week
E. Serial urine βhCG assays with the next test 48 hours later

Answer [ ]

47. A 47-year-old woman presents with a six-month history of regular heavy menstrual bleeding. She has had normal smears in the past and pelvic examination is unremarkable. Histology on a 'pipelle' sample of the endometrium and ultrasound scan are reported as normal. She had a DVT following a long-haul flight in the past but is otherwise healthy. Which of the following is the most appropriate treatment option for her menorrhagia?

A. Combined oral contraceptive pill
B. Hysterectomy
C. Levonorgestrel releasing IUS (Mirena®)
D. Norethisterone 15 mg daily from day 5–26 of menstrual cycle
E. Tranexamic acid

Answer [ ]

48. In the Teenage Family Planning Clinic you meet a 14-year-old schoolgirl requesting emergency contraceptive help after a mid-cycle condom breakage. Her parents are unaware of her sexual activity and do not approve of the relationship with her 22-year-old partner because he has another girlfriend who is currently pregnant. You decide that she is Fraser-competent and the recommended action in this situation would be:

A. Referral to police because of underage sexual activity
B. Referral to social services to investigate her sexual relationship with an adult
C. Referral to GUM clinic for full sexually transmitted disease screening
D. Refuse to supply contraception until the parents' consent
E. Supply contraception and arrange follow-up appointment

Answer [   ]

Mock exam paper 1: Answers

EXTENDED MATCHING QUESTIONS

A.	Anomaly scan at 20 weeks gestation
B.	Laparoscopy
C.	Midstream urine specimen for culture
D.	Repeat ultrasound scan in one week
E.	Repeat ultrasound scan in one month
F.	Routine booking scan
G.	Serum βhCG assay
H.	Serum lactate
I.	Serum progesterone levels
J.	Thyroid function test
K.	Viability scan

These pregnant women have been admitted to hospital with excessive vomiting. For each patient select an appropriate investigation.

Each option may be used once, more than once or not at all.

1. A 39-year-old primigravid woman is admitted to hospital with vomiting at eight weeks gestation. Her ultrasound scan shows a 'snowstorm' appearance.

    G. Serum βhCG assay

    This ultrasound appearance is typical of hydatidiform mole, which should be dealt with surgically. The baseline βhCG level helps the trophoblastic centre plan her subsequent follow-up and management.

2. A primigravid woman is admitted to hospital with intractable vomiting for the first time at 16 weeks gestation. She has seen her midwife a few times during the pregnancy already and everything seemed to be fine.

    C. Midstream urine specimen for culture

    It is unusual for hyperemesis to start in the second trimester so it is more likely that her symptoms are caused by urinary tract infection. She will already have had a booking scan which will have excluded molar pregnancy and twins.

3. Having been treated for hyperemesis twice before, a primigravid woman is readmitted with further vomiting at 13 weeks gestation. She is very

dehydrated and her urine contains a lot of ketones but nothing else. On her first admission at eight weeks she had a scan which showed a twin pregnancy.

A. Anomaly scan at 20 weeks gestation

Although she has had recurrent admissions, this is not unusual with twin pregnancies and there is no need to worry about underlying causes such as UTI especially as her urine only shows ketones. Her next scan should be the anomaly scan at 20 weeks and she does not need another one before then.

A.	Chorioamnionitis
B.	Pelvic girdle pain
C.	Placental abruption
D.	Preterm labour
E.	Pyelonephritis
F.	Red degeneration of fibroid
G.	Torsion of ovarian cyst
H.	Urinary tract infection
I.	Uterine rupture

The following clinical scenarios relate to women experiencing pain in pregnancy. For each case suggest the single most likely diagnosis from the list above.

Each option may be used once, more than once or not at all.

4. A 35-year-old African woman presents at 34 weeks gestation with severe continuous abdominal pain. There is no vaginal bleeding or history suggestive of ruptured membranes and fetal movements are normal. On examination the uterus is irregular, large for dates and tender. The cardiotocograph is reassuring.

F. Red degeneration of fibroid

The salient feature here is her ethnic origin; fibroids are more common in African women, and the uterus is irregular. You will know from your revision that fibroids can undergo red degeneration in pregnancy even if you've never seen a case. Since the pain is continuous it makes the option of preterm labour unlikely even though it is a more common condition.

5. A woman presents at 28 weeks gestation feeling unwell with generalized abdominal pain for the last 12 hours. She gives a history of losing fluid per vaginam intermittently over the preceding three days. Fetal movements are present but reduced. On examination she is apyrexial and normotensive but has a tachycardia of 120 bpm. On examination the uterus is tender and the symphysis–fundal height is 24 cm.

A. Chorioamnionitis

The salient features in this case are the history suggestive of prolonged rupture of the membranes (PROM) and the significant tachycardia. The PROM is a major risk factor for ascending infection and in pregnant women a tachycardia usually precedes the pyrexia and is always a worrying sign. The pain is described as 'generalized' rather than intermittent (intermittent pain might suggest preterm labour). The small for dates uterus would fit with oligohydramnios due to ruptured membranes.

6. A 20-year-old woman in her first pregnancy presents to the labour ward complaining of a sudden onset of severe abdominal pain six hours ago. She hasn't felt any fetal movements since the pain started. There is no history of vaginal loss or bleeding. On examination her blood pressure is 170/110 mmHg, pulse 100 bpm and she is apyrexial. Urinalysis shows protein ++++. On abdominal palpation the uterus is hard and tender and the fetal heart cannot be detected.

   C. Placental abruption

   The salient features in this case are the severe hypertension and proteinuria suggesting pre-eclampsia, the lack of fetal movements and absent fetal heart suggesting an intrauterine death and the hard uterus suggesting the Couvelaire uterus of a large abruption. From your revision you know that abruption is a complication of pre-eclampsia and don't be distracted by the absence of vaginal bleeding as even large abruptions can be concealed.

A.	Await result of fetal anomaly scan at 20 weeks gestation
B.	Inform the woman that Down syndrome is confirmed
C.	Inform the woman that Down syndrome is excluded
D.	Inform the woman that the risk for this pregnancy is low
E.	Nuchal translucency scan at 11–13 weeks gestation
F.	Offer amniocentesis
G.	Offer chorionic villus sampling
H.	Offer cordocentesis
I.	Serum screening at 15–17 weeks gestation

These clinical scenarios relate to women seeking prenatal testing for Down syndrome. For each woman select the most appropriate option.

Each option may be used once, more than once or not at all.

7. A 38-year-old woman has a nuchal translucency test at 11 weeks of gestation and the risk of Down syndrome is calculated at 1 in 80. She requests a diagnostic test to be done as soon as possible.

   G. Offer chorionic villus sampling

   The patient is keen on a diagnostic test, which narrows the selection down to F, G or H. The quickest result would be obtained by chorionic villus sampling because active placental cells will be dividing quickly enough to obtain a karyotype within 24–48 hours. Cordocentesis is reserved for later in pregnancy to investigate serious and rare conditions like fetal anaemia.

8. A primigravid 40-year-old woman is ten weeks pregnant after many years of fertility investigations and she consults an obstetrician in private practice for antenatal care. She is concerned about the risk of having a baby affected by Down syndrome and wishes to have a diagnostic test with lowest possible risk of miscarriage.

F. Offer amniocentesis

The patient wants a diagnostic test and the one with lowest risk of pregnancy loss is amniocentesis.

9. A 36-year-old woman presents late for antenatal care at 15 weeks gestation in her first pregnancy because she was unaware that she was pregnant on account of irregular cycles. She has serum screening only done for Down syndrome and the result shows a 1 in 5000 risk of the pregnancy being affected.

D. Inform the woman that the risk for this pregnancy is low

Screening tests do not exclude Down syndrome but this low risk result is reassuring.

A.	Delivery by caesarean section at 37 weeks gestation is recommended
B.	Elective caesarean section carries less fetal risks than vaginal birth
C.	Emergency caesarean section in labour is as safe as elective section
D.	Induction of labour is contraindicated
E.	Induction of labour is recommended at 40 weeks of gestation
F.	Pregnancy could continue to await spontaneous labour
G.	The risk of scar rupture/dehiscence in labour is 10%
H.	Vaginal delivery is contraindicated for maternal reasons
I.	Vaginal delivery is only possible if expected fetal weight is < 4000 g

Each of these pregnant women is seeking advice about the management of their delivery. Select the most appropriate advice in each case.

Each option may be used once, more than once or not at all.

10. A 22-year-old woman attends antenatal clinic at 36 weeks gestation in her second pregnancy, worried about her mode of delivery. Her current pregnancy is uncomplicated and she previously had an elective caesarean section for placenta praevia.

F. Pregnancy could continue to await spontaneous labour

The reason for her previous section is non-recurrent so she should be able to have a vaginal birth this time. We would normally have a full discussion about the risks and benefits of VBAC (vaginal birth after caesarean) and go through them again in the third trimester. Spontaneous labour is preferable to induced labour in this situation because the drugs we use to induce labour – prostaglandin and oxytocin – increase the risk of scar rupture. Induction is not completely contraindicated, just less safe but you could induce if there were good maternal reasons, e.g. pre-eclampsia.

11. A 25-year-old woman attends your clinic at 37 weeks gestation in her first pregnancy to discuss mode of delivery. She is anxious because scan confirms a breech presentation and she refuses to consider external cephalic version.

B. Elective caesarean section carries less fetal risks than vaginal birth

The best option is external cephalic version because it reduces the incidence of breech presentation at term. If she won't accept this then the 'Term Breech Trial' showed that section is safer for the breech baby than vaginal delivery.

12. A 34-year-old primigravid woman with a singleton uncomplicated pregnancy attends your clinic wishing to discuss mode of delivery. She is 38 weeks pregnant, having conceived following her third cycle of IVF. She has no complications and the baby is well grown.

F. Pregnancy could continue to await spontaneous labour

Although this woman has had difficulty getting pregnant, she should now be treated like any other mother. There is no indication to interfere.

A.	Anorexia nervosa
B.	Anovulatory cycles
C.	Asherman syndrome
D.	Haematocolpos
E.	Juvenile-type granulosa cell tumour of the ovary
F.	Kallman syndrome
G.	Munchausen syndrome by proxy
H.	Polycystic ovarian syndrome
I.	Pregnancy
J.	Sheehan syndrome

These teenage patients are referred by their GPs to gynaecology outpatients with amenorrhoea. For each patient select the most likely diagnosis based on the clinical information given.

Each option may be used once, more than once or not at all.

13. Six months of secondary amenorrhoea in a 19-year-old professional model with a BMI of 16. Examination of the abdomen and pelvis is normal.

A. Anorexia nervosa

The distractor is pregnancy, which is the most common cause of secondary amenorrhoea in teenagers, but the normal examination makes this less likely. Her BMI is extremely low and she is probably not ovulating. Disappearance of periods is an indication that anorexia is becoming very serious.

14. Secondary amenorrhoea of four months duration followed by a week of intermittent light vaginal bleeding in a shy 18-year-old shop worker who weighs 68 kg. She has a mass palpable in the suprapubic region arising from the pelvis.

I. Pregnancy

The mass could be an ovarian cyst but a granulosa cell tumour of the ovary is more likely to cause irregular bleeding than amenorrhoea and in any case they are extremely rare. Haematocolpos can also present with a lower abdominal mass, but the patient would have primary amenorrhoea, not secondary. Pregnancy is the most likely option.

15. A 15-year-old girl who has not yet started menstruating complains of lower abdominal pain for three days. You note that she has been admitted to hospital twice already during the previous three months with pain and suspect that she is avoiding school as exams are imminent. Her younger sister also has frequent episodes of pain but attained menarche recently at the age of 14 years.

D. Haematocolpos

Imperforate hymen can cause cyclical pain as the haematocolpos gets bigger and it is not unusual to find a couple of hospital admissions have occurred before the diagnosis is reached. Many teenagers have anovulatory cycles but this causes irregular periods and menorrhagia rather than primary amenorrhoea.

A.	Admission to isolation ward
B.	Admission to maternity ward
C.	Advise termination of pregnancy
D.	Prescribe antibiotics
E.	Prescribe acyclovir
F.	Reassurance that no action necessary
G.	Send blood for varicella zoster IgG levels
H.	Varicella zoster immunoglobulin (VZIG)
I.	Varicella zoster vaccination

These clinical scenarios relate to chickenpox in pregnancy. For each pregnant woman select the most appropriate management option.

Each option may be used once, more than once or not at all.

16. A woman whose first pregnancy is 28 weeks advanced is in the surgery for a routine check with the midwife. She sees a poster about chickenpox in pregnancy on the surgery wall and realizes that she was exposed to a toddler with chickenpox six weeks ago at a birthday party. She had chickenpox herself as a child and is currently well.

F. Reassurance that no action necessary

The incubation period for varicella is one to three weeks so she would have developed it herself by now. As VZIG is only effective if given within ten days of exposure, it is too late to consider that for this woman anyway. A personal history of chickenpox is 99% predictive of the presence of serum varicella antibodies, so this woman does not even need testing for zoster IgG levels.

17. A newly qualified teacher is exposed to chickenpox at 20 weeks gestation when a child in her class is sent home from school unwell with a fever and a rash. She did have some routine screening tests when she started her job six months ago but was not given any results. She visits her GP that afternoon, who contacts occupational health and discovers that the teacher is not immune to varicella zoster.

H. Varicella zoster immune globulin (VZIG)

There was a window of opportunity to vaccinate this woman against varicella before she got pregnant but now the only option is to give her VZIG to try and prevent her getting chickenpox (if that is what is wrong with the child in her class). It is still not recommended as part of a national screening programme to check antibody status and vaccinate all women in the UK like we do for rubella, but some occupational health departments do undertake this in high-risk groups such as teachers. If a woman contracts varicella in pregnancy she can become very ill with serious problems such as pneumonia and of course we worry about fetal varicella syndrome and infection of the newborn.

18. A woman whose current pregnancy is 15 weeks advanced takes her three-year-old daughter to the GP because the child is unwell with a maculopapular rash. The GP diagnoses chickenpox and checks in her own medical notes in the surgery to discover that the patient may have had it herself as a child.

G. Send blood for varicella zoster IgG levels

If the woman had had chickenpox herself she is likely to be immune so it is reasonable to check her antibody levels rather than prescribing VZIG. The VZIG is manufactured from the plasma of blood donors and is a limited and expensive resource. If her antibodies are negative, there is still an opportunity to give VZIG up to ten days.

Source: RCOG Green-top guideline number 13. *Chickenpox in Pregnancy.*

A.	CT scan of the pelvis
B.	Barium enema
C.	Diagnostic laparoscopy
D.	Erythrocyte sedimentation rate
E.	Faecal occult bloods
F.	Laparoscopy and dye test
G.	MRI scan of the pelvis
H.	Serum estradiol levels
I.	Transvaginal ultrasound scan
J.	Triple swabs

Each of these clinical scenarios describes a woman presenting in primary care with pain which is likely to be gynaecological in origin. For each patient pick the most appropriate investigation given the clinical information provided.

Each option may be used once, more than once or not at all.

19. An 18-year-old woman presents to her GP with cyclical pain for the previous nine months. She is not yet sexually active and her mother had similar problems before starting a family.

C. Diagnostic laparoscopy

If she is not sexually active she will not have pelvic inflammatory disease so the most likely diagnosis here is endometriosis, especially as it can run in families. Laparoscopy is the gold standard investigation as scan will not show up small deposits of endometriosis. An MRI is sometimes used to investigate endometriosis but only looking for deep deposits in sites such as the rectovaginal septum in a patient where you already know the diagnosis.

20. An 18-year-old biology student presents to the University Student Health Centre for contraceptive advice. She mentions that she has experienced severe deep dyspareunia for several weeks and wishes to stop using depot medroxy progesterone acetate as she has read that it can cause low estrogen levels, which she thinks is responsible for her problem.

J. Triple swabs

It is more likely that she is suffering from pelvic inflammatory disease as a cause of her symptoms rather than vaginal atrophy so triple swabs would be the first investigation, especially as speculum examination would allow you to reassure her about the state of her vaginal skin at the same time. She does not need scan or laparoscopy unless her pain becomes chronic and a definite diagnosis is necessary.

21. When she attends the surgery for a routine smear a 51-year-old woman mentions to the practice nurse that she has had lower abdominal pain for several months associated with bloating and episodes of diarrhoea. Her symptoms have not responded to mebeverine, which one of your colleagues has prescribed recently. The nurse arranges for her to have a CA125 blood test and the result is 66 IU/l.

I. Transvaginal ultrasound scan

GPs are urged to do CA125 blood tests on women presenting with new onset of symptoms similar to irritable bowel after the age of 50 years and this result is raised. The next step is ultrasound, although there are many other conditions apart from ovarian cancer that can cause raised CA125. A thorough careful history and examination is recommended to avoid missing other pathology such as inflammatory bowel disease. The distractors in this question are the bowel investigation modalities such as barium enema, and CT scan which is more expensive than ultrasound and involves a dose of ionizing radiation.

A.	Cervical biopsy
B.	Cervical smear at three months postpartum
C.	Colposcopy within four weeks
D.	Counselling regarding increased risk of preterm labour
E.	High vaginal swab
F.	Large loop excision of the transformation zone (LLETZ)
G.	Repeat cervical smear in 12 months

H.	Routine colposcopy
I.	Routine smear for liquid-based cytology
J.	Urgent smear for liquid-based cytology
K.	Urine or endocervical swab for *Chlamydia trachomatis* screen

These scenarios relate to women who have presented for cervical screening. For each woman select the most appropriate management plan based on the clinical information given.

Each option may be used once, more than once or not at all.

22. A 26-year-old nulliparous woman recently had her first cervical smear which is reported as showing severe dyskaryosis. She tells you she is delighted to have discovered that she is about eight weeks pregnant.

C. Colposcopy within four weeks

Although this woman will have to wait until after she has delivered for treatment, someone must look at her cervix urgently to make sure that she is not one of the women with severe dyskaryosis who actually has cervical cancer already. Biopsy is possible in pregnancy if it is necessary.

23. A 26-year-old nulliparous woman complains of postcoital bleeding for the last three weeks. She has been recently assessed at the colposcopy clinic because her second smear showed mild dyskaryosis.

K. Urine or endocervical swab for *Chlamydia trachomatis* screen

One of the most common causes of postcoital bleeding is chlamydia. As her cervix has recently been inspected at colposcopy, the smear history is irrelevant.

24. A 26-year-old nulliparous woman attends for contraceptive advice. She has never had a cervical smear but as the whole family attend your GP practice you are aware that her sister had a hysterectomy for cervical cancer at the age of 28 years.

G. Repeat cervical smear in 12 months

The family history is not relevant as cervical cancer is not genetic. However, this woman has reached the age at which she should be enrolled on the screening programme and this seems like a good opportunity. Ethically the GP cannot mention the sister's medical history while trying to persuade her because of the confidentiality issue.

A.	Abdominal x-ray (KUB) to look for calculus
B.	Creatinine clearance
C.	Flexible cystoscopy
D.	FSH and LH levels
E.	Intravenous urogram (IVU)
F.	Micturating cystogram

G.	Renal perfusion study
H.	Serum urea and electrolytes
I.	Three early-morning urine specimens for culture
J.	Urodynamics (bladder pressure study)

Each of these clinical scenarios describes a woman presenting in primary care with urinary symptoms. For each patient pick the most appropriate investigation based on the clinical information given.

Each option may be used once, more than once or not at all.

25. A perimenopausal woman who is seeing you for hormone replacement therapy complains of urge and stress incontinence which is beginning to affect her social life as she cannot leave home without a pad.

    J. Urodynamics (bladder pressure study)

    The diagnosis is likely to be either detrusor instability or genuine stress incontinence and urodynamics will help you differentiate between them.

26. Since arriving in the country three months ago, a 47-year-old immigrant agricultural worker has experienced urinary frequency and urgency. She is at risk of losing her job as she cannot continue to work in the fields on account of her symptoms. She is still menstruating regularly but wonders if she is menopausal because she has night sweats. Pelvic examination reveals a minor cystocoele and a tender bladder.

    I. Three early-morning urine specimens for culture

    Tuberculosis of the urinary tract is uncommon in the UK but possibly not in the country she has come from. It will not be picked up on routine MSU – you need to send the whole of a morning void to the lab and specify TB testing.

27. The nurse running your smoking cessation programme sends a 61-year-old woman to see you on account of longstanding urinary incontinence, which is made worse by her chronic cough. On testing her urine you find microscopic haematuria.

    C. Flexible cystoscopy

    Smoking is a risk factor for transitional cell carcinoma of the bladder which should be excluded first before the incontinence is addressed, especially in view of the haematuria.

A.	Arrange to see the woman on her own to ask her about domestic abuse
B.	Arrange an independent translator and ask about domestic abuse
C.	Ask the relatives if she is experiencing domestic abuse
D.	Ask the community midwife to visit her at home
E.	Contact the adult safeguarding team
F.	Contact the police

G.	Discuss child protection issues with the on-call social work team
H.	Encourage the woman to confide in a close relative if she is being abused
I.	Give the woman a card with contact numbers of agencies and refuges
J.	Offer immediate admission to hospital

You are concerned about the possibility of domestic violence in each of these women who are attending the hospital for antenatal care. In each case select the best course of action.

Each option may be used once, more than once or not at all.

28. While performing an anomaly scan at 20 weeks gestation, the ultrasonographer notices several bruises of different colours on the abdomen of a timid 17-year-old primigravid woman. Her 25-year-old boyfriend is also present to watch the scan and when she is asked questions (such as her address and date of birth) he supplies the answers.

A. Arrange to see the woman on her own to ask her about domestic abuse

Controlling behaviour can be a marker for domestic violence and the bruises of different ages need an explanation. She is not likely to disclose anything if he is present, so you will have to get her on her own to ask the question.

29. At 02.30 hours in the morning a 19-year-old primigravid woman presents to labour ward with postcoital bleeding. Her pregnancy is 32 weeks gestation and she is unaccompanied. On examination you notice that she has a 'black eye' and some circular bruises on her arms. Speculum examination reveals a tear in the posterior vaginal fornix which is not actively bleeding and the cervix is healthy. The baby is moving well, the uterus is not tender and the cardiotocograph is normal.

J. Offer immediate admission to hospital

This young woman has presented alone with clear signs of domestic violence (DV) in the small hours of the morning and if discharged home will most likely have to return to her abuser. The reality is that DV services are not available 24 hours a day so contacting the safeguarding team is not applicable at 2.30 am. This scenario does not mention any existing children so there would be no indication to involve the on-call social work team who are responsible for arranging emergency foster care. The option of encouraging the woman to confide in a close relative is inappropriate as they may be involved in the abuse or be being abused themselves by a controlling family member and therefore be in no position to help. Asking a midwife to visit is reasonable if there is low-level concern about abuse in the long term but the mode of presentation suggests that this woman has reached crisis point and needs help to remove herself from the abusive situation. The hospital is a place of safety and admission would allow the DV services to become involved and possibly arrange for her removal from the abusive situation in the morning. Therefore the reasons for admission are not clinical as fetal wellbeing has been confirmed; however, in the holistic approach to the patient, admission is justified.

30. A 26-year-old immigrant woman attends antenatal clinic at 34 weeks with her sister-in-law who translates for her, as she speaks no English at all. This is her first pregnancy and she is having growth scans on account of recurrent antepartum haemorrhage. The growth of the baby is fine, but when you are auscultating the fetal heart you notice some circular lesions on the maternal abdomen which look like cigarette burns.

B. Arrange an independent translator and ask about domestic abuse

Domestic violence is a common problem which crosses social boundaries and sometimes results in extreme outcomes, i.e. the death of the woman. In some areas of the country up to a quarter of women booking for antenatal care will have experienced some sort of domestic abuse which can take many forms: violence, sexual abuse, psychological abuse, control of her finances etc.

Obstetricians and GPs should have some knowledge of this issue as they are well placed to identify the problem in the first place. Clinicians should be aware of the existence of agencies and facilities able to help protect the woman and be able to discuss the subject with a patient at short notice.

Women should be asked about the possibility of domestic abuse at some stage in their antenatal care without any other family members or acquaintances being present, in case they are part of the problem. If necessary translators paid by the NHS such as 'language-line' should be used.

If a woman discloses that she is being subjected to violence, you may need to arrange admission to a place of safety such as hospital. There could be child protection issues if he is harming the children as well so if there are children in the equation, don't forget their needs.

SINGLE BEST ANSWER QUESTIONS

31. A woman who has three children has unfortunately conceived while wearing a copper coil for contraception. She comes to see you in surgery having had a positive pregnancy test at the chemists and reports that she is probably seven weeks gestation. Having talked to her husband, she is not too upset and is intending to keep the pregnancy.

    Select the most appropriate course of action:

    A. Perform a full STI screen as infection is likely to cause miscarriage
    B. Prescribe a course of antibiotics prophylactically
    C. Remind the midwife that the coil needs removing at her postnatal appointment
    D. Send her for a routine booking scan mentioning the coil on the scan request form
    E. Take the coil out as there is a risk of septic miscarriage

    Although removing the coil may cause miscarriage, leaving it in the uterus is more likely to result in pregnancy loss. Not only that, miscarriage is more likely to be complicated by infection if the coil is still present, so the advice is to remove it.

    There is a risk of ectopic pregnancy when a woman conceives with the coil in situ so an earlier scan than 12 weeks is indicated.

32. As she is completing the hospital discharge paperwork for a recently delivered mother on the maternity ward one of the midwives accidentally puts her copy of the list of current patients on the ward into the hand-held notes, so that the woman takes the list home with her. Which of these options is the most appropriate course of action for the midwife in charge of the ward to take?

    A. Ask the woman's community midwife to visit and retrieve the list
    B. Complete an incident form and inform the Information Governance Lead
    C. Send the police to retrieve the list from the patient's house

D.   Telephone the woman and ask her to shred the list

E.   Write to the woman and ask her to return the list

This is a serious breach of confidentiality and the person responsible for information governance will have to be informed. The action to be taken is their decision.

33.   A 26-year-old primigravid woman has a routine appointment with her community midwife at 32 weeks gestation. Her ankles and feet are so swollen that she has had to wear sandals instead of shoes to work and can no longer wear her rings. Her BP at booking was 120/70 and it is now 130/80. Urinalysis is negative. On examination she does have bilateral varicose veins and both ankles are mildly oedematous but there is no redness or tenderness in either leg. Which is the most appropriate management option?

A.   Advise the use of compression stockings

B.   Arrange lower limb venous Doppler studies

C.   Commence low-dose aspirin

D.   Refer to an obstetrician

E.   Request serum U&E and urate testing

This patient does not have pre-eclampsia although it would be prudent to recheck her BP earlier than normal. Her oedema is likely to be physiological, related to pregnancy, and is not a problem (apart from the discomfort) unless she does develop pre-eclampsia. As she has varicose veins too, some of her discomfort may be alleviated by compression stockings.

34.   A 20-year-old woman is admitted to the gynaecology ward over a bank holiday weekend with lower abdominal pain, deep dyspareunia, vaginal discharge and a fever of 38 °C. She has no gastrointestinal symptoms, is using the pill for contraception and is half way through a packet. On examination there is suprapubic tenderness and bimanual pelvic examination elicits cervical motion tenderness. Urinalysis is negative as is her pregnancy test. Which of the following is the most appropriate management plan?

A.   Take triple swabs and prescribe appropriate antibiotics according to sensitivities

B.   Prescribe doxycycline 100 mg twice daily for 14 days

C.   Prescribe metronidazole 400 mg and cefalexin 50 mg tds for 14 days

D.   Prescribe metronidazole and ofloxacin 400 mg bd for 14 days

E.   Administer azithromycin 1 g intramuscular injection and refer to the GUM clinic

Broad-spectrum antibiotics which will cover chlamydia infections and possibly gonorrhoea as well as anaerobes are needed. You should not wait for the culture results as the sequelae of not treating acute PID are serious (pelvic abscess, tubal damage, infertility and ectopic).

If the culture reveals gonorrhoea you might need to change the ofloxacin because of increasing resistance to quinolones in the UK.

Source: RCOG Green-top guideline number 32. *The Management of Acute Pelvic Inflammatory Disease.*

35.   The reason that obstetric units utilize a 'maternity dashboard' which describes items such as the caesarean section rate and the number of third-degree tears in the month is:

A. To keep track of the costs incurred on labour ward
B. To reduce the risk of litigation in relation to labour
C. To check on the performance of individual obstetricians for revalidation
D. To present the data to the CNST inspectors
E. **To compare the outcomes of their maternity services with other units**

Maternity dashboards were introduced a few years ago to give the obstetricians and midwives working in a hospital some idea of how their services were performing in relation to neighbouring hospitals. Obviously the demographics of the local population will have some effect on the outcomes, but sometimes problems are flagged up which can be solved by changing protocols and guidelines, e.g. reducing the induction rate will produce a fall in the caesarean section rate.

36. Following the realization that suicide is an important cause of maternal death, GPs are expected to be aware of issues concerning the mental health of pregnant women. Which one of the following statements is true?

A. A previous history of puerperal psychosis carries a recurrence risk of 5%
B. A woman with a history of depression should always be referred for a formal psychiatric opinion during pregnancy
C. The risk of suicide increases during pregnancy
D. **New mothers who commit suicide are more likely to die by violent means rather than overdose**
E. The Edinburgh Depression Scale may be used to screen for the risk of a psychotic depressive illness occurring

The Edinburgh scale is used to screen for postnatal depression symptoms and is of no use in predicting serious psychotic illness which, in relation to pregnancy, is usually a serious delusional state with a rapid onset 'out of the blue' and swift deterioration.

The risk of a psychotic illness recurring after the next pregnancy is frighteningly high and these women should be offered prenatal counselling so that they are aware of the risk. These issues were highlighted by the 2000–2002 Confidential Enquiries.

The recurrence risk for a major depressive illness, e.g. bipolar disorder, is similarly high at about 50% and there should be a plan of care written in conjunction with a psychiatrist which is available in all the woman's clinical notes.

The actual risk of suicide is lower in pregnancy but there is a massive increase following delivery and maternal suicide features as a leading cause of death in the triennial maternal mortality reports.

Because suicide is often associated with psychotic illness the attempt is much more likely to be serious and irretrievable, i.e. death by hanging, stabbing or jumping rather than the usual 'female' method of overdose.

37. Following a ward round with the registrar on labour ward you are left with a list of tasks to do. Which job takes priority over the rest?

A. Inserting an IV line for a patient labouring with a previous caesarean scar
B. **Performing a fetal blood sample on account of late decelerations on the CTG at 5 cm dilatation**
C. Clerking a new patient admitted with raised blood pressure at 39 weeks gestation
D. Discharging a patient who has been treated for severe postpartum haemorrhage to the postnatal ward

E. Obtaining consent for postmortem from a mother who is waiting to be discharged, having delivered her stillborn baby six hours ago

Checking for fetal distress in the abnormal CTG situation is the most pressing item on this list. The hypertensive new patient may actually have pre-eclampsia and be at risk of fitting so this would be the next priority. The IV access for the patient undergoing vaginal birth after caesarean is on account of the risk of scar rupture and not that urgent.

38. Six days after a hysterectomy operation, one of your patients presents to the surgery with right loin pain. She reports that she felt 'tired and shivery' when she was discharged from hospital three days before but now looks very unwell with a temperature of 38 °C. There is no vaginal bleeding or discharge. On examination she is tender in the right renal angle and right hypochondrium. You send off a midstream urine specimen and can see that she needs readmission for antibiotic treatment, but what will be the most appropriate investigation to make a diagnosis when she gets to hospital?

A. Intravenous urogram

B. Laparoscopy

C. Serum amylase

D. Three-swab test with methylene blue in the bladder

E. MRI scan of the gallbladder and liver

The suspicion is that she has ureteric damage, although a similar picture could occur with UTI or an abscess. The three-swab test is to look for vesicovaginal fistula.

39. You are clerking a new patient in gynaecology clinic with pelvic pain and trying to sort out a differential diagnosis. Which one of the following is a recognized symptom of endometriosis?

A. Abdominal bloating

B. Postcoital bleeding

C. Secondary dysmenorrhoea

D. Superficial dyspareunia

E. Weight loss

Endometriosis patients get secondary dysmenorrhoea, not primary dysmenorrhoea. There is no reason for the cervix to bleed so postcoital bleeding is not usually caused by endometriosis. If they do get dyspareunia, it is deep dyspareunia rather than superficial (as superficial means that there is something wrong in the vagina or vulva).

40. Two years after her last menstrual period a woman aged 51 is referred to a menopause clinic because of severe dyspareunia which is so bad that she can no longer tolerate intercourse. She was glad to see the end of her periods because they were becoming increasingly troublesome and has not experienced any vasomotor symptoms. On speculum examination the vulva and vagina look very atrophic and opening the speculum causes a small amount of bleeding by splitting the skin at the introitus. What is the most appropriate treatment in her case?

A. Fenton's operation to enlarge the vaginal introitus

B. Oral combined sequential estradiol and progesterone

C. Psychosexual counselling

D. Transdermal estradiol gel 1mg daily

E. Vaginal estradiol pessaries

As her symptoms are confined to the genital tract she only needs local treatment, not systemic HRT. Sequential therapy would bring a return of her bleeding which she would not be keen on, having been glad to get rid of her periods. Transdermal gel on its own is contraindicated anyway as she still has her uterus and would be at risk of endometrial cancer because of unopposed estrogen. There is no point in doing a Fenton's operation to enlarge the introitus before restoring the vaginal skin as without estrogen the skin would just continue to split.

41. In a postmenopausal patient presenting to gynaecology clinic with an advanced uterovaginal prolapse, which of the following clinical problems is **not** likely to be attributable to the prolapse?

A. Bleeding

B. Constipation

C. Digitation

D. Recurrent cystitis

E. Ulceration of the vaginal walls

Digitation means having to reduce the prolapse with a finger to facilitate defaecation. Women with procidentia often have pressure sores on the vaginal walls because of trauma. Although bleeding may be coming from ulceration of the vaginal walls, it would be prudent to exclude more sinister causes such as endometrial cancer.

42. You are seeing a woman in antenatal clinic who has developed obstetric cholestasis in her second pregnancy at 34 weeks gestation. She wishes to discuss her birth plan as she wanted a home birth with 'everything as natural as possible', having had a lot of medical intervention with a forceps delivery in her first labour. Which of the following plans is **not** correct or appropriate advice for her?

A. Continuous electronic fetal monitoring is advisable in labour

B. Daily fetal monitoring with CTG until delivery will predict the possibility of stillbirth

C. She may be offered induction of labour after 37 weeks to avoid the risk of stillbirth

D. She should deliver in the consultant unit rather than at home

E. She should have repeat liver function tests done a couple of weeks postpartum

The risk of stillbirth in cholestasis cannot be predicted using CTG and is the main reason for offering induction – although this increases the maternal and fetal morbidity due to iatrogenic prematurity. Meconium and fetal distress in labour are likely.

Source: RCOG Green-top guideline number 43. *Obstetric Cholestasis.*

43. The main purpose of organizing a bladder pressure (urodynamic) study for a woman presenting with a mixed picture of stress and urge incontinence with nocturia is:

A. To check for urinary fistula

B. To differentiate detrusor instability from genuine stress incontinence

C. To find out whether her symptoms are due to uterovaginal prolapse

D. To gauge the results of anticholinergic treatment

E. To prevent subsequent medicolegal problems if she does not respond to treatment

Some women develop 'de novo' bladder instability following operations for stress incontinence (which increase the pressure at the bladder neck). Requesting a bladder pressure study prior to a stress incontinence operation may be advisable to protect the gynaecologist against the accusation that they got the initial diagnosis wrong; but the main reason is to sort out the patients with unstable bladder in the first place who need anticholinergics and bladder drill, not surgery.

44. A primigravid woman presents to labour ward at 32 weeks gestation with vaginal bleeding. She is stable and the baby is well, but she is known to be Rhesus negative. Her clinical notes confirm that she had her prophylactic anti-D injection at 28 weeks gestation administered by her midwife.

Select the most appropriate management option:

A. Administer 250 IU anti-D and perform Kleihauer test
B. Administer 500 IU anti-D
C. Administer 500 IU anti-D and perform Kleihauer test
D. Ask the lab to check for residual anti-D from her prophylactic injection
E. No action necessary

She still needs anti-D in view of the recent bleed because the prophylactic dose will not cover this new event. There will be residual anti-D in her circulation, so you need to let the lab know about her prophylactic dose. She needs 500 IU because you have to make sure that the dose is enough to cover the amount of feto-maternal haemorrhage that has occurred.

45. One of the following is **not** a fetal risk factor for intrauterine growth restriction:

A. Congenital rubella infection
B. Chromosomal abnormalities
C. Cytomegalovirus infection in utero
D. Female sex
E. Multiple gestation

Syndromes such as Down and Edward syndrome may give rise to early onset IUGR and may prompt karyotyping if growth problems are noted early in pregnancy.

Placental insufficiency is more common in multiple pregnancies and can be more difficult to diagnose in the absence of regular growth scans.

46. A 25-year-old woman presents to the Early Pregnancy Unit with brown vaginal discharge. She is unsure of her last menstrual period but thinks the gestational age might be about seven weeks. The ultrasound scan has shown a small sac in the uterus with no contents. On vaginal examination you find no pelvic tenderness. What is the most suitable management plan?

A. Booking scan at 12 weeks gestation
B. Evacuate the uterus and send the contents for histological examination
C. Laparoscopy
D. Repeat ultrasound scan in one week
E. Serial urine βhCG assays with the next test 48 hours later

As she is unsure of the gestation there is still a chance that she has an intrauterine pregnancy (of lesser gestation than she estimates from her unsure last menstrual period). A decidual ring in the uterus can look like a gestation sac on scan however, so you still have not ruled out ectopic pregnancy. Serial hCG titres every 48 hours will help but it is serum, not urine.

47. A 47-year-old woman presents with a six-month history of regular heavy menstrual bleeding. She has had normal smears in the past and pelvic examination is unremarkable. Histology on a 'pipelle' sample of the endometrium and ultrasound scan are reported as normal. She had a DVT following a long-haul flight in the past but is otherwise healthy. Which of the following is the most appropriate treatment option for her menorrhagia?

A. Combined oral contraceptive pill

B. Hysterectomy

C. Levonorgestrel releasing IUS (Mirena®)

D. Norethisterone 15 mg daily from day 5–26 of menstrual cycle

E. Tranexamic acid

She cannot use either tranexamic acid or the combined pill because of the DVT risk and she is too old for the pill anyway. Hysterectomy is not first-line management and cyclical norethisterone is no longer recommended for dysfunctional uterine bleeding.

48. In the Teenage Family Planning Clinic you meet a 14-year-old schoolgirl requesting emergency contraceptive help after a mid-cycle condom breakage. Her parents are unaware of her sexual activity and do not approve of the relationship with her 22-year-old partner because he has another girlfriend who is currently pregnant. You decide that she is Fraser-competent and the recommended action in this situation would be:

A. Referral to police because of underage sexual activity

B. Referral to social services to investigate her sexual relationship with an adult

C. Referral to GUM clinic for full sexually transmitted disease screening

D. Refuse to supply contraception until the parents consent

E. Supply contraception and arrange follow-up appointment

There is a duty of care to this teenager to help her prevent an unwanted pregnancy which is reasonable as you have decided that she understands the issues and is competent to make a decision for herself. You should be concerned about the age discrepancy between the teenager and her partner and there are overtones of possible child abuse or exploitation which need addressing on a separate occasion. The best course of action regarding that would be to discuss her case with your local child protection agency but we have not given you this option. Involving her parents is a good idea and you should encourage her to do so, but you cannot do this yourself without her consent because of confidentiality. Informing the police, while legally correct, is not an appropriate first response to this situation as her contraceptive needs outweigh all other considerations.

Mock exam paper 2: MCQs

1. A primigravid woman has been in labour all day and on an oxytocin drip for the previous eight hours. A decision is made for assisted vaginal delivery on account of delay in the second stage. There is no caput or moulding of the fetal head and the maternal condition is satisfactory. Which of the following factors are essential before undertaking the delivery?

A. Fetal head not palpable per abdomen   [T] [F]
B. Arranging theatre as a difficult delivery is anticipated   [T] [F]
C. Adequate analgesia   [T] [F]
D. Fully dilated cervix   [T] [F]
E. Normal fetal heart rate on the cardiotocograph   [T] [F]

2. Regarding consent issues in contraceptive practice:

A. Written consent and verbal consent are equally valid   [T] [F]
B. Consent may be implied (non-verbal)   [T] [F]
C. Implied consent is sufficient for insertion or removal of intrauterine devices   [T] [F]
D. Expressed (written or verbal) consent is needed for removal of subdermal implants   [T] [F]
E. If a married woman is seeking sterilization, her husband's consent should also be obtained   [T] [F]

3. A primigravid woman has been admitted two hours ago bleeding heavily from placenta praevia at 30 weeks gestation and emergency caesarean section under general anaesthetic is proposed. A dose of dexamethasone has been administered, maternal observations are stable in spite of the continued bleeding and the cardiotocograph is satisfactory. When discussing the situation with the attending paediatrician which of these statements is correct?

A. The use of general anaesthetic may result in the baby needing resuscitation   [T] [F]
B. The baby may be anaemic because the surgeon might cut through the placenta   [T] [F]
C. Respiratory distress is less likely in this case because of the steroids   [T] [F]
D. The lie of the baby in the uterus is not relevant   [T] [F]
E. Delivery may be traumatic because there is no lower uterine segment   [T] [F]

4. Polycystic ovaries and polycystic ovarian syndrome can lead to the following problems:

A. A higher risk of first-trimester miscarriage   [T] [F]

B.	Short stature	[T]	[F]
C.	Obesity	[T]	[F]
D.	Endometrial hyperplasia	[T]	[F]
E.	Increased risk of diabetes in later life	[T]	[F]

5. One of your patients is going into hospital for a hysterectomy operation at the age of 34 years. She has always been excessively concerned about her appearance and spends a lot of money on spray tans. She had a 'tummy tuck' operation last year and she wishes to discuss the surgical scar before going into hospital.

A.	If the hysterectomy is being done for cancer she is more likely to have a longitudinal scar	[T]	[F]
B.	Transverse (Pfannenstiel) incisions are more likely to dehisce than longitudinal	[T]	[F]
C.	The choice of suture material for the skin depends on the surgeon's preference rather than whether the scar is longitudinal or transverse	[T]	[F]
D.	A Pfannenstiel incision is not likely to compromise her previous cosmetic surgery	[T]	[F]
E.	Unless she has uterine prolapse the hysterectomy cannot be done vaginally	[T]	[F]

6. Regarding the use of an intrauterine contraceptive device:

A.	There is a risk of infection within the first three weeks following insertion	[T]	[F]
B.	Insertion may provoke a seizure in a woman with epilepsy	[T]	[F]
C.	For maximum effectiveness standard devices carry at least 380 mm of copper	[T]	[F]
D.	They are contraindicated in nulliparous women	[T]	[F]
E.	They can be inserted within 48 hours in the immediate postpartum period	[T]	[F]

7. A woman aged 35 years consults you about continuing to use the combined oral contraceptive pill (COC) rather than changing her method of contraception. When assessing her risk factors and the benefits of the COC, in which circumstances would you suggest that she stop using the pill?

A.	Her BMI is 40 kg/m²	[T]	[F]
B.	She smokes 20 cigarettes per day	[T]	[F]
C.	She has developed migraine with aura	[T]	[F]
D.	Her mother has been diagnosed with breast cancer	[T]	[F]
E.	She has just been treated for CIN 3	[T]	[F]

8. Women with Turner syndrome:

A.	Are of shorter stature unless they have mosaic karyotype	[T]	[F]
B.	Should be investigated for congenital renal tract abnormality	[T]	[F]
C.	Do not usually have a uterus	[T]	[F]
D.	Are at risk of osteoporosis at an early age	[T]	[F]
E.	Could have a baby with oocyte donation	[T]	[F]

9. You have to complete a consent form with a recently delivered mother who has retained her placenta. Which of these risks and complications is correct and relevant to a woman about to undergo manual removal of placenta?

A. Blood transfusion may be needed because of primary haemorrhage [T] [F]

B. She will be given antibiotics because of the risk of introducing infection [T] [F]

C. She is likely to be offered a pudendal nerve block for analgesia [T] [F]

D. It is possible to perforate the uterus [T] [F]

E. Uterine inversion is an extremely rare but serious complication [T] [F]

10. Chorionic villus sampling:

A. Can only be done in the first trimester of pregnancy [T] [F]

B. Has a miscarriage risk of 2 to 3% [T] [F]

C. Is able to detect neural tube defects [T] [F]

D. Can be used to detect sex-linked inherited conditions [T] [F]

E. Carries a small risk of limb reduction defects in the fetus [T] [F]

11. A woman who has suffered recurrent miscarriages has been found to have a normal karyotype, as has her partner. The following management plans can be recommended for this couple as they have been shown to increase the chances of successful term pregnancy:

A. Screening for antiphospholipid syndrome and prescribing aspirin and heparin if positive [T] [F]

B. Prescribing progesterone during the first half of the pregnancy [T] [F]

C. Refer for preimplantation genetic diagnosis at the local fertility clinic [T] [F]

D. Regular scans during the first trimester in Early Pregnancy Unit [T] [F]

E. Human chorionic gonadotrophin supplements until 12 weeks gestation [T] [F]

12. In women relying on progesterone-only pills (POP) that do not contain desogestrel for contraception:

A. They should take their POP at the same time each day [T] [F]

B. The efficacy is reduced if the woman weighs over 75 kg [T] [F]

C. The bleeding pattern is likely to be unpredictable or absent in over half the women [T] [F]

D. 50% of women will stop taking the POP within a year because of unpredictable bleeding [T] [F]

E. They have a 12-hour window in which to take a pill they have missed [T] [F]

13. The UK National Maternal Mortality Report:

A. Presents data relating to all maternal deaths over a five-year period of time [T] [F]

B. Uses information from maternal deaths to recommend changes to obstetric practice [T] [F]

C. Includes information about mothers who have committed suicide postpartum [T] [F]

D. May suggest referral of a clinician to the GMC where care is found to be substandard [T] [F]

E. Covers deaths relating to early pregnancy problems such as abortion [T] [F]

14. With regard to classical caesarean section:

A. It must be performed under general anaesthetic [T] [F]

B. May be preferred over lower segment caesarean if the fetus is less than 30 weeks gestation [T] [F]

C. Placenta praevia with transverse lie of the fetus is an indication [T] [F]

D. The chance of the scar rupturing in the next pregnancy is 50% [T] [F]

E. It involves the surgeon making a longitudinal incision on the uterus [T] [F]

15. With regard to premenstrual syndrome:

A. It can occur in anovulatory cycles [T] [F]

B. Women have a symptom-free interval of at least one week following menstruation [T] [F]

C. It is defined by the onset of symptoms prior to ovulation [T] [F]

D. It may include weight gain in the latter part of the menstrual cycle [T] [F]

E. Symptoms will resolve if ovarian function is pharmacologically suppressed [T] [F]

16. In a woman over 40 years of age who needs contraception:

A. FSH measurement in the pill-free interval can be used to diagnose ovarian failure in a woman taking the combined pill [T] [F]

B. depot medroxy progesterone acetate has been shown to reduce bone density [T] [F]

C. She should continue using contraception for two years after her last period if she is under 50 years old [T] [F]

D. Mirena® has a licence for seven years contraception if inserted into a woman when she is over the age of 45 years [T] [F]

E. Sequential hormone replacement therapy formulations can be prescribed as contraception [T] [F]

17. The following factors in a woman's medical history increase her risk of ectopic pregnancy:

A. Previous surgery for reversal of sterilization [T] [F]

B. Conception in spite of current use of the Progesterone only pill [T] [F]

C. Ovulation induction treatment [T] [F]

D. Conception using in vitro fertilization [T] [F]

E. Treated chlamydial infection [T] [F]

18. You are called to labour ward to see a primigravid woman whose obstetric care has been midwifery-led until she presented in advanced labour at 39 weeks gestation and her BP on admission was noted to be 165/105 (booking level 115/60). She has only been on the labour ward for 20 minutes but appears to be actively pushing and the midwife tells you that she has a fully dilated cervix. Which of these actions are correct and appropriate in this case?

A. Draw up an ampoule of syntometrine ready for the third stage of labour [T] [F]

B. Insert an IV cannula and take blood samples [T] [F]

C. Obtain a sample of urine for protein testing [T] [F]
D. Repeat the blood pressure in between contractions [T] [F]
E. Ask the midwife to commence electronic fetal monitoring [T] [F]

19. Regarding the Mirena® intrauterine system:

A. It releases a steady dose of etonogestrel from the sheath enveloping the stem [T] [F]
B. It can be used to oppose estrogen-only hormone replacement therapy [T] [F]
C. Whatever the indication the licence lasts five years before replacement [T] [F]
D. It is licensed to treat endometrial hyperplasia [T] [F]
E. Irregular bleeding can be expected after insertion for many months [T] [F]

20. In a man seeking vasectomy:

A. The operation should be deferred if he has an inguinal hernia [T] [F]
B. The operation is contraindicated if he has no children at all [T] [F]
C. The operation is more risky in patients with Von Willebrand's disease [T] [F]
D. The operation cannot be done if he has a hydrocoele on examination [T] [F]
E. The operation can be relied on for contraception after the next ejaculation [T] [F]

21. Regarding prolapse of the uterus:

A. A shelf pessary should be offered as first-line treatment if a woman is very unfit [T] [F]
B. Surgical treatment usually involves hysterectomy [T] [F]
C. Can be treated successfully with pelvic floor exercises in younger patients [T] [F]
D. May be related to habitual straining due to constipation [T] [F]
E. May become symptomatic because of a pelvic tumour [T] [F]

22. An ultrasound scan is necessary for a patient seeking termination of pregnancy in the following situations:

A. If the uterus is larger than expected for the gestational age [T] [F]
B. If the patient has experienced vaginal bleeding while pregnant [T] [F]
C. The patient is undecided whether to have a medical or surgical method [T] [F]
D. The doctor is hoping to persuade her against termination [T] [F]
E. The patient refuses vaginal examination [T] [F]

23. An 84-year-old woman presents to the surgery complaining of recent onset of cystitis symptoms and urinary frequency. She has also noticed haematuria on several occasions but had ignored it until the discomfort prompted her to seek an appointment. As an afterthought as she is leaving the room she mentions 'something coming down' and on examination you are surprised to find a complete procidentia. Testing her urine reveals protein and a lot of blood. Which of the following investigations are appropriate given the clinical findings?

A. Cystoscopy [T] [F]

B. Serum urea and electrolytes   [T]   [F]

C. Cystogram x-ray   [T]   [F]

D. Midstream specimen of urine   [T]   [F]

E. Scan of kidneys and bladder   [T]   [F]

24. Sepsis related to the genital tract in pregnant women:

A. Is the leading direct cause of maternal death in the 2006–2008   [T]   [F]
UK Mortality Report

B. Is excluded if the woman has a temperature $< 37\,°C$ on   [T]   [F]
admission

C. May be associated with a streptococcal sore throat   [T]   [F]

D. Is more likely following a vaginal birth rather than a caesarean   [T]   [F]

E. Is not likely to be the diagnosis if the patient's white cell   [T]   [F]
count $< 4 \times 10^9/l$

25. Venous thromboembolism is more likely in pregnant patients with:

A. Hyperemesis gravidarum   [T]   [F]

B. Pre-eclampsia   [T]   [F]

C. Ovarian hyperstimulation syndrome   [T]   [F]

D. Asymptomatic gallstones   [T]   [F]

E. Thrombocytopaenia   [T]   [F]

26. Regarding the duties of a doctor:

A. When treating a patient for a sexually transmitted infection, you   [T]   [F]
always have a duty to inform the spouse regardless of the
patient's consent

B. A chaperone is needed for gynaecological pelvic examinations   [T]   [F]
only if the doctor is male

C. When consenting a patient for a surgical procedure, only   [T]   [F]
common complications need to be discussed

D. If you see a child with a proven sexually transmitted infection   [T]   [F]
this must always be reported

E. Consent is not required for anomaly scans performed at 20 weeks   [T]   [F]
gestation

27. Characteristic features of physiological jaundice in the newborn include:

A. Onset after the first 24 hours of life   [T]   [F]

B. Disappearance by the fourth day   [T]   [F]

C. Associated anaemia   [T]   [F]

D. Could lead to kernicterus if not treated   [T]   [F]

E. Occurs more frequently in preterm infants   [T]   [F]

28. A 41-year-old woman has always attended for regular cervical screening and all her tests so far have been normal. It would be appropriate to take a smear from her in the following circumstances:

A. She presents with a new diagnosis of genital warts   [T]   [F]

B. She discovers a family history of cervical cancer   [T]   [F]

C. She presents with a history of postcoital bleeding   [T]   [F]

| D. | She is noted on examination to have a cervical polyp | [T] | [F] |
| E. | She had her previous cervical screen three years ago | [T] | [F] |

29. With regard to human papilloma virus vaccines:

A.	It is pointless giving the vaccine if the woman is already sexually active	[T]	[F]
B.	A full course provides lifelong immunity against cervical cancer	[T]	[F]
C.	They contain live virus	[T]	[F]
D.	They are contraindicated in males	[T]	[F]
E.	A woman who has been vaccinated does not need smears	[T]	[F]

30. If a pregnant woman is infected with German measles (rubella) in the first trimester, her baby has an increased risk of:

A.	Cataract	[T]	[F]
B.	Short limbs	[T]	[F]
C.	Congenital heart lesions	[T]	[F]
D.	Conductive deafness	[T]	[F]
E.	Facial clefts	[T]	[F]

31. With regard to bacterial vaginosis diagnosed in pregnancy:

A.	It is thought to cause pelvic inflammatory disease after termination	[T]	[F]
B.	It should be treated if detected in pregnancy	[T]	[F]
C.	It is associated with a two-fold increase in preterm delivery	[T]	[F]
D.	It is a risk factor for second-trimester miscarriage	[T]	[F]
E.	It may be treated with oral clindamycin	[T]	[F]

32. Mothers who smoke cigarettes:

A.	Are more likely to suffer placental abruption	[T]	[F]
B.	Are more likely to have a postpartum haemorrhage	[T]	[F]
C.	Are more likely to be referred to antenatal clinic by their midwife for a growth scan	[T]	[F]
D.	Are more likely to develop cervical cancer	[T]	[F]
E.	Are more likely to experience sudden infant death syndrome	[T]	[F]

33. Surgically removing the ovaries at the time of hysterectomy:

A.	Is usually done if the woman has endometrial cancer	[T]	[F]
B.	Could result in loss of libido	[T]	[F]
C.	Will eliminate premenstrual syndrome	[T]	[F]
D.	Is not usually done if the hysterectomy is performed vaginally	[T]	[F]
E.	Is referred to as a total hysterectomy	[T]	[F]

34. If a woman presents to the GP with postmenopausal bleeding:

A.	She is most likely to have endometrial cancer	[T]	[F]
B.	She should stop taking hormone replacement therapy	[T]	[F]
C.	It is defined as vaginal bleeding more than six months after her last menstrual period	[T]	[F]

D. She could be treated with estrogen cream initially if speculum [T] [F]
exam reveals atrophic vaginitis

E. She does not need hysteroscopy if her endometrium is 7 mm [T] [F]
thick on ultrasound scan

35. With regard to *Chlamydia trachomatis* infection:

A. It may cause neonatal conjunctivitis and pneumonia [T] [F]
B. It is usually asymptomatic in women [T] [F]
C. It may lead to infertility [T] [F]
D. It is treated with mebendazole [T] [F]
E. It can cause epididymo-orchitis in men [T] [F]

36. Regarding group B streptococcus colonization in pregnancy:

A. Group B streptococcus bacteriuria in this pregnancy is an [T] [F]
indication for intrapartum antibiotics

B. The antibiotic of choice for prophylaxis is clindamycin [T] [F]
C. Oral benzylpenicillin is indicated in labour if there is known [T] [F]
group B streptococcal colonization

D. Routine screening using high vaginal swabs is common in UK [T] [F]
practice

E. Prophylaxis is required for high-risk women having planned [T] [F]
caesarean sections

37. Regarding haemorrhagic disease of the newborn:

A. It is a risk because vitamin K stores in neonates are low [T] [F]
B. It only occurs in the first few days of life [T] [F]
C. Prevention with IM injection is more effective than oral vitamin K [T] [F]
D. It is more common in wholly breastfed babies [T] [F]
E. There is a better outlook for babies with the late-onset form [T] [F]

38. Regarding a woman who has undergone female genital mutilation (also
known as female circumcision or infibulation) as a child:

A. Caesarean section will be necessary if she decides to have a baby [T] [F]
B. The infibulation cannot be surgically undone during pregnancy [T] [F]
C. The operation is illegal in the UK [T] [F]
D. She is more likely to subject her daughters to the same procedure [T] [F]
E. The husband can legally insist on the infibulation being restored [T] [F]

39. Pregnancy has an adverse effect on:

A. Iron deficiency anaemia [T] [F]
B. Pulmonary tuberculosis [T] [F]
C. Mitral stenosis [T] [F]
D. Crohn's disease [T] [F]
E. Rheumatoid arthritis [T] [F]

40. Regarding cervical cerclage (suturing the cervix closed) in pregnancy:

A. It is indicated in a woman with a history of recurrent painless [T] [F]
late miscarriages

B. The suture is inserted after the first trimester is completed   [T]   [F]

C. Removal of the suture requires general or spinal anaesthetic   [T]   [F]

D. The suture is usually inserted abdominally, requiring a laparotomy   [T]   [F]

E. The procedure can be done as a 'rescue' operation if the cervix starts dilating   [T]   [F]

Mock exam paper 2: Answers

1. A primigravid woman has been in labour all day and on an oxytocin drip for the previous eight hours. A decision is made for assisted vaginal delivery on account of delay in the second stage. There is no caput or moulding of the fetal head and the maternal condition is satisfactory. Which of the following factors are essential before undertaking the delivery?

A.	Fetal head not palpable per abdomen	T
B.	Arranging theatre as a difficult delivery is anticipated	F
C.	Adequate analgesia	T
D.	Fully dilated cervix	T
E.	Normal fetal heart rate on the cardiotocograph	F

This should be an easy delivery as the baby's head is well engaged and there is no sign of cephalopelvic disproportion. We would only plan to do an assisted delivery in theatre if we thought there was a good chance of having to proceed to caesarean section. There should be adequate analgesia, e.g. epidural or pudendal block may be sufficient. The factors that must be in place for a successful assisted delivery are that the fetal head is not palpable abdominally, the bladder and bowel are empty, the cervix is fully dilated and the position of the head is known. Therefore most of the statements are prerequisites for safe assisted delivery except for 'normal CTG' – we might be doing the assisted delivery because we are worried about the baby's condition. Even if the fetal heart trace is not perfect, assisted delivery in this instance is to bring the second stage to an end quickly.

2. Regarding consent issues in contraceptive practice:

A.	Written consent and verbal consent are equally valid	T
B.	Consent may be implied (non-verbal)	T
C.	Implied consent is sufficient for insertion or removal of intrauterine devices	T
D.	Expressed (written or verbal) consent is needed for removal of subdermal implants	F
E.	If a married woman is seeking sterilization, her husband's consent should also be obtained	F

If a woman attends a clinic seeking contraceptive advice and chooses the intrauterine device or implant methods, submitting herself to the insertion procedure implies consent. Most clinics seek verbal or written consent.

3. A primigravid woman has been admitted two hours ago bleeding heavily from placenta praevia at 30 weeks gestation and emergency caesarean section under general anaesthetic is proposed. A dose of dexamethasone has been administered, maternal observations are stable in spite of the continued bleeding and the cardiotocograph is satisfactory. When discussing the

situation with the attending paediatrician which of these statements is correct?

A. The use of general anaesthetic may result in the baby needing resuscitation   T

B. The baby may be anaemic because the surgeon might cut through the placenta   T

C. Respiratory distress is less likely in this case because of the steroids   F

D. The lie of the baby in the uterus is not relevant   F

E. Delivery may be traumatic because there is no lower uterine segment   T

When a general anaesthetic is administered to a mother, the baby is often anaesthetized too – so we scrub and get ready to start immediately she is asleep so that the baby gets as little anaesthetic as possible. If the placenta is anterior we sometimes have to cut through it to reach the baby and some of the blood lost will belong to the baby. She has only had one dose of steroids – and that only recently – so it is not likely to make a difference to the incidence of respiratory distress. Because the placenta occupies the lower part of the uterus the baby is likely to be lying transversely, which can make it really difficult to deliver, so that it will be in need of resuscitation. The lower uterine segment often does not form until 30 weeks, so it can be difficult to extract the baby through a transverse incision and sometimes we perform a classical incision in premature situations.

4. Polycystic ovaries and polycystic ovarian syndrome can lead to the following problems:

A. A higher risk of first-trimester miscarriage   T

B. Short stature   F

C. Obesity   T

D. Endometrial hyperplasia   T

E. Increased risk of diabetes in later life   T

Polycystic ovaries (PCO) is a multisystem disorder of the pituitary–ovarian axis which has widespread effects in addition to anovulation. PCO leads to metabolic syndrome characterized by obesity and increased risk of type 2 diabetes as it is an insulin-resistant state. Unfortunately we cannot do much about the increased risk of miscarriage and in fact we do not usually counsel patients about that. Endometrial hyperplasia is a risk because of unopposed estrogen stimulation due to anovulation.

The exact mechanism whereby PCO causes miscarriage is uncertain, but may be related to insulin resistance, hyperinsulinaemia and hyperandrogenaemia.

5. One of your patients is going into hospital for a hysterectomy operation at the age of 34 years. She has always been excessively concerned about her appearance and spends a lot of money on spray tans. She had a 'tummy tuck' operation last year and she wishes to discuss the surgical scar before going into hospital.

A. If the hysterectomy is being done for cancer she more likely to have a longitudinal scar   T

B. Transverse (Pfannenstiel) incisions are more likely to dehisce than longitudinal   F

C. The choice of suture material for the skin depends on the surgeon's preference rather than whether the scar is longitudinal or transverse   T

D. A Pfannenstiel incision is not likely to compromise her previous cosmetic surgery   T

E. Unless she has uterine prolapse the hysterectomy cannot be done vaginally   F

Most gynaecological surgery is done through Pfannenstiel incisions because they give good access to the pelvis, unless there is a large pelvic mass such as an ovarian cyst or fibroid. If there is a suspicion of cancer, we normally use longitudinal incisions to get access to the upper abdomen and because the incision can be extended in order to remove masses intact without spilling contents.

Longitudinal incisions are not as robust as transverse and because they are more likely to dehisce, we use non-absorbable or very slowly absorbed material on the rectus sheath (where the strength of the wound is), whereas we can get away with absorbable sutures in Pfannenstiel incisions. Surgeons can use what they like on the skin because it is not the skin that holds the abdominal wall together.

Patients who have had the fatty 'pannus' removed previously usually have a massive transverse scar right across their lower abdomen, which can be used again to perform the hysterectomy. Even if the scar is longitudinal it does not interfere with the cosmetic result from her 'tummy tuck'.

In many patients it is possible to remove the uterus vaginally even if there is no prolapse, except if the hysterectomy is being done for cancer, ovarian cysts or for large fibroids. If the ovaries are to be removed as well, it is not easy to reach the ovaries from below but this is not likely to be considered in someone aged 34 years (except if the operation is being done for cancer).

6. Regarding the use of an intrauterine contraceptive device:

A. There is a risk of infection within the first three weeks following insertion   T

B. Insertion may provoke a seizure in a woman with epilepsy   T

C. For maximum effectiveness standard devices carry at least 380 mm of copper   T

D. They are contraindicated in nulliparous women   F

E. They can be inserted within 48 hours in the immediate postpartum period   T

If infection occurs it is most likely within 20 days of insertion likely due to intrauterine carriage of existing STIs from the cervix. Standard devices also have banded copper on the arms to increase efficacy. Dilating the cervix in epileptic women may give rise to a fit.

The method is suitable for women of all ages regardless of parity. Postpartum fitting within 48 hours has been shown to be safe but after this time fitting should be deferred to four weeks following confinement.

7. A woman aged 35 years consults you about continuing to use the combined oral contraceptive pill (COC) rather than changing her method of contraception. When assessing her risk factors and the benefits of the COC, in which circumstances would you suggest that she stop using the pill?

A. Her BMI is 40 kg/m²   T

B. She smokes 20 cigarettes per day   T

C. She has developed migraine with aura   T

D. Her mother has been diagnosed with breast cancer   F

E. She has just been treated for CIN 3   F

The use of the COC in women aged 35 or over who smoke is not recommended. The risks of using COC in women with a BMI ≥ 35 kg/m² usually outweighs the benefits (UKMEC 3). Migraine with aura is a condition for which the COC presents an unacceptable risk to health (UKMEC 4).

Studies have demonstrated an increased risk of breast cancer with COC use that disappears within ten years of stopping the COC. However, no studies have demonstrated any increased risk of death from breast cancer. Any woman with a family history of breast cancer is at increased risk from the condition; this risk does not appear to be increased as a result of taking the COC. However, for women with a proven BRCA1 or BRCA2 mutation current UKMEC 3 guidance suggests that the theoretical or proven risks generally outweigh the advantages of using the method.

Sources: *Sexual and Reproductive Health for Individuals with Inflammatory Bowel Disease. Faculty of Sexual & Reproductive Healthcare Guidance, June 2009.*

Combined Hormonal Contraception. Faculty of Sexual & Reproductive Healthcare Guidance, October 2011.

8.   Women with Turner syndrome:

A.   Are of shorter stature unless they have mosaic karyotype   T
B.   Should be investigated for congenital renal tract abnormality   T
C.   Do not usually have a uterus   F
D.   Are at risk of osteoporosis at an early age   T
E.   Could have a baby with oocyte donation   T

Women with karyotype 45XO are usually of short stature but women with a mosaic karyotype (some cell lines with 45XO and some with 46XX) can be of normal height. They have streak ovaries but normal pelvic organs otherwise and can have children using donated eggs as long as they have received enough estrogen to grow the uterus to normal proportions at puberty.

They are at risk of osteoporosis because of low estrogen levels and need HRT until normal menopausal age.

9.   You have to complete a consent form with a recently delivered mother who has retained her placenta. Which of these risks and complications is correct and relevant to a woman about to undergo manual removal of placenta?

A.   Blood transfusion may be needed because of primary haemorrhage   T
B.   She will be given antibiotics because of the risk of introducing infection   T
C.   She is likely to be offered a pudendal nerve block for analgesia   F
D.   It is possible to perforate the uterus   T
E.   Uterine inversion is an extremely rare but serious complication   T

Pudendal nerve block is not enough analgesia for manual removal, which involves the operator inserting their whole hand into the uterine cavity. It is normally done under spinal or general anaesthetic. Uterine inversion of the fundus of the uterus appearing at the vaginal introitus could happen if the surgeon pulls on the placenta before detaching it from the uterus and is a possibility if there is placenta accreta.

10.   Chorionic villus sampling (CVS):

A.   Can only be done in the first trimester of pregnancy   F
B.   Has a miscarriage risk of 2 to 3%   T
C.   Is able to detect neural tube defects   F
D.   Can be used to detect sex-linked inherited conditions   T
E.   Carries a small risk of limb reduction defects in the fetus   T

Chorionic villus sampling (CVS) refers to taking a biopsy of the placenta and can be done at any gestation but tends to be called placental biopsy when performed later in pregnancy. The idea is that women can get a diagnosis early enough in pregnancy to allow surgical termination but the earlier it is done, the more chance of harm to the fetus. The risk of limb reduction defects is the main reason that it is deferred until 11 weeks rather than being done earlier in pregnancy.

11. A woman who has suffered recurrent miscarriages has been found to have a normal karyotype, as has her partner. The following management plans can be recommended for this couple as they have been shown to increase the chances of successful term pregnancy:

A. Screening for antiphospholipid syndrome and prescribing aspirin and heparin if positive T

B. Prescribing progesterone during the first half of the pregnancy F

C. Refer for preimplantation genetic diagnosis at the local fertility clinic F

D. Regular scans during the first trimester in Early Pregnancy Unit T

E. Human chorionic gonadotrophin supplements until 12 weeks gestation F

This is a difficult situation for couples to face and they are usually desperate to pursue any form of treatment that might increase their chances of a successful pregnancy. However, the only manoeuvres that have been proved to work are the identification and treatment of antiphospholipid syndrome and regular reassurance scans during the first trimester (can't explain why this should work).

Source: RCOG Green-top guideline number 17. *The Investigation and Treatment of Couples with Recurrent Miscarriage.*

12. In women relying on progesterone-only pills (POP) that do not contain desogestrel for contraception:

A. They should take their POP at the same time each day T

B. The efficacy is reduced if the women weighs over 75 kg F

C. The bleeding pattern is likely to be unpredictable or absent in over half the women T

D. 50% of women will stop taking the POP within a year because of unpredictable bleeding F

E. They have a 12-hour window in which to take a pill they have missed F

There is no evidence that the efficacy of POPs is reduced in women with a high BMI although many practitioners prescribe double doses for them.

The POP is well known for producing an unpredictable bleeding pattern: 20% amenorrhoea, 40% irregular and 40% of women with a normal pattern. This leads to discontinuation of the method in between 10 and 25% of users within the first year of use.

Cerazette® which contains desogestrel has a 12-hour window; the others only have three hours.

13. The UK National Maternal Mortality Report:

A. Presents data relating to all maternal deaths over a five-year period of time F

B. Uses information from maternal deaths to recommend changes to obstetric practice T

C. Includes information about mothers who have committed suicide postpartum T

D. May suggest referral of a clinician to the GMC where care is found to be substandard F

E. Covers deaths relating to early pregnancy problems such as abortion T

The UK National Maternal Mortality Report – 'Saving Mothers' Lives' – is triennial, i.e. it covers a three-year period. The latest before the publication of this book was 2006–2008 and was published in March 2011. It gives learning points to allow the readers to understand why these deaths occur and to assist them to make changes to their practice, including a list of their 'top ten recommendations'. The report considers all deaths of women up to 364 days following delivery, but concentrates on deaths from any pregnancy-related problems. Substandard care is identified in each case, but only with regard to making improvements in service delivery in the future, not as a reason for referral to the regulating body.

14. With regard to classical caesarean section:

A. It must be performed under general anaesthetic   F

B. May be preferred over lower segment caesarean if the fetus is less than 30 weeks gestation   T

C. Placenta praevia with transverse lie of the fetus is an indication   T

D. The chance of the scar rupturing in the next pregnancy is 50%   F

E. It involves the surgeon making a longitudinal incision on the uterus   T

Classical caesarean section involves making a longitudinal incision on the uterus regardless of the orientation of the skin incision. It is used when it is difficult to get the baby out through the lower segment, for example if the baby is lying transversely or if there is a fibroid in the way. There is no lower segment under 32 weeks gestation so sometimes classical section is necessary in extreme preterm situations. The scar is more likely to rupture in a subsequent pregnancy than a lower segment scar but the risk is 2 to 9% not 50%.

Source: RCOG Green-top guideline number 45. *Birth after Previous Caesarean Birth.*

15. With regard to premenstrual syndrome:

A. It can occur in anovulatory cycles   F

B. Women have a symptom-free interval of at least one week following menstruation   T

C. It is defined by the onset of symptoms prior to ovulation   F

D. It may include weight gain in the latter part of the menstrual cycle   T

E. Symptoms will resolve if ovarian function is pharmacologically suppressed   T

Premenstrual syndrome (PMS) is generally thought to be a situation where a woman is very sensitive to normal levels of progesterone in the second half of the cycle after ovulation. It does not occur in anovulatory cycles. There are psychological and physical symptoms which are similar to the side effects of progestogen therapy.

16. In a woman over 40 years of age who needs contraception:

A. FSH measurement in the pill-free interval can be used to diagnose ovarian failure in a woman taking the combined pill   F

B. depot medroxy progesterone acetate has been shown to reduce bone density   T

C. She should continue using contraception for two years after her last period if she is under 50 years old   T

D. Mirena® has a licence for seven years contraception if inserted into a woman when she is over the age of 45 years   F

E. Sequential hormone replacement therapy formulations can be prescribed
as contraception   F

*The FSH is an unreliable indicator of ovarian failure in women on the COC but
can be used to diagnose early menopause in women using progesterone methods.
Mirena® only has a license for five years contraception at any age but can be used
off-licence in women over 45 years. Hormone replacement therapy (HRT) is not
contraceptive.*

Source: *Faculty of Family Planning guidance on contraception for women aged
over 40 years (2010).*

17. **The following factors in a woman's medical history increase her risk of
ectopic pregnancy:**

A. Previous surgery for reversal of sterilization   T

*The ectopic is held up at the site of the scar from the reanastomosis
operation.*

B. Conception in spite of current use of the Progesterone only pill   T

*Progesterone slows down the action of the cilia in the fallopian tubes so that the
conceptus is wafted down the tube at a slower rate and has a greater chance of
implanting there.*

C. Ovulation induction treatment   F

This should have no effect on the ectopic risk.

D. Conception using in vitro fertilization   T

*There is a substantial risk of ectopic with IVF (up to 10%), which seems
counterintuitive as the embryos are replaced directly into the uterus.*

E. Treated chlamydial infection   T

*Adhesions and scarring after pelvic inflammatory disease are a main cause of
ectopic pregnancy.*

18. **You are called to labour ward to see a primigravid woman whose obstetric
care has been midwifery-led until she presented in advanced labour at
39 weeks gestation and her BP on admission was noted to be 165/105 mmHg
(booking level 115/60 mmHg). She has only been on the labour ward for 20
minutes but appears to be actively pushing and the midwife tells you that she
has a fully dilated cervix. Which of these actions are correct and appropriate
in this case?**

A. Draw up an ampoule of syntometrine ready for the third stage
of labour   F

*She can't be given syntometrine because it might cause an elevation in her blood
pressure, which is already extremely high.*

B. Insert an IV cannula and take blood samples   T

*Although she is about to deliver, you should take blood for pre-eclampsia
biochemistry.*

C. Obtain a sample of urine for protein testing   T

You might need to catheterize her in order to get an uncontaminated sample.

D. Repeat the blood pressure in between contractions   T

*As well as repeating the measurement, her blood pressure needs treating,
otherwise she is at risk of having a stroke as her diastolic is > 160 mmHg.*

E. Ask the midwife to commence electronic fetal monitoring   T

There is likely to be placental insufficiency if she has pre-eclampsia.

19. **Regarding the Mirena® intrauterine system:**

A. It releases a steady dose of etonogestrel from the sheath enveloping
the stem   F

B. It can be used to oppose estrogen-only hormone replacement therapy   T

C. Whatever the indication the licence lasts five years before replacement   F

D. It is licensed to treat endometrial hyperplasia   F

E. Irregular bleeding can be expected after insertion for many months   T

*Mirena® contains levonorgestrel and if it is being used to oppose estrogen the
license is only for four years. It is not licensed to treat endometrial hyperplasia at the
current time.*

*It is primary treatment for menorrhagia and the patient should be warned
about the bleeding pattern, otherwise they will visit their GP to have it removed
after only a few months.*

20. **In a man seeking vasectomy:**

A. The operation should be deferred if he has an inguinal hernia   F

B. The operation is contraindicated if he has no children at all   F

C. The operation is more risky in patients with Von Willebrand's disease   T

D. The operation cannot be done if he has a hydrocoele on examination   F

E. The operation can be relied on for contraception after the next ejaculation   F

An inguinal hernia is not a reason to defer vasectomy.

*Although a man may be sterilized if he has not fathered any children, great care
must be taken during the counselling procedure, particularly with men under
30 years of age.*

*Bleeding disorders such as Von Willebrand's lead to an increased risk of
postoperative haematoma formation and this in turn may lead to increased
infection risk.*

*The presence of a hydrocoele can make it difficult to palpate the vas; a single
operation when the hydrocoele is repaired at the same time as the vasectomy is likely
to decrease the complication rate.*

*The operation is not counted as successful until semen samples are clear of
spermatozoa, which can vary. There is no clear rationale for taking two tests but
this is the convention in the UK, usually at 12 and 16 weeks. In some areas of the
world the number of ejaculations postoperatively is used as a marker, e.g. 20
ejaculations, particularly where no semen testing can be done.*

Source: RCOG Evidence-based clinical guideline number 4. 2004 – *Male and
Female Sterilization.*

21. **Regarding prolapse of the uterus:**

A. A shelf pessary should be offered as first-line treatment if a woman is
very unfit   F

B. Surgical treatment usually involves hysterectomy   T

C. Can be treated successfully with pelvic floor exercises in younger patients   F

D. May be related to habitual straining due to constipation   T

E. May become symptomatic because of a pelvic tumour   T

*We usually choose ring pessaries as first-line treatment and reserve shelf pessaries
for use in women where we cannot get a ring to stay in the vagina, as they are more
difficult to insert and remove. If the prolapse involves the uterus, it is usual to
perform a vaginal hysterectomy often combined with pelvic floor repair. Uterine
prolapse is due to stretching of the transverse cervical and uterosacral ligaments*

which are supposed to support the uterus but do not contain muscle so cannot be exercised. Chronic constipation is associated with prolapse and sometimes a woman may present acutely with a new prolapse because it is being pushed down by a tumour in the pelvis. Careful abdominal and vaginal examination is necessary in the initial assessment.

22. An ultrasound scan is necessary for a patient seeking termination of pregnancy in the following situations:

A.	If the uterus is larger than expected for the gestational age	T
B.	If the patient has experienced vaginal bleeding while pregnant	T
C.	The patient is undecided whether to have a medical or surgical method	F
D.	The doctor is hoping to persuade her against termination	F
E.	The patient refuses vaginal examination	T

If the uterus is large for dates she may have a multiple pregnancy, a molar pregnancy or the dates may be wrong. If there has been bleeding she may already have miscarried or may have an ectopic pregnancy. Ultrasound does not usually aid the choice of method and should definitely not be used to upset the patient or pressurize her not to go ahead with termination, which must be her decision having weighed up the pros and cons. Counselling should be non-judgemental.

If she refuses vaginal examination you will not be sure of the gestation (and also lose the opportunity for STI screening).

23. An 84-year-old woman presents to the surgery complaining of recent onset of cystitis symptoms and urinary frequency. She has also noticed haematuria on several occasions but had ignored it until the discomfort prompted her to seek an appointment. As an afterthought as she is leaving the room she mentions 'something coming down' and on examination you are surprised to find a complete procidentia. Testing her urine reveals protein and a lot of blood. Which of the following investigations are appropriate given the clinical findings?

A.	Cystoscopy	T
B.	Serum urea and electrolytes	T
C.	Cystogram x-ray	F
D.	Midstream specimen of urine	T
E.	Scan of kidneys and bladder	T

Procidentia can result in kinking of the ureters and subsequent mild chronic renal failure, which resolves when the prolapse is treated. However, she has haematuria which needs investigating anyway and she should be referred to a fast-track haematuria clinic where they will look at both upper and lower urinary tracts. Although UTI is the most likely cause of her symptoms, they may also be due to bladder tumour.

24. Sepsis related to the genital tract in pregnant women:

A.	Is the leading direct cause of maternal death in the 2006–2008 UK Mortality Report	T
B.	Is excluded if the woman has a temperature < 37 °C on admission	F
C.	May be associated with a streptococcal sore throat	T
D.	Is more likely following a vaginal birth rather than a caesarean	F
E.	Is not likely to be the diagnosis if the patient's white cell count $< 4 \times 10^9 /l$	F

UK obstetricians were surprised to find the leading cause of maternal death in this report was sepsis because it had been many years since sepsis was a major problem. The 'new' bug was streptococcus pyogenes related to sore throats and we had to develop new protocols for dealing with it (mostly known as the 'sepsis bundle' in hospitals). Some of these women become extremely sick very quickly and the finding of a low temperature and white cell count can be an ominous sign.

25. **Venous thromboembolism (VTE) is more likely in pregnant patients with:**

A.	Hyperemesis gravidarum	T
B.	Pre-eclampsia	T
C.	Ovarian hyperstimulation syndrome	T
D.	Asymptomatic gallstones	F
E.	Thrombocytopaenia	F

Pregnancy predisposes women to VTE anyway but the risks are increased if they become dehydrated (as in hyperemesis, pre-eclampsia and hyperstimulation syndrome). The other two conditions are not risk factors, unless she develops cholecystitis as a result of her gallstones.

26. **Regarding the duties of a doctor:**

A.	When treating a patient for a sexually transmitted infection, you always have a duty to inform the spouse regardless of the patient's consent	F
B.	A chaperone is needed for gynaecological pelvic examinations only if the doctor is male	F
C.	When consenting a patient for a surgical procedure, only common complications need to be discussed	F
D.	If you see a child with a proven sexually transmitted infection this must always be reported	T
E.	Consent is not required for anomaly scans performed at 20 weeks gestation	F

Confidentiality prevents you from informing a spouse about a sexually transmitted infection without consent although it is your duty to try and persuade them to allow disclosure. However, if the benefit to the spouse's health outweighs the patient's confidentiality such as with HIV infection the situation may be different. You would be well advised to discuss with your defence/protection society.

It is good practice to offer a chaperone for consultations whatever the sex of the doctor. Complications which are rare but of important consequence to the patient must be discussed when obtaining consent.

If you diagnose a child with a sexually transmitted infection the child protection services must be informed as the age of consent is 16 years in England and Wales, under the Sexual Offences Act 2003.

Anomaly scans do require consent although this can be verbal or written.

27. **Characteristic features of physiological jaundice in the newborn include:**

A.	Onset after the first 24 hours of life	T
B.	Disappearance by the fourth day	F
C.	Associated anaemia	F
D.	Could lead to kernicterus if not treated	T
E.	Occurs more frequently in preterm infants	T

Physiological jaundice usually peaks at two to four days of life and resolves within two weeks. If the baby is also anaemic there could be a more sinister cause associated

with haemolysis and further investigation is warranted. Phototherapy is very
effective at reducing bilirubin levels so kernicterus is a rare event.

28. **A 41-year-old woman has always attended for regular cervical screening and all her tests so far have been normal. It would be appropriate to take a smear from her in the following circumstances:**

A.	She presents with a new diagnosis of genital warts	F
B.	She discovers a family history of cervical cancer	F
C.	She presents with a history of postcoital bleeding	F
D.	She is noted on examination to have a cervical polyp	F
E.	She had her previous cervical smear three years ago	T

Genital warts are a different virus from CIN so this would not be an indication for an opportunistic smear, neither is there a genetic component. Postcoital bleeding could be due to cervical cancer but she needs a speculum examination not a smear. Cervical polyps are irrelevant. At the age of 41, she will be on a three-yearly screening programme.

29. **With regard to human papilloma virus vaccines:**

A.	It is pointless giving the vaccine if the woman is already sexually active	F
B.	A full course provides lifelong immunity against cervical cancer	F
C.	They contain live virus	F
D.	They are contraindicated in males	F
E.	A woman who has been vaccinated does not need smears	F

Vaccines against the HPV virus 16 and 18 (those that are clearly linked to the development of cervical cancer) are designed to be effective before sexual activity starts to protect women from exposure to the virus. To date the duration of protection has not been fully established although studies suggest that protection is maintained for at least six years after a complete course. The vaccines are produced using recombinant DNA techniques. The quadrivalent vaccine available also protects against HPV 6 and 11 which cause genital warts. This vaccine can be given to males. The vaccines available do not protect against all strains of HPV and hence women should still have regular cervical cytology at present.

30. **If a pregnant woman is infected with German measles (rubella) in the first trimester, her baby has an increased risk of:**

A.	Cataract	T
B.	Short limbs	F
C.	Congenital heart lesions	T
D.	Conductive deafness	T
E.	Facial clefts	F

Congenital rubella syndrome includes developmental delay and intellectual disability as well as cataracts and deafness. Heart defects include pulmonary artery stenosis and patent ductus. Babies can also have microcephaly and neonatal seizures. These risks are maximal if the mother contracts rubella within the first three months of pregnancy.

31. **With regard to bacterial vaginosis diagnosed in pregnancy:**

A.	It is thought to cause pelvic inflammatory disease after termination	T
B.	It should be treated if detected in pregnancy	T
C.	It is associated with a two-fold increase in preterm delivery	T

D. It is a risk factor for second-trimester miscarriage   T

E. It may be treated with oral clindamycin   T

There is evidence that bacterial vaginosis, far from being a harmless irritant, is related to second-trimester miscarriage and preterm delivery.

Source: RCOG Green-top guideline number 17. *The Investigation and Treatment of Couples with Recurrent Miscarriage.*

32. Mothers who smoke cigarettes:

A. Are more likely to suffer placental abruption   T

B. Are more likely to have a postpartum haemorrhage   F

C. Are more likely to be referred to antenatal clinic by their midwife for a growth scan   T

D. Are more likely to develop cervical cancer   T

E. Are more likely to experience sudden infant death syndrome   T

Mothers who smoke are likely to have a smaller baby and so referral for a growth scan is usual. Cigarette smoking is known to be a co-factor in the development of cervical cancer. Babies exposed to smoke in the home are more likely to die from sudden infant death syndrome (SIDS).

33. Surgically removing the ovaries at the time of hysterectomy:

A. Is usually done if the woman has endometrial cancer   T

When a hysterectomy is performed for endometrial cancer, the ovaries will be removed for histology and peritoneal washings will be taken for cytology in order to stage the cancer.

B. Could result in loss of libido   T

Removal of the ovaries reduces the production of testosterone, which a woman requires for libido.

C. Will eliminate premenstrual syndrome   T

Symptoms of PMS are eliminated because there is no longer an ovarian cycle.

D. Is not usually done if the hysterectomy is performed vaginally   T

When the hysterectomy is performed vaginally it is technically much more difficult to remove the ovaries safely and so it is not a usual part of such an operation.

E. Is referred to as a total hysterectomy   F

Total hysterectomy refers to the complete removal of the uterus – i.e. the body of the uterus and the cervix.

34. If a woman presents to the GP with postmenopausal bleeding:

A. She is most likely to have endometrial cancer   F

B. She should stop taking hormone replacement therapy   T

C. It is defined as vaginal bleeding more than six months since her last menstrual period   F

D. She could be treated with estrogen cream initially if speculum exam reveals atrophic vaginitis   F

E. She does not need hysteroscopy if her endometrium is 7 mm thick on ultrasound scan   F

There is a 10% chance of the diagnosis being endometrial cancer but she should stop taking HRT until investigations are complete as this is a hormone-dependent cancer. Likewise it is not safe to treat atrophic vaginitis with estrogen until the uterus has been investigated as she may have endometrial cancer as well as an atrophic vagina. Bleeding becomes postmenopausal bleeding if it is more than 12 months since her last period. If the endometrial thickness is > 5 mm on scan, she requires a hysteroscopy.

35. With regard to *Chlamydia trachomatis* infection:

A.	It may cause neonatal conjunctivitis and pneumonia	T
B.	It is usually asymptomatic in women	T
C.	It may lead to infertility	T
D.	It is treated with mebendazole	F
E.	It can cause epididymo-orchitis in men	T

Chlamydia can affect the baby if it is contracted during labour, and causes an eye infection called ophthalmia neonatorum. One of the most serious consequences of undiagnosed infection, which is not uncommon because there are often no symptoms, is fallopian tube blockage.

36. Regarding group B streptococcus colonization in pregnancy:

A.	Group B streptococcus bacteriuria in this pregnancy is an indication for intrapartum antibiotics	T
B.	The antibiotic of choice for prophylaxis is clindamycin	F
C.	Oral benzylpenicillin is indicated in labour if there is known group B streptococcal colonization	F
D.	Routine screening using high vaginal swabs is common in UK practice	F
E.	Prophylaxis is required for high-risk women having planned caesarean sections	F

We don't have a screening programme in the UK at the moment but we do have guidelines that offer suggestions for the care of women where group B streptococcus colonization has been diagnosed in pregnancy. The incidence is said to be 0.5 per 1000 births and is the same in the UK (where there is no screening programme) as in the USA (where there is an active screening and prevention programme).

The antibiotic of choice is benzylpenicillin, intravenous rather than oral, unless the woman is allergic to penicillin when clindamycin is used instead.

Source: RCOG Green-top guideline number 31. *The Prevention of Early-onset Neonatal Group B Streptococcal Disease.*

37. Regarding haemorrhagic disease of the newborn:

A.	It is a risk because vitamin K stores in neonates are low	T
B.	It only occurs in the first few days of life	F
C.	Prevention with IM injection is more effective than oral vitamin K	T
D.	It is more common in wholly breastfed babies	T
E.	There is a better outlook for babies with the late-onset form	F

Vitamin K does not easily cross the placenta and neonates have low stores at delivery. It usually occurs on the first few days of life but there is a late-onset form seen in babies who did not receive vitamin K at birth (which is offered routinely in the UK). The late-onset form is more likely to lead to intracranial bleeding. There is not as much vitamin K in breast milk as in formula milk so breastfed babies are at more risk.

38. Regarding a woman who has undergone female genital mutilation (also known as female circumcision or infibulation) as a child:

A.	Caesarean section will be necessary if she decides to have a baby	F

B.	The infibulation cannot be surgically undone during pregnancy	F
C.	The operation is illegal in the UK	T
D.	She is more likely to subject her daughters to the same procedure	T
E.	The husband can legally insist on the infibulation being restored	F

This operation is done for cultural rather than religious reasons and is common in immigrants from North Africa. It is illegal in this country but families may take their small girls back to their country of origin to have it done before puberty. Vaginal delivery is possible if the operation is reversed before labour and will save the woman an unnecessary caesarean section.

39. Pregnancy has an adverse effect on:

A.	Iron deficiency anaemia	T
B.	Pulmonary tuberculosis	T
C.	Mitral stenosis	T
D.	Crohn's disease	F
E.	Rheumatoid arthritis	F

There is an increased demand for iron in pregnancy.

Pregnancy often improves the symptoms of diarrhoea in Crohn's patients and joint swelling in rheumatoid patients because of suppression of the immune system.

Conversely TB may get worse because of immune suppression.

The increased cardiac output in pregnancy can result in pulmonary oedema in patients with mitral stenosis, with the outlook being worse with increasing severity of the stenosis.

40. Regarding cervical cerclage (suturing the cervix closed) in pregnancy:

A.	It is indicated in a woman with a history of recurrent painless late miscarriages	T
B.	The suture is inserted after the first trimester is completed	T
C.	Removal of the suture requires general or spinal anaesthetic	F
D.	The suture is usually inserted abdominally, requiring a laparotomy	F
E.	The procedure can be done as a 'rescue' operation if the cervix starts dilating	T

The suture is normally put in when it is clear that the pregnancy is not going to miscarry, i.e. after the first trimester, and removed at 37 weeks. Inserting the stitch does require an anaesthetic of some sort but removing it is normally not painful. The outcome for emergency sutures is not as successful as elective sutures but the patients have to be selected carefully to be sure that you are dealing with cervical incompetence, which can only really be determined by assessing the history of events during the late miscarriages, i.e. painless bleeding or ruptured membranes followed by rapid delivery with few or no contractions. Abdominal sutures are rarely indicated but can be inserted via a laparotomy incision, e.g. if the cervix is amputated for cancer (trachelectomy) but in this case the suture is normally left in and the baby delivered by caesarean section.

Source: RCOG Green-top guideline number 60. *Cervical Cerclage.*

Useful web addresses

www.bashh.org for Genitourinary Medicine guidance

www.bhiva.org for clinical guidance about HIV

www.cancerscreening.nhs.uk for information on cervical screening and human papilloma virus vaccination

www.fetalanomaly.screening.nhs.uk for details of the NHS fetal anomaly screening programme (FASP)

www.fpa.org.uk for information on contraception and sexual health

www.frsh.org for Faculty of Reproductive and Sexual Health clinical guidance

www.gmc-uk.org for *Duties of a Doctor*, ethical issues and consent

www.nice.org.uk for NICE guidance

www.rcog.org.uk for Green-top guidelines

Glossary

A&E	Accident and Emergency
AIDS	Acquired Immunodeficiency Syndrome
BMI	Body Mass Index
BP	Blood Pressure
CBT	Cognitive Behavioural Therapy
CNST	Clinical Negligence Scheme for Trusts
COC	Combined Oral Contraceptive Pill
CT	Computerized Tomography
CTG	Cardiotocograph
DVT	Deep Vein Thrombosis
EMQ	Extended Matching Question
FGM	Female Genital Mutilation
FSH	Follicle Stimulating Hormone
GA	General Anaesthetic
GMC	General Medical Council
GnRH	Gonadotrophin Releasing Hormone
GUM	Genitourinary Medicine
hCG	Human Chorionic Gonadotrophin
HIV	Human Immunodeficiency Virus
HPV	Human Papilloma Virus
HRT	Hormone Replacement Therapy
IM	Intramuscular
IUCD	Intrauterine Contraceptive Device
IUD	Intrauterine Device
IUGR	Intrauterine Growth Restriction
IUS	Intrauterine System
IV	Intravenous
IVF	In Vitro Fertilization
IVP	Intravenous Pyelogram
IVU	Intravenous Urogram
KUB	Kidney, Ureter and Bladder (x-ray)
LFT	Liver Function Test

LH	Luteinizing Hormone
LHRH	Luteinizing Hormone Releasing Hormone
LLETZ	Large Loop Excision of the Transformation Zone (of the Cervix)
LMP	Last Menstrual Period
MCQ	Multiple Choice Question
MDT	Multidisciplinary Team
MRI	Magnetic Resonance Imaging
MSU	Midstream Specimen of Urine
NHS	National Health Service
OA	Occipito-Anterior
OP	Occipito-Posterior
OSCE	Objective Structured Clinical Examination
PCO	Polycystic Ovary
PCR	Polymerase Chain Reaction
SARC	Sexual Assault Referral Centre
SBA	Single Best Answer
SSRI	Selective Serotonin Reuptake Inhibitor
STI	Sexually Transmitted Infection
TOP	Termination of Pregnancy
TVS	Transvaginal Scan
TVT	Tension-Free Vaginal Tape
U&E	Urea and Electrolytes
USS	Ultrasound Scan
VBAC	Vaginal Birth After Caesarean section
VZIG	Varicella Zoster Immunoglobulin

Index

279